EMS Special Operations

Jeffrey T. Lindsey, PhD, PM, EFO, CFO
Distance Education Coordinator
for the Fire and Emergency Services Programs
University of Florida
Gainesville, Florida

EMS Management Series

SERIES EDITOR, *Jeffrey T. Lindsey, PhD, PM, EFO, CFO*

PEARSON

Boston Columbus Indianapolis New York San Francisco Upper Saddle River
Amsterdam Cape Town Dubai London Madrid Milan Munich Paris Montreal Toronto
Delhi Mexico City São Paulo Sydney Hong Kong Seoul Singapore Taipei Tokyo

Publisher: Julie Levin Alexander
Publisher's Assistant: Regina Bruno
Editor-in-Chief: Marlene McHugh Pratt
Product Manager: Sladjana Repic
Program Manager: Monica Moosang
Development Editor: Allison Murray, iD8-TripleSSS
Editorial Assistant: Kelly Clark
Director of Marketing: David Gesell
Executive Marketing Manager: Brian Hoehl
Marketing Specialist: Michael Sirinides
Project Management Lead: Cynthia Zonneveld
Project Manager: Julie Boddorf
Full-Service Project Manager: Munesh Kumar, Aptara®, Inc.
Editorial Media Manager: Amy Peltier
Media Project Manager: Ellen Martino
Creative Director: Jayne Conte
Cover Image: Shutterstock/B Calkins
Composition: Aptara®, Inc.
Text Font: Times Ten LT Std

Credits and acknowledgments borrowed from other sources and reproduced, with permission, in this textbook appear on the appropriate pages within the text.

Library of Congress Cataloging-in-Publication Data

Lindsey, Jeffrey, author.
EMS special operations / Jeffrey T. Lindsey.
p. ; cm. – (EMS management series)
Includes bibliographical references.
ISBN-13: 978-0-13-610002-7
ISBN-10: 0-13-610002-3
I. Title. II. Series: EMS management series.
[DNLM: 1. Emergency Medical Services–organization & administration–Handbooks. 2. Mass Casualty Incidents–Handbooks. 3. Rescue Work–Handbooks. WX 39]
RA975.5.E5
362.18–dc23 2013034478

10 9 8 7 6 5 4 3 2 V092 14

PEARSON

ISBN 13: 978-0-13-610002-7
ISBN 10: 0-13-610002-3

Contents

Dedication

I want to dedicate this book to the three best kids in the world—Natasha, Melissa, and Matthew Lindsey—who have always supported me, and in memory of their mother Kandace. I also acknowledge and thank my stepson, Austin Wolfangel, and hope his career ambitions in fire and EMS come true. I also dedicate this to my wife, Sue Wolfangel-Lindsey, with gratitude for her love and understanding. And in gratitude to my parents, Thomas and Janet Lindsey, for always encouraging me in everything I do, I also dedicate this work.

Chapter 3

Mass Gatherings and Special Events 31

Chapter 4

Tactical Response 51

Chapter 7

Structural Collapse 110

David Harrington

Chapter 8

Confined-Space Rescue 149

David Harrington

Chapter 11

Chapter 12

Chapter 13

Chapter 14

Chapter 15

Preface

INTRODUCTION

EMS special operations consists of a variety services an EMS agency may consider providing for those situations to which personnel may not respond to on a regular basis but that have a potential for occurring in their jurisdiction. Unless you are a large agency with a very diverse geographic range of responses, an agency will typically never be prepared to create a specialized response team for all of the various needs in the community or topics in this text.

This text was written not to be exhaustive in each of the topic areas but, rather, to give the reader—who in most cases is or will be an EMS manager—a solid foundation of understanding of each of the topic areas. Although there are specialized courses for responders to train to the level needed to respond effectively for each of the topics, EMS managers may not have this level of training; however, they must have at least an understanding of each of the specialized areas.

Examples are offered throughout this text. They richly illustrate the concepts presented. An agency does not need to create a specialized team for every potential specialized event; however, the agency does need to have a plan in place for its community should that hundred-year event hit.

ORGANIZATION OF THIS TEXT

Chapter 1 provides an overview of special operations as it relates to EMS. It provides the foundation for the rest of the text. The text is addressed to the EMS manager, not to provide specific training for each topic but, rather, to provide an overview to educate an EMS manager on each specialty area.

Chapter 2 discusses mass casualty incidents (MCIs). It includes an overview on the triage, treatment, and transport of an MCI. It includes the incident management system as it pertains to EMS at an MCI. This topic can affect every EMS agency.

Chapter 3 addresses EMS at mass gatherings or special events. Whether you are a small or large agency, at times your agency will be called to do a standby or respond to an event. Many agencies have specialized units to address such events. This chapter gives an overview of what to expect and how to handle such events.

Chapter 4 provides an overview of tactical medicine. This specialty has become more known. It is somewhat controversial whether EMS should be involved or not. This chapter looks at the components of and what a tactical EMS team does.

Chapter 5 discusses pandemics. Recent years have shown how predisposed we in the United States are to a pandemic. For both small and large agencies, a pandemic can create havoc. This chapter provides insight on how pandemics affect an EMS agency.

Chapter 6 covers vehicle extrication. Vehicle extrication is typically performed in the United States by either EMS or fire departments. Regardless, EMS will be on the scene of a vehicle crash at least to perform medical care.

Chapter 7 covers structural collapse. This topic can be very complex. Some EMS agencies are part of the specialized team that responds to such incidents. A structural collapse can occur anywhere. However, depending on its resources, it may or may not be prudent for an EMS agency to have a specialized team.

Chapter 8 discusses confined-space rescue. As with many of the topics in this text, this topic can affect virtually any community. In order to function at the scene of a confined-space rescue, personnel must be specially trained and certified.

Chapter 9 reviews above- and below-grade rescue. This covers many types of rescue. Your geographic area will determine the kinds of rescues you may face.

Chapter 10 provides insight on and for the technical rescue safety officer. The term *technical rescue safety officer* can be interchanged with *incident safety officer*; however, in this text it is designated for technical rescues since the text is devoted to specialized rescues. In these situations it is important to have a safety officer who understands the complexities of the rescue.

Chapter 11 highlights hazardous materials incidents. EMS can be involved in hazardous materials at various levels. This chapter looks at the various levels EMS can be involved in at a hazardous materials incident from the viewpoint of an EMS manager.

Chapter 12 discusses water rescue and dive medicine. This chapter is a specialized topic that may not involve your agency unless you have a body of water in your response area. Diving is also an area that tends to be very specialized.

Chapter 13 covers land-based search and rescue. The chapter looks at rescues involving wilderness areas, among others. Depending on the area an agency covers, the information may not all be relevant. However, the chapter covers various topics so the EMS manager can gain an appreciation of this specialized area.

Chapter 14 provides an insight on incidents of national consequence. These can occur anywhere. The plane crash in a field in Pennsylvania on September 11, 2001, illustrates this point, although such incidents are more prevalent in larger cities. This chapter also looks at some past incidents.

Chapter 15 focuses on developing a special operations team. This chapter provides the EMS manager with an overview of the process of developing a special operations team. Regardless of the type of team, it needs to be developed in the proper way.

FEATURES

Chapter Objectives: Objectives are identified at the beginning of each chapter and outline the material the reader should understand upon completion of the chapter.

Key Terms: Key terms are listed at the beginning of each chapter and are bold upon introduction in the chapter. Each chapter's terms are defined at the end of the chapter, and all terms are included in the comprehensive glossary at the end of the book.

What Would You Do? Case Study: Every chapter starts with an EMS manager tackling some issue related to special operations that is related to the content of the chapter. How he resolved the issue based on information in the chapter is presented in the **What Would You Do? Reflection** feature at the end of the chapter.

Best Practice: Every chapter includes a real-world example that illustrates information from the chapter having been used successfully by an EMS agency.

Side Bars: This feature relates interesting information that corresponds very closely to text discussion.

Review Questions: Students are required to draw on the knowledge presented in the chapter to answer the questions.

References: A list of bibliographical references appears at the end of each chapter.

ROAD MAP/HOW TO USE THIS TEXT

This text is designed to be used as a reference and how-to manual for EMS managers seeking to develop or manage an EMS special operations team. Each chapter focuses on a special topic specific to a certain area. The EMS manager can use this text to gain an appreciation for each topic area. The text is used for informing the EMS manager, not to make them an expert.

TEACHING AND LEARNING RESOURCES

For information on instructor resources, including PowerPoint presentations, assessment tools, and student resources, please contact your Brady sales representative.

Acknowledgments

A text with this level of specialty cannot be effectively written by one person. The contributors for this text were a special group of experts in the field. The text would have been incomplete without their contribution. A special thank you to all the contributors:

Ray Whatley
Eric Powell
Sam Bradley
Randy Kearns
James Logan
David Harrington
Scott Chappell
Kevin Spratlin
Frank DeFrancesco
Raphael Barishansky

To the wonderful staff at Brady—Marlene Pratt, Lois Berlowitz, Sladjana Repic-Bruno, Kelly Clark, Julie Boddorf, and Monica Moosang—and to the developmental editors Kay Peavey and Allison Murray.

To all the reviewers for their feedback and encouragement to make this a great text!

To all those who read this text, thanks for taking the time. It is my desire that your efforts will make an impact in the EMS profession for the betterment of all.

Reviewers

Chris Prutzman, CCNRP-T
Clinical Services Coordinator
Emergency Medical Services Authority
Oklahoma City, OK

Lawrence A. Nelson, MS, NMCEM, EMT-P (ret.)
Director, EMS/Emergency Management BAAS Program
Eastern New Mexico University
Portales, NM

Douglas Skinner, BS, NREMTP, NCEE
EMS Education Coordinator
Physicians Transport Service
Herndon, VA

George Hettenbach, BBA, MS
Adjunct Professor
Delaware County Community College
Havertown, PA

Donald Walsh, Ph.D., EMT-P, I/C
EMS Chief (Ret.)
Chicago Fire Department EMS
Chicago, IL

Jeff Lewis, BS Business Administration
Captain II / VATF1 – Medical Co-Section Lead, Adjunct Faculty
Fairfax County Fire and Rescue / Fairfax County Urban Search and Rescue Program, Northern Virginia Community College
Fairfax, VA

Sam Bradley, BS, EMT-P
EMS QI and Training
Livermore-Pleasanton Fire Department
Pleasanton, CA

Rintha Simpson
Program Director
SnS Training Specialists, LLC
Pride, LA

About the Author

Jeffrey T. Lindsey, Ph.D., EMT-P, EFO, CFO

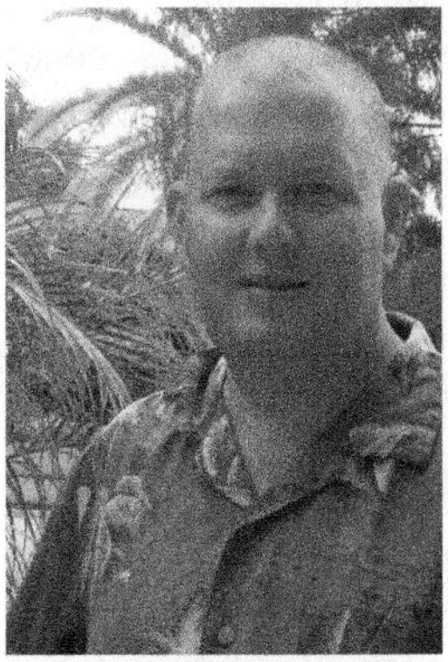

Dr. Jeffrey Lindsey has served in a variety of roles in the fire and EMS arena for the past 30 years. He has held positions of firefighter, paramedic, dispatcher, educator, coordinator, deputy chief, and chief. He started his career in Carlisle, Pennsylvania, as a volunteer firefighter/EMT. In 1985 Dr. Lindsey pioneered the first advanced life support service in Cumberland County, Pennsylvania. He is retired as the Fire/EMS Chief for Estero Fire Rescue, where he served as the South Division Incident Commander during major events. He was also part of the Area Command for Lee County EOC. Currently he is the Distance Education Coordinator for the Fire and Emergency Services Programs at the University of Florida.

He has served as an inaugural member on the National EMS Advisory Council, representing fire-based EMS, and is a past member of the State of Florida EMS Advisory Council, where he served as the firefighter/paramedic representative. He currently serves as representative to the Fire and Emergency Services Higher Education EMS degree committee. He has been active in the IAFC, serving as liaison to ACEP and attending various meetings representing fire-based EMS, and as the inaugural chair of the Community Paramedic committee, and he is an associate member of the Prehospital Research Forum.

He was a monthly columnist on product reviews for 3 years for *The Journal of Emergency Medical Services (JEMS)*, a national EMS journal. He is a columnist for Firerehab.com and has authored numerous fire and EMS texts for Brady/Pearson. He is currently the Chief Learning Officer for the Health and Safety Institute, which produces *24-7 EMS* and *24-7 Fire* videos. He also was an EMS professor for St. Petersburg College (Florida).

Dr. Lindsey has been involved in a number of large events and has served within the incident command system at the upper level, including during a number of wildland fires and Hurricane Charley. He has also been involved in the preparations for a number of other hurricanes and tropical storms.

He holds an associate's degree in paramedicine from Harrisburg Area Community College, a bachelor's degree in Fire and Safety from the University of Cincinnati, a master's degree in Instructional Technology from the University of South Florida, and a Ph.D. in Instructional Technology/Adult Education from the University of South Florida.

In addition, Dr. Lindsey has completed the Executive Fire Officer Program at the National Fire Academy. He has designed and developed various courses in fire and EMS. Dr. Lindsey is accredited with the Chief Fire Officer Designation. He also is a certified Fire Officer II, Fire Instructor III, and paramedic in the state of Florida; holds a paramedic certificate for the state of Pennsylvania; and is a certified instructor in these and a variety of other courses.

Dr. Lindsey has an innate interest in alternative health. He is a certified nutritional counselor, a master herbalist, and a holistic health practitioner.

About the Chapter Authors

The following individuals served as chapter authors for this textbook. It is their work that brings value to it, for they are truly subject matter experts.

Raymond C. Whatley, Jr., M.B.A., NREMT-P, is an EMS Supervisor who serves with the Alexandria (Virginia) Fire Department. His experience began as a volunteer paramedic in Prince William County (Virginia) with the Occoquan Woodbridge Lorton Volunteer Fire Department. Currently he has more than 25 years of experience in EMS. During his career he has served as a hazardous materials medic, tactical medic, EMS training officer, and EMS field supervisor. Mr. Whatley has also served with the Office of Emergency Management. In addition, he serves as the Training Center Coordinator for the Northern Virginia EMS Council, the Virginia American Heart Association Emergency Cardiovascular Care Committee, and as a regional member. In 2011, he was recognized by the George Washington Chapter of the Sons of the American Revolution and was awarded the Emergency Medical Services Commendation Medal.

Eric Powell, Ph.D., FF/NRP, has been involved in emergency medical services, law enforcement, and the fire service for 28 years. He is active with numerous national public-safety educational and policy-making organizations and is a research co-investigator with emergency medicine and disaster management projects for the Tennessee Department of Health/Office of EMS and the Tennessee EMS for Children/Committee on Pediatric Emergency Care.

Dr. Powell holds baccalaureate degrees from Western Carolina University and Colorado State University; a master's degree from the Medical University of South Carolina; a doctorate from the University of Tennessee at Knoxville; and two postdoctoral endeavors through the United States Naval Postgraduate School's Department of National Security Affairs and the University of South Florida's College of Public Health. He is also enrolled at the National Fire Academy's Executive Fire Officer Program. He is currently the Paramedic and Fire Science Program Director at Walters State Community College in Morristown, Tennessee.

(Sandra) Sam Bradley, BS, EMT-P, has been in EMS for 34 years as a paramedic, clinical and educational services coordinator, and ambulance company field supervisor. She is currently the EMS/QI Specialist at the Livermore-Pleasanton Fire Department in Northern California, and functions as a QI consultant and EMS educator for another fire department and a fire-based communications center. She has taught primary paramedic and EMT courses for most of her career. A prolific writer, she does freelance work for EMS-related journals, online publications, and textbook publishers. In addition, she has published a number of fiction stories and is very involved in social media and blogging. Following her passion for photography, videography, and disaster EMS, she functions as a producer and photographer for the First Responders Network (FRNtv) and is currently working on producing a disaster-related podcast for the Promed Network. Ms. Bradley is the Training Officer for the federal Disaster Medical Assistance Team (DMAT) CA-6 and worked for the State of California to create the state-level

disaster medical team (CALMAT). Service work includes the position of CEO for the Interstate Disaster Medical Services Consortium (ISDMC), and board member and secretary for the Coalition for Tactical Medicine (CTM).

Randy D. Kearns, DHA, MSA, CEM, NREMT-P ret., is a Clinical Assistant Professor and holds faculty appointments in both the Department of Surgery and the Department of Emergency Medicine at the University of North Carolina, School of Medicine. He serves as the Program Director for the North Carolina and Southern Burn Disaster Programs as well as certificate programs in EMS Leadership and Medical Disaster Management. He also serves as the Administrator for the EMS Performance Improvement Center.

Dr. Kearns has worked as a paramedic; taught paramedic programs; led fire, rescue, and EMS organizations; served in hospital administration; and worked at the local, state, and federal levels of emergency management. Dr. Kearns was one of the first 100 paramedics in North Carolina and has been involved in emergency services for 38 years.

Dr. Kearns completed a bachelor's degree in Disaster Management and Human Services (BSHS) from Thomas Edison State College, a master's degree in Administration (MSA) from Central Michigan University, a doctorate in Health Administration (DHA) from the Medical University of South Carolina, and is an education doctorate (EdD) student at the University of St. Augustine for Health Sciences.

Dr. Kearns has authored more than 30 peer-reviewed articles, textbook chapters, and other materials regarding medical disaster preparedness and response to a mass casualty incident. Recently, he was a contributor to the National Burn Bed Surge Strategy Roundtable conducted by the US DHHS ASPR Hospital Preparedness and Public Health Preparedness Programs; served as a panelist for the Food and Drug Administration Medical Counter Measures Response to a Burn Disaster; and served as a panelist for the Institutes of Medicine, Medical Surge Capacity workgroup.

J. Harold "Jim" Logan, BS, EMT-P/IC, is a 29-year veteran of fire-based EMS and serves as an acting Chief Officer and Paramedic for the Memphis Fire Department in an EMS administration capacity, specializing in EMS Consequence Management, Emergency Preparedness, Quality Improvement, and Education. He is a nationally known author with regular publications in *EMS World Magazine*, *Journal of Emergency Medical Services* (JEMS), *Firehouse*, *Fire Engineering*, and other trade journals and emergency service industry textbooks. He is an EMS instructor coordinator and fire instructor for the Memphis Fire Department and the State of Tennessee.

Mr. Logan has also received national attention and awards for innovation in EMS education. He holds a bachelor's degree in health and safety from the University of Memphis. For more than a decade, he has also served as a Rescue/Medical Specialist and a Medical Coordinator for FEMA's Tennessee Task Force One Urban Search and Rescue Team and is Co-Chair of the Memphis Shelby County Metropolitan Medical Response System Steering Committee.

David Harrington, AA, TN-EMTP, NREMTP, Mr. Harrington has been involved in emergency services for over 30 years. He got his start in 1982 as a volunteer with the Knoxville Volunteer Rescue Squad where he is still a member and instructor. There he served as a shift officer, Assistant Chief, and Chief. Currently, Mr. Harrington is the Deputy Chief of Fire Operations as well as the Ambulance Director for the City of Oak Ridge (Tennessee) Fire Department, where he has worked since 1991. He is a Hazardous Materials Specialist, USAR Type III All Hazards Incident Commander, Task Force Leader, Operations

Section Leader, Logistics Section Leader, and Planning Section Leader. He is also a former adjunct faculty with Roane State Community College in Knoxville, Tennessee, where he has instructed on both the EMT and Paramedic levels. He is a member of NAEMSA, TARS, IAAI, IAFF, and IAFC.

Scott Chappel, is the US&R and Haz Mat Program Coordinator for the State Fire Marshal at the Florida State Fire College. He entered the fire service in 1993 and has been teaching at the Florida State Fire College since 2000. He has a bachelor's degree in Philosophy from the University of Florida as well as a master's degree in Public Administration from Barry University. He served as the Program Coordinator for Central Florida Community College's Fire Science Program and is on various committees and work groups for US&R, Haz Mat, and the State Homeland Security Grant Program (SHSGP). In addition to his responsibilities as the State Fire Marshal, Mr. Chappel is a Lieutenant with Marion County Fire Rescue (MCFR) and is active on MCFR's Technical Rescue Team, Hazardous Materials Team, and Florida US&R Task Force 8.

Charles Kevin Spratlin, BPS, NREMT-P, has been involved in EMS since 1995, beginning his career with the Grenada Lake Medical Center ambulance service in Grenada, Mississippi. He currently serves as a firefighter/paramedic and EMS Training instructor with the Memphis Fire Department in Memphis, Tennessee. Mr. Spratlin is also a Medical Specialist with Tennessee Task Force One, one of 28 FEMA Urban Search and Rescue teams in the United States, and is a partner with Prehospital Education Associates LLC. He received a bachelor's degree in Fire Administration from the University of Memphis in 2010 and is nearing completion of a Master of Science degree from the University of Arkansas in Operations Management with a focus on Safety and Health Administration.

Frank DeFranceso, CFO started in fire service in 1975 as a junior firefighter for East Farmingdale, New York, and has progressed through the ranks to Assistant Chief of Hernando County Fire Rescue in Hernando County, Florida. In 1984, he was a charter member of the Pinellas County Hazardous Materials Team, in Largo, Florida. He has an associate of science degree in Emergency Medical Services, a bachelor of science in Fire Science, and a bachelor of science in business administration. He is currently working on a master's degree in Public Administration. Mr. DeFrancesco has served on various local and state committees to enhance the state's hazardous materials response capabilities, such as the Local Emergency Planning Committee, State Emergency Response Committee's Training Task Force, and the Florida Fire Chief's Association of Hazardous Materials Responders.

Raphael M. Barishansky, MPH, MS, is the Director of the Office of Emergency Medical Services (OEMS) for the Connecticut Department of Public Health. Prior to holding this position, he served as Chief of Public Health Emergency Preparedness and Response for the Prince George's County (Maryland) Health Department.

Mr. Barishansky holds a bachelor of arts degree from Touro College, a master of public health degree in Health Policy and Management from New York Medical College, and a master of science degree in Homeland Security Studies from Long Island University. He is also a graduate of the Senior Executives in State and Local Government program held at the John F. Kennedy School of Government at Harvard University (2006) and the Healthcare Leadership and Administrative Decision Making class held at the Center for Domestic Preparedness in Anniston, Alabama (2009).

Mr. Barishansky has served as adjunct faculty at New York Medical College, Yeshiva University, and Westchester Community

College and has been a guest lecturer at the George Washington University EMS degree program, the Philadelphia University Disaster Medicine and Management graduate degree program, and the George Mason Biodefense graduate degree program.

In addition, Mr. Barishansky has written extensively. His articles have been featured in *EMS World Magazine*, *Journal of Emergency Medical Services* (JEMS), *EMS Insider*, *Domestic Preparedness Journal*, *Journal of Homeland Security and Emergency Management*, *Emergency Management Magazine*, *Public Safety Communications*, and *Crisis Response Journal* (United Kingdom). He is a regular presenter at regional, state, and national EMS and public health conferences.

About FESHE

FESHE (Fire and Emergency Services Higher Education) is a dedicated group of individuals from around the country. It is hosted by the United States Fire Administration through the National Fire Academy. The mission of this group is to develop a uniform model curriculum for associates, bachelor, and masters degree. In December 2006 a group of EMS educators convened as the inaugural EMS committee for FESHE. The mission was to develop a model curriculum in EMS management at the bachelor level. It was the consensus of the leaders across the country that the committee focus on the management issues of EMS. The clinical portion of the industry is addressed through the National EMS Education Standards and is mainly focused at the associate's level.

This text is written to meet the needs of the national model curriculum for EMS management at the bachelor's level. The EMS management curriculum includes six core courses and seven elective courses. Following are titles in Brady's *EMS Management Series*, designed to meet the FESHE curriculum.

CORE

- Foundations of EMS Systems
- Management of EMS
- EMS Community Risk Reduction
- EMS Quality Management and Research
- Legal, Political and Regulatory Environment in EMS
- EMS Safety and Risk Management

ELECTIVE

- Management of Ambulance Services
- Foundations for the Practice of EMS Education
- EMS Special Operations
- EMS Public Information and Community Relations
- EMS Communications and Information Technology
- EMS Finance
- Analytical Approaches to EMS

Introduction to Special Operations

1 CHAPTER

JEFFREY LINDSEY

Objectives

After reading this chapter, the student should be able to:

1.1 Describe the role of special operations in EMS.
1.2 Discuss the various special operations involving EMS.
1.3 Discuss the importance of EMS personnel trained in special operations.

Key Terms

basic rescue teams
disaster medical assistance teams (DMATs)
light and medium tactical rescue task forces
special operations
strike team
task force
typing of incidents
urban search and rescue (USAR)

WHAT WOULD YOU DO?

An EMS department in your county experienced a structure collapse with multiple victims. The service had to call in a specialized rescue team from 30 miles away to assist at the scene. Your board of directors wants to know what would happen if the same thing were to occur in your response area. You know that the special response team would take another 30 minutes to reach you from where the structure collapse occurred, for a total response time of 1 hour. In the same respect, the financial cost to start a team is not within the budget. The board of directors wants a presentation at the next meeting in 2 weeks in response to this scenario.

Questions

1. What factors should you consider when putting together your presentation?
2. What would be your response to establishing a special operations team for structural collapse?
3. What would be your recommendation?

INTRODUCTION

When you hear the word *special*, you think of something outside the norm or something of importance. EMS special operations are no different. Numerous, if not all, departments throughout the United States offer some special operations service. Special operations, which can assume many forms, took the forefront after the September 11, 2001, terrorist events. Because of these events, homeland security became the center of attention in the United States and the president initiated several directives, including the following:

> Homeland Security Presidential Directive 8 (HSPD-8), "National Preparedness," issued December 17, 2003, tasked the Secretary of Homeland Security, in coordination with the heads of other appropriate Federal departments and agencies and in consultation with State and local governments, to strengthen the preparedness of the United States to prevent and respond to threatened or actual domestic terrorist attacks, major disasters, and other emergencies. It requires:
>
> - a national domestic preparedness goal;
> - mechanisms for improved delivery of federal preparedness assistance to state and local governments; and
> - actions to strengthen preparedness capabilities of federal, state, and local entities. (The White House, 2003)
>
> HSPD-21, "Public Health and Medical Preparedness," was released on October 18, 2007. It establishes a National Strategy for Public Health and Medical Preparedness (Strategy), which builds upon principles set forth in *Biodefense for the 21st Century* (April 2004) and will transform our national approach to protecting the health of the American people against all disasters. (The White House, 2007)

EMS special operations have many faces. This chapter introduces the special operations concept for EMS teams.

SPECIAL OPERATIONS

As pertaining to EMS, **special operations** can be divided into three areas: patient care, technical rescue, and specialized services. Patient care includes advanced triage and transportation, mass gatherings and special events, tactical medicine, and pandemics. Technical rescue includes vehicle extrication, structural collapse, confined space rescue, above- and below-grade rescue, and a technical rescue safety officer. Specialized operations include hazardous materials, water rescue and dive medicine, land-based search and rescue, incidents of national consequence, and developing a special operations team.

A special operation is simply an operation that is not an everyday call for which you are prepared to respond and mitigate. Special operations require special training, equipment, and personnel. The types of incidents vary from jurisdiction to jurisdiction. As an EMS manager, it is your responsibility to determine what specialized operation is required for your jurisdiction. Table 1.1 lists some emergency support functions (ESFs) that a special operations team may fulfill.

TABLE 1.1 ■ Emergency Support Functions

Support Function	***Responsibility***
ESF #1 Transportation	Assess transportation capabilities and provide transportation assistance
ESF #2 Communications	Ensure internal and external communications
ESF #3 Public Works and Engineering	Provide engineering and public works technical assistance for infrastructure
ESF #4 Firefighting	Coordinate deployment of fire suppression resources
ESF #5 Emergency Management	Provide core management and administrative functions
ESF #6 Mass Care, Emergency Assistance, Housing and Human Services	Arrange for the opening, staffing, and operation of shelters
ESF #7 Logistics Management and Resource Support	Provide logistical and resource support
ESF #8 Public Health and Medical Services	Provide for medical care, emergency medical services (EMS) operations, and resources
ESF #9 Urban Search and Rescue	Coordinate search-and-rescue operations, including ground, collapse, and confined space searches
ESF #10 Oil and Hazardous Materials Response	Coordinate the response to releases or potential releases of hazmats
ESF #11 Agriculture and Natural Resources	Provide for food and water that then may be distributed through ESF #6 Mass Care
ESF #12 Energy	Coordinate power establishment
ESF #13 Public Safety and Security	Facility and resource security planning and support access to traffic and crowd control
ESF #14 Long-Term Recovery	Social and economic impact assessments, long-term recovery assistance
ESF #15 External Affairs	Emergency and public information, media and community relations, congressional and internal affairs
ESF #16 Law Enforcement and Security	Establish procedures for the command, control, and coordination of all county law enforcement personnel and equipment to support local law enforcement agencies

INCIDENT TYPING

Typing of incidents is a means to define a "major incident" and is based on many factors, including the number of resources and the time span or number of operational periods. The size and capacity of the jurisdiction experiencing the incident are also factors in determining incident complexity. Typically, Type 1, Type 2, and Type 3 incidents are considered "major or complex." A mass casualty incident is relative to the capacity of the agency that responds to the incident. What may be overwhelming for one agency may be a typical, everyday call for another agency. Hence, incident typing can assist in determining the resources necessary to mitigate the situation.

An incident can become major in two ways. It can start as a small incident, such as smoke in the building, and escalate to a major fire causing evacuation of an entire nursing facility or a hazardous material spill that becomes a major incident as a result of wind or surface conditions. A delay in responding to the scene, poor incident management, and/or a lack of resources could escalate the incident to a major event. Alternatively, an incident such as a tornado outbreak, hurricane, flood, or aircraft incident may be major incident from the beginning of the event. These incidents start out as complex and can quickly become overwhelming.

Incidents such as an earthquake or tornado outbreak can be distributed over a large geographic area. They can also be isolated to an area, such as in the event of a mass shooting at a school or business.

Side Bar

Definition Review of Incident Command Nomenclature

Division. That organizational level having responsibility for operations within a defined geographic area.

Group. Groups are established to divide the incident into functional areas of operation.

Branch. That organizational level having functional, geographic, or jurisdictional responsibility for major parts of the incident operations.

Task Force. A group of resources that is sent to or formed at an incident and that has common communications and a possibly preestablished leader.

Strike Team. Specified combinations of the same kind and type of resources, with common communications and a leader.

Single Resources. An individual piece of equipment and its personnel complement, or an established crew or team of individuals, with an identified work supervisor, that can be used on an incident.

AMBULANCE STRIKE TEAMS AND EMERGENCY MEDICAL TASK FORCES

When using Incident Command Services, resources are commonly assembled into functional units known as *task forces* and *strike teams*. These terms are not used interchangeably, but rather have specific meanings.

A **task force** is defined as a group of resources (generally mixed in type) that is sent to or formed at an incident and that has common communications and a possibly pre-established leader. Task forces are established to perform a specific function. For example, a wildland fire suppression task force might consist of two brush trucks, one engine, one water tender, and a supervisor. This task force could be requested from a neighboring community (or communities) and respond as a group, or it could be assembled from resources already in a staging area.

To apply the concept of task forces to the EMS arena, a community might predefine an emergency medical task force consisting of three advanced life support ambulances with two paramedics each, two engines with EMTs or even medical first responders, and a supervisor. Once deployed at an incident, the resources brought with these units could be reassembled to form a functioning group of six treatment teams of one paramedic and one EMT each. These treatment teams could then function together to treat a large number of casualties or even support the medical needs of a casualty collection point. By assembling resources in a modular fashion, the treatment capability of three ambulances has increased at least twofold.

A **strike team** is a specified combination of the same type and kind of resources (generally three to five similar units), with common communications and a leader. The concept of a strike team is that of mustering quantity. Examples would be five engines and a chief officer, all operating on a common radio frequency at a major fire or structural collapse; or five police cruisers with two officers each and a supervisor working together to provide scene security.

As with the task force, we also can apply this concept to EMS through the establishment of ambulance strike teams comprising three to five advanced life support or basic life support ambulances with a supervisor providing medical care and transportation in a specific area of a community ravaged by tornadoes. This strike team could receive assignments through its supervisor and function as a resource within a certain geographic area.

Regardless of the concepts applied to a specific community, the single most important factor is defining the resources in advance. The best procedure would be to follow the national or state typing model for national and state resources in order to maintain consistency. Therefore, when disaster strikes and an ambulance strike team or medical task force is called, the exact physical and human resources that will be available are known.

A major incident requires a large number of resources. As a result of this need, strike teams and task forces are designed to aid in bringing a set number of resources to the scene. An incident commander wants to know that when an ambulance strike team is requested, all members of the team will consistently receive a set number of resources with certain capabilities. The following describes the resources that will be received when an ambulance strike team is requested:

Ambulance Strike Team

- Five advanced life support ambulances
- Two crews for each ambulance
- One supervisor
- Common communications

Likewise, a debris removal task force will provide the following:

Removal Task Force

- One front-end loader
- One backhoe
- Five- to six-cubic-yard dump trucks
- Two crews for each piece
- Two forepersons
- One supervisor

Responding units should have a means of common communication between units capable of working outside their home jurisdictions.

ROLE OF EMS PROVIDERS

EMS providers may have the opportunity to train to be an essential part of a special team. **Urban search and rescue (USAR)** and **disaster medical assistance teams (DMATs)** are the two most common teams in which EMS

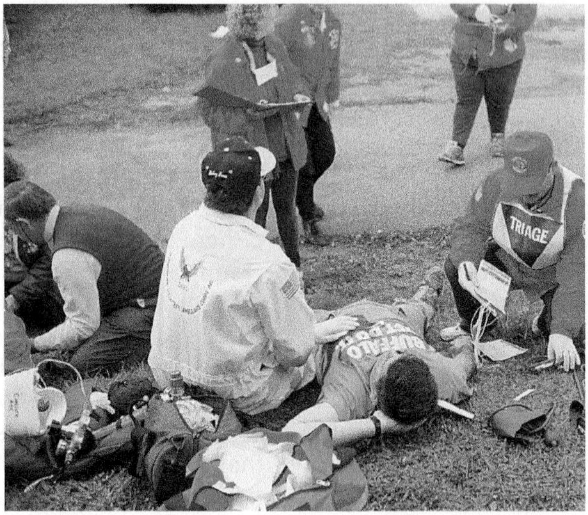

FIGURE 1.1 A DMAT typically consists of medical personnel who perform triage and provide treatment at the scene of an incident or at multiple sites over a wide geographic area.

personnel participate. (See Figure 1.1.) USAR teams comprise a multitude of skilled personnel who perform search and rescue during natural or manmade events. The teams respond to incidents from earthquakes to flooding to tornados to explosions. Typically, the events are large with mass causalities or the potential of mass causalities whereby specialized teams are needed to perform search and rescue.

A DMAT typically consists of medical personnel who perform triage and provide treatment at the scene of an incident or at multiple sites over a wide geographic area. Although the team is functionally medical, it also includes communications, logistics, command, and emergency medical records specialists.

MEDICAL RESERVES CORP

Another group that is available for volunteers to be part of is the Medical Reserves Corp (MRC). MRC units are community based and function to locally organize and utilize volunteers who want to donate their time and expertise to prepare for and respond to emergencies and to promote healthy living throughout the year. MRC volunteers supplement existing emergency and public health resources.

MRC volunteers include medical and public health professionals such as physicians, nurses, pharmacists, dentists, veterinarians, and epidemiologists. Many community members—interpreters, chaplains, office workers, legal advisors, and others—can fill key support positions.

MRC units are provided by the U.S. Surgeon General to specific areas in the country to strengthen the public health infrastructure of that community. The overarching goal is to improve health literacy, and in support of this, the U.S. Surgeon General wants to work toward increasing disease prevention, eliminating health disparities, and improving public health preparedness.

MRC volunteers can choose to support communities in need nationwide. When the U.S. Southeast was battered by hurricanes in 2004,

Best Practice

Urban search and rescue (USAR) has a long history. It is the foundation of specialized teams designed to respond and mitigate incidents requiring specialized personnel and equipment.

In the early 1980s, the Fairfax County Fire and Rescue and Metro-Dade County Fire Department created elite search-and-rescue teams trained for rescue operations in collapsed buildings. Working with the U.S. State Department and Office of Foreign Disaster Aid, these teams provided vital search-and-rescue support for catastrophic earthquakes in Mexico City, the Philippines, and Armenia.

The Federal Emergency Management Agency (FEMA) established the National Urban Search and Rescue Response System in 1989 as a framework for structuring local emergency services personnel into integrated disaster response task forces. Then, in 1991, FEMA incorporated this concept into the Federal Response Plan (now the National Response Plan), sponsoring twenty-five national urban search-and-rescue task forces.

Events such as the 1995 bombing of the Alfred P. Murrah building in Oklahoma City, the Northridge (California) earthquake, the Kansas grain elevator explosion in 1998, and earthquakes in Turkey and Greece in 1999 underscore the need for highly skilled teams to rescue trapped victims.

The terrorist attacks on the World Trade Center and the Pentagon on September 11, 2001, thrust FEMA's urban search-and-rescue teams into the spotlight. Their important work transfixed the world and brought a surge of gratitude and support.

Today, there are twenty-eight national task forces staffed and equipped to conduct round-the-clock search-and-rescue operations following earthquakes, tornados, floods, hurricanes, aircraft accidents, hazardous materials spills, and catastrophic structure collapses. These task forces, complete with necessary tools and equipment, and required skills and techniques, can be deployed by FEMA for the rescue of victims of structural collapse.

Source: FEMA (2012).

MRC volunteers in the affected areas and beyond helped communities by filling in at local hospitals, assisting their neighbors at local shelters, and providing first aid to those injured by the storms. During this 2-month period, more than thirty MRC units worked as part of the relief efforts, including those who were volunteers called in from across the country to assist the American Red Cross and the Federal Emergency Management Agency (FEMA).

CONCEPT AND MISSION OF THE NATIONAL DISASTER MEDICAL SYSTEM

The National Disaster Medical System (NDMS) is a federally coordinated system designed to provide emergency medical assistance to large numbers of casualties from either a domestic disaster or a conventional overseas war. It usually is activated when a catastrophic disaster or other major emergency overwhelms both local and state resources.

The NDMS is designed to supplement other resources and is oriented primarily to large-scale disasters in which local medical care capabilities are severely overwhelmed. It has two primary missions:

1. To supplement state and local medical resources during major domestic natural and technological catastrophic disasters and emergencies

2. To provide backup medical support to the Department of Defense (DoD) and the Department of Veterans Affairs (VA) medical systems in providing care for U.S. Armed Forces personnel who become casualties during overseas conventional conflicts

In peacetime activation, which generally consists of domestic natural or technological catastrophic disasters, the NDMS has three objectives:

1. To provide health, medical, and related social service response to a disaster area in the form of medical response units or teams and medical supplies and equipment
2. To evacuate patients who cannot be cared for in the affected area to designated locations elsewhere in the country
3. To provide hospitalization in federal hospitals and a voluntary network of nonfederal, acute care hospitals that have agreed to accept patients in the event of a national emergency

Organizational Resources

To carry out these three objectives, the NDMS has three organizational resources.

Voluntary Teams. DMATs are voluntary medical personnel units organized and equipped to provide austere medical care in a disaster area, or medical services at transfer points or reception sites associated with patient evacuation. Hospitals, volunteer agencies, or health and medical organizations may participate in DMATs and recruit interested medical and paramedical personnel to participate. DMATs are classified into three readiness levels, as follows:

Level 1	Fully Operational
Level 2	Operational
Level 3	Augment Type I or II

The deployment ready time is relevant to whether the team is on call, on standby, or advisory. This time can range between 4 and 24 hours. The specifics concerning operation capabilities and training can be found in the National Incident Management System *Health and Medical Resource Typing Document.*

Casualty Evacuation System. Movement of patients from disaster sites to locations where definitive medical care can be provided is administered through the DoD. Casualty tracking is conducted by the Armed Services Medical Regulating Office, and the U.S. Air Force provides airlift through the Air Mobility Command, which can be supplemented by civilian resources through the Civil Reserve Air Fleet. Other types of transportation such as specially outfitted Amtrak trains can be called into service through this system.

Definitive Medical Care Network. The NDMS has enrolled more than 110,000 reserve beds in 1,818 participating civilian hospitals to receive casualties from disaster areas. The DoD and the VA can provide additional beds, if required. These hospitals are located in 107 metropolitan areas. Maintaining this network is the responsibility of the DoD and VA under the current concept of NDMS operations.

The entire NDMS, or selected components, can be activated in a number of ways. The governor of a state can request assistance from the president of the United States, who, in turn, can either declare a disaster or order activation of federal assistance to that state. Currently, such activations are authorized under the Stafford Act of 1988 and administered through the National Response Framework of 2008. The Public Health Service Act also authorizes the Secretary of Health and Human Services to provide emergency medical assistance on request of state or local authorities, and the NDMS is an authorized vehicle for such assistance. The Secretary of

Defense also can activate the NDMS in situations of national emergency. In practice, the Director of the Office of Emergency Preparedness would be the principal operating agent for the NDMS in all of these cases.

TRAINING

EMS special operations call for EMS providers to serve in many different roles. As a result, training programs vary. Each discipline requires various levels of training. In many instances, such as with hazardous materials, a basic EMS provider will be required to complete an awareness-level training program. Table 1.2 provides the requirements for level of search-and-rescue teams. Every special operations team has a chart that depicts the requirements for the typing prescribed for that level of capability.

Basic rescue teams require minimal additional training to perform these functions. These types of rescues are ideally suited for community emergency response teams and virtually all levels of public safety responders, law enforcement, EMS, and fire service.

Prior to the occurrence of a disaster, basic rescue teams should be located throughout the community. These teams should have predefined objectives and search patterns. A basic rescue team can join with a debris-clearing team in order to increase effectiveness and accomplish search goals.

Beginning with the light rescue teams, a progressively higher and higher level of training and equipment is required. This progression culminates with the Type 1 Heavy Rescue, which is exemplified by FEMA's urban search-and-rescue teams. Communities need to analyze the potential resource needs with regard to rescue teams and determine what team levels are necessary based on potential hazards and vulnerabilities. As the necessary resources become more complicated and equipment more expensive, individual communities may want to develop these resources jointly on a regional basis, rather than on an individual community basis.

Light and medium tactical rescue task forces are teams of trained first responders that can be placed into action after a natural disaster and, if warning allows, should be predeployed. The role of these specially equipped teams is to locate victims rapidly in affected areas, ensure the safety of injured or stranded citizens, and reduce system service delays by the expedient clearance of critical roadways and facilities, which will allow for movement of essential services and relief efforts. See Table 1.3 for examples of a light and medium tactical rescue task force as well as typical vehicles and equipment this type of team will use.

Light and medium search-and-rescue task forces can be developed using available local

TABLE 1.2 ■ Levels and Capabilities of Search-and-Rescue Teams

	Level			
	Type 1 Heavy	***Type 2 Medium***	***Type 3 Light***	***Type 4 Basic***
Capabilities	Reinforced concrete structural collapse Steel structures Confined space rescue Trench rescue	Reinforced and unreinforced masonry Tilt-up construction Heavy-timber construction	Light-frame construction Basic rope rescue	Surface rescue Nonstructural entrapment Noncollapsed structures

TABLE 1.3 ■ Light and Medium Search-and-Rescue Task Forces

Law Enforcement	*EMS*	*Fire Suppression*	*Public Works*	*Utilities*
Four officers	One paramedic Two emergency medical technicians	One officer Three firefighters	Six public works employees	One telephone service technician Two power company linepersons

Vehicles and Equipment for Each Team

One four-wheel-drive truck	Cellular phone	Three plug wrenches/six files/one guide
One front-end loader	Portable radio (TF to EOC)	Two 24-inch bolt cutters
One dump truck	Portable radio (TF to TF)	One 36-inch bolt cutter
One 2½ -ton flatbed truck	Two 16-inch chainsaws	Three 6-foot pry bars
One power company trouble truck with bucket	One 24-inch chainsaw	Three axes
One fire engine (1,000+ gpm, 750-gallon, National Fire Protection Association equipped)	Six extra chains for saws	Two flat shovels
One school bus	5 gallons bar lube	One K-12 power saw
One advanced life support ambulance	Two 12-foot, $\frac{3}{8}$-inch chains with grab hooks	One generator
One spotlight, 5,000 candlepower	Five 2½ -gallon cans fuel fix for saws	One Hurst tool

Personal equipment to include food and water for each team member for 1 to 3 days of operations, depending on anticipated relief schedule

resources with little additional capital expenditure. These teams comprise approximately twenty multidisciplinary personnel representing fire, EMS, public works, law enforcement, and utilities. Although the teams can be assembled in any fashion deemed necessary by the community, a suggested arrangement is provided here. As you review this arrangement, bear in mind that this particular task force's primary goal is to perform rescue and clear major transportation routes.

HAZARDOUS MATERIALS RESPONSE TEAMS

A hazard materials (hazmat) response team is a group of generally no less than eight specially trained and equipped personnel who can perform offensive operations while wearing specialized chemical protective clothing. Next to EMS, hazmat is one of the most heavily regulated emergency response functions performed. Both the U.S. Environmental Protection Agency (EPA) and the Occupational Safety and Health Administration (OSHA) have established mandatory standards to which these specialized units must train and operate. In addition to EPA and OSHA regulations, numerous consensus standards exist to guide their operations.

During hazmat emergencies, EMS will play one of three specific roles: (1) medical surveillance of responders, (2) treatment of patients generated by the event, and (3) treatment of responders who are injured inadvertently during operations. Specialized training is required for EMS personnel who are interested in performing hazmat-specific roles.

CHAPTER REVIEW

Summary

The number of EMS special operation teams has increased across the country. To be a specialized team, personnel need to be trained at the level of capability for the team. In addition, the proper equipment will need to be purchased. It can be an expensive endeavor to create an EMS special team. Careful analysis of risk and benefit is needed to determine whether a team is needed and what level of team should be established.

An EMS manager on the scene of an incident needs to be aware of incident typing in order to know what to expect when a special team is requested to report to the incident scene. In addition, knowing the difference between various levels of teams will provide advance knowledge of the team's capabilities before it even arrives at the scene.

WHAT WOULD YOU DO? Reflection

When preparing your presentation, you want to include the historical perspective of teams and why agencies create a team. Include past incidents in which the team could have been used. Identify risks in your community that would be affected in a major event. Use these risks as a model for the development of your presentation. Be sure to include alternatives for establishing a team in your agency. One option to present for a special operations team for structural collapse may be to provide a lower level of training until a specialized team can arrive.

Your presentation should include the plan for a similar response and training of personnel until a specialized team arrives. Explain the ongoing costs of a team and how it is beneficial to establish a mutual aid agreement with another team. Begin training with the team so there is a smooth transition on the scene of an incident.

Review Questions

1. List as many different specialized teams as you have read about or seen.
2. Which ESF unit provides medical care, EMS operations, and resources?
3. What are the components of an ambulance strike team?
4. What level of search-and-rescue teams would include the following capabilities: reinforced and unreinforced masonry; tilt-up construction; and heavy-timber construction?
5. What three specific roles will EMS play in a hazardous material emergency?
6. What task forces can be developed using available local resources with little additional capital expenditure?

References

FEMA. (2012). "About Urban Search and Rescue." See the organization website.

The White House. (2003, December 17). "Homeland Security Presidential Directive/

HSPD-8—Subject: National Preparedness." See the organization website.
The White House. (2007, October 18). "Homeland Security Presidential Directive/HSPD-21—Subject: Public Health and Medical Preparedness." See the organization website.

Key Terms

basic rescue teams A group of individuals that provides rescue at incidents and that has a minimal level of education and training to perform said services.

disaster medical assistance teams (DMATs) Voluntary medical personnel units organized and equipped to provide austere medical care in a disaster area or medical services at transfer points or reception sites associated with patient evacuation.

light and medium tactical rescue task forces Teams of trained first responders that can be placed into action after a natural disaster and, if warning allows, should be predeployed.

special operations Teams that provide patient care, technical rescue, and specialized services at major events, specialized incidents, and mass casualty incidents.

strike team A specified combination of the same type and kind of resources (generally three to five similar units), with common communications and a leader.

task force A group of resources (generally mixed in type) with common communications and a leader that may be preestablished and sent to or formed at an incident.

typing of incidents A way of defining a major incident.

urban search and rescue (USAR) The location, rescue (extrication), and initial medical stabilization of victims trapped in confined spaces.

2 CHAPTER

Mass Casualty Incidents: Triage, Treatment, and Transport

JEFFREY LINDSEY

RAY WHATLEY

Objectives

After reading this chapter, the student should be able to:

2.1 Discuss the placement and functions of the medical branch in an incident management system.

2.2 Describe the functions of the triage, treatment, and transport groups in the medical branch.

2.3 Discuss the importance of a post-incident review following a mass casualty incident.

2.4 Discuss what constitutes a mass casualty incident.

2.5 Describe the START, JumpSTART and SALT triage processes.

2.6 Describe considerations in determining the transport destination for patients in a mass casualty incident.

2.7 Describe the implementation of incident command for a mass casualty incident.

2.8 Acknowledge the importance of adhering to principles of triage in mass casualty incidents.

Key Terms

mass casualty incident (MCI)
medical ambulance bus
National Response Framework
persons with special needs (PSNs)
post-incident review (PIR)
primary triage
secondary triage
task force
triage

WHAT WOULD YOU DO?

You have been dispatched for a possible vehicle crash. The following resources were dispatched: one engine company and one medic unit. Further information revealed that the caller did not witness the crash but only heard what sounded like a large crash in a residential neighborhood. As you arrive on the scene, you see a yellow school bus on its side with another vehicle that seems to be entangled with the underside of the bus. You give your on-scene report and assume or pass command. Immediately, you request additional resources and have communications activate the Regional Hospital Coordination Center. Once on scene, you do your size-up. If any hazards are present, they must be secured lest they impair your ability to begin triage. As you listen to the sounds around your crew, you hear the screams and shouts of the patients. You see small children crying and calling out for someone to help them. Triage must be started, and you have two vehicles involved. As you begin the process to triage, you remember that JumpSTART is better suited for younger children. As one of the initial resources on the scene, your actions set the tone for this event.

Questions

1. What is the most critical element for a smooth incident scene?
2. What does every responder have the obligation to know and understand?
3. What sections should be added after completion of triage?

INTRODUCTION

A **mass casualty incident (MCI)** is an event in which there are more patients than there are resources immediately available. The term *mass casualty incident* is relative to the geographic location of the incident; that is, managing an MCI is defined by the local agencies based on their capabilities. Regardless of the location, managing an MCI taxes the resources on hand. Training and preplanning are important pre-event considerations to prepare for an MCI.

Operations at an MCI can be overwhelming in the early minutes of the incident. EMS personnel must be familiar with a systematic approach to managing an MCI. In many situations, the first-arriving EMS personnel will be the sole provider(s) on the scene of the incident. Beginning the triage process establishes the plan of action for the treatment and, eventually, the transport of patients from the scene.

COMMAND AND CONTROL OF A MASS CASUALTY INCIDENT

As resources arrive on the scene of an MCI, focus on a single role versus wearing multiple hats. In many instances, the initial incident is chaotic and

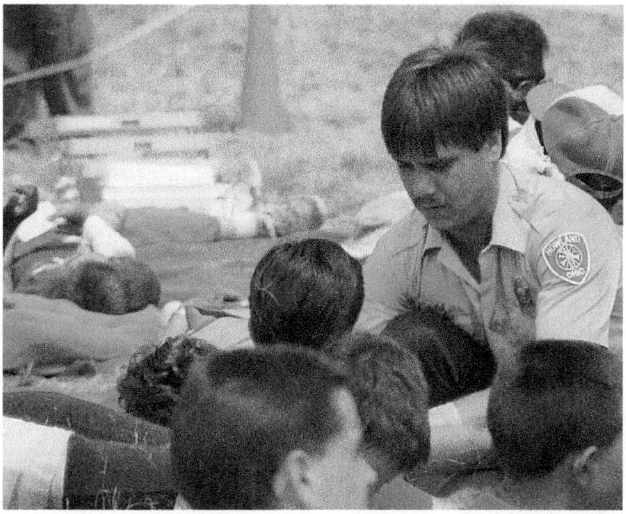

FIGURE 2.1 The first-arriving EMS personnel are responsible for the initial triage effort.

confusing, but knowing the steps that need to be taken will help organize the situation.

Triage is the first step. Once triage is completed, patients should be moved to the treatment area and then transported off the scene in order of their priority. (See Figure 2.1.) It takes personnel to manage the incident, hence the need to request resources early on.

TRIAGE AREA

The first-arriving EMS personnel are responsible for the initial triage effort. **Triage** is conducted quickly and identifies critical patients. Victims are tagged according to the priority of their condition. Once the initial triage is complete, personnel should be assigned to another area. Triage is ongoing; however, personnel assigned to the treatment and transport areas also conduct secondary triage as part of their responsibilities.

TREATMENT AREA

The treatment area is the next step in the process after the patient leaves the triage group and begins treatment of life-threatening treatment as determined by the triage area. As soon as the number of personnel on the scene allows for it, the treatment area must be established. This may occur after triage is under way or as soon as more personnel arrive.

Treatment units are designated in coordination with the triage system. For example, if your agency uses the system that denotes red, yellow, green, and black, you would establish red, yellow, and green treatment units. Patients would be distributed to the respective units based on their triage priority. Patients may be moved from one unit to another as their conditions change. Typically, there is no "black" treatment unit, as these victims are deceased and require no additional treatment. A temporary morgue is established, and a morgue officer is assigned to the unit.

TRANSPORT AREA

The transport area is set up in order to move patients from the treatment units to the receiving facility. This unit is responsible for maintaining the status of all hospitals and for distributing the patients according to the treatment needs and patient load capabilities of each facility. In many regions or counties across the United States, the dispatch center maintains the status of the area's hospital capacity. It is also responsible for coordinating the number of units needed from staging in order to transport patients to the receiving facilities.

The transport supervisor should consider local transport options such as buses and other fleet vehicles. Aeromedical transportation should be reserved for critical patients or for patients who need transportation to facilities outside the immediate area of the incident. Do not rely on aeromedical transport because weather, scene conditions, and number of patients all play roles in the type of transport being used.

The transport area is also responsible for patient tracking. Hospital destinations should be based on the severity of the patients' conditions. Regardless of the method of transportation, the transport area should keep a log of the destination of each transported patient. One of the greatest concerns at the scene of an MCI is where patients ultimately are transported. At a minimum, the log should contain the patient's name, what unit transported the patient, the patient's triage category, and where the patient was transported. This information is crucial to patient tracking at an MCI.

STAGING

The need for resources is typically great for an MCI. Depending on the incident and number of victims, many resources may be needed. A staging area is established as a holding area for these resources. All resources responding to the scene should go to the staging area unless they are part of the initial response. If all units arrived at the incident, the scene would become congested and difficult to manage. As resources are needed, the staging officer will send them to the scene.

Supervisors on the scene will make requests for resources as they deem necessary. For example, there may be fifteen transport units responding to the incident scene, but only three ambulances can be accommodated at a time. As patients are transported off the scene, the transportation supervisor will request additional transport units from staging to come to the scene.

Staging creates a cache of resources that are available and ready to come to the scene. If resources are sent only when needed from their home base, the response time would be great in many instances. Staging helps reduce the time necessary to get additional resources directly on scene at the incident. (See Figure 2.2.)

SUPERVISION

The medical area officer is assigned to command of the medical area. He reports to the incident commander or to the operations section chief, if that position has been established. At an MCI event, each of these areas will have a supervisor. For example, the treatment area has a treatment supervisor who is responsible for the treatment area and reports to the medical area officer. If the incident is large enough and multiple treatment areas are using the color code (see the "Triage Tags" section), then each color would have a supervisor.

TRIAGE

The French word *triage* means "to sort out." In a medical context, triage entails determining the priority of a patient by considering the physiologic state of the patient. Patients who are not able to compensate and who are physiologically comprised are identified as high-priority patients.

The concept of triage is not new; in fact, it is hundreds of years old. Dominique Jean Larrey, Napoleon's field surgeon, helped give birth to the use of triage after modeling his

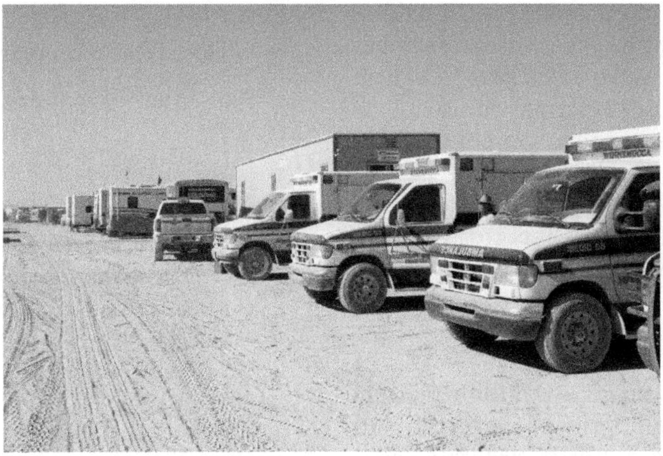

FIGURE 2.2 A staging area is established to hold resources. *Source:* © *Dr. Bryan E. Bledsoe.*

ambulance corps during French warfare after the fast-moving artillery sections, or "flying artillery," that moved quickly about the battlefield (Dible, 1959). He took this same idea and introduced "flying ambulances" with the goal of removing injured soldiers, regardless of their nationality, from the battlefield in less than 15 minutes. So impressed was the Duke of Wellington with the bravery of the French ambulance workers at the Battle of Waterloo that he directed his men not to fire in their direction.

Part of the first-arriving EMS provider's responsibility is to determine the priority of each patient on scene. By doing so, the EMS provider will also know how many patients need to be treated. Triage is an ongoing evaluation and is divided into primary and secondary triage.

PRIMARY TRIAGE

Similar to the primary and secondary assessment, **primary triage** is the first contact with the patients. Primary triage rapidly identifies the critically injured patients on scene, and gives the basis to formulate the action plan to treat and transport patients from the scene of the incident. Personnel should document the location and transport needs of each patient. In addition, the priority level of all patients should be identified with a triage tag or label. Some agencies like to use a ribbon to identify the initial priority assigned to the patient.

Performing the primary triage quickly to sort out the patients, identify the number of patients, and determine the level of severity of patients is critical to management and performance at an MCI. Triage is not the time to treat patients—it is a time to classify and establish a plan to treat patients.

SECONDARY TRIAGE

Patients' conditions change; therefore, continuously performing **secondary triage** until all patients are transferred to the appropriate receiving facility is critical in the care of patients on the scene of an MCI.

Three different events at an MCI can trigger secondary assessment:

1. When the patient is moved to the treatment area
2. When the patient is moved to the transport area
3. When the patient arrives at the hospital

A paper tag or document is completed and attached to every patient. This allows other providers to re-triage or administer treatment with a foundation of information about the patient. Patient care reports are not practical for use in an MCI until the patient is designated for transport. Once the patient is moved to transport, a patient care report is easier to establish and keep with the patient.

TRIAGE TAGS

Different triage systems use different methods to identify the priority of the victim during the initial triage. Cardboard and paper tags used as a temporary medical record are popular and serve as a visual signal to the treatment crews who provide care to the patient once they reach the treatment area. The Simple Triage and Rapid Treatment (START) triage system is used during initial triage; this is when the tag indicating the triage category of the patient is placed on the patient. The portion of the color-coded tag used to identify the patient's condition must be removed.

Some EMS personnel like to use a system to easily identify the number of patients at the scene without having to do a complete head count. For example, personnel can bundle triage tags in a set of ten, making sure that everyone in the agency knows that triage tags are bundled in sets of ten. At the scene of an MCI, count the remaining tags in a packet and deduct that number from ten. Adding the number of complete sets of ten used gives the total number of patients triaged. (See Figure 2.3.)

The international agreement on color coding and priorities standardizes the priority levels of patients in an MCI. They are as follows:

- Immediate Red Priority-1 (P-1)
- Delayed Yellow Priority-2 (P-2)
- Hold Green Priority-3 (P-3)
- Deceased Black Priority-0 (P-0)

Examples of patient priorities are as follows:

- Immediate
  - Airway and breathing difficulties
  - Uncontrolled or severe bleeding
  - Decreased mental status
  - Patients with severe medical problems
  - Shock (hypoperfusion)
  - Severe burns
- Delayed
  - Burns without airway problems
  - Major or multiple bone or joint injuries
  - Back injuries with or without spinal cord damage
- Hold
  - Minor painful, swollen, deformed extremities
  - Minor soft tissue injuries
- Deceased

TRIAGE PRINCIPLES

There is no recommended or standardized triage and treatment system in the United States for EMS. No mass casualty triage system has been validated by any post-incident data (Wiseman, Ellenbogen, and Shaffrey, 2002). Different systems exist that universally use the color-coded categories of red (immediate/critical), yellow (delayed), green (minor), and black (dead/unsalvageable).

TRIAGE SYSTEMS

A limited number of triage systems are available for the prehospital setting. Lerner, Schwartz, Coule, and Pirrallo (2010) conducted a research study that compared the various commercial triage systems. The START triage system received the highest overall evaluation. As a result of the study,

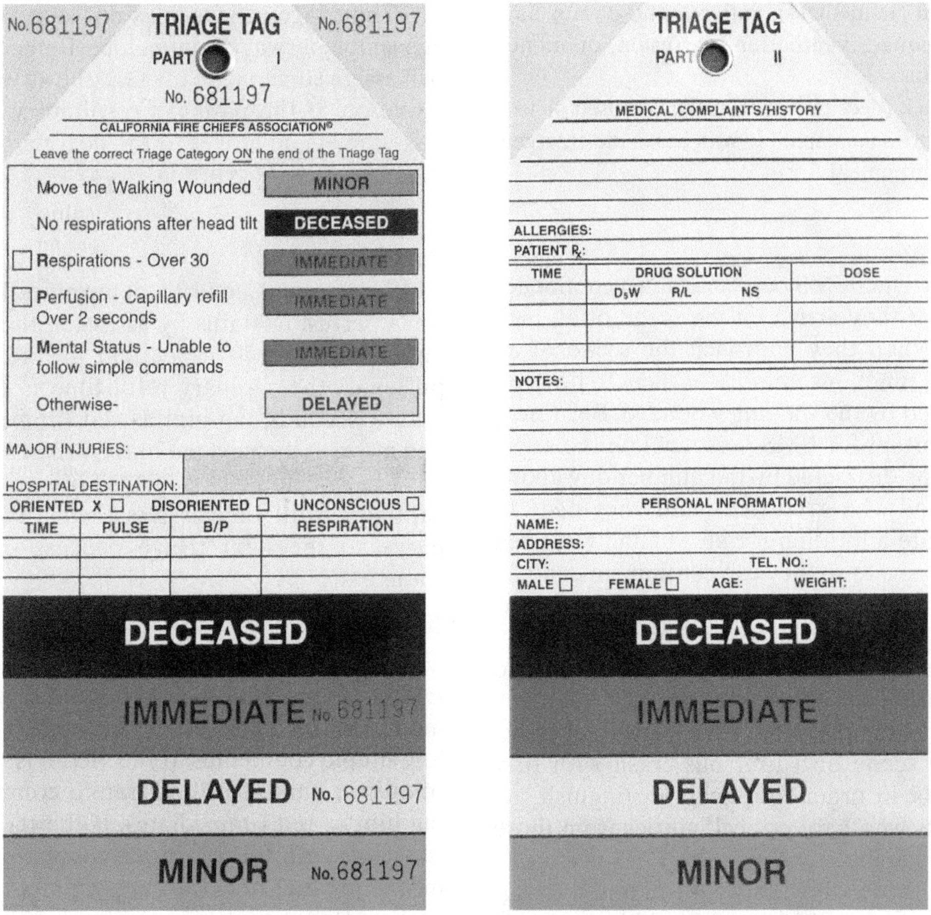

FIGURE 2.3 ■ This is one example of a triage tag used in an MCI. (*Source: "A Typical Triage Tag" from EMT COMPLETE: A Comprehensive Worktext, 2E by C. LeBaudour, D. Batsie, E. T. Dickinson, D. Limmer. Copyright © 2014, p. 1161. Reprinted and Electronically reproduced by permission of Pearson Education, Inc., Upper Saddle River, New Jersey.*)

another system called the SALT triage system was developed.

THE START SYSTEM

The START triage system is the triage system used in many EMS agencies. It was developed by Hoag Hospital and the Newport Beach Fire Department in the 1980s (Pullum and Kaull, 2001). Designed for the adult patient, the system takes into account four different variables: ambulation, respirations, perfusion, and mental status. It is rapidly performed in the prehospital setting and helps the responder quickly assign a priority to the patient.

START triage is designed to complete the primary triage process in as little as 30 seconds for each patient. It uses a color-coded designator for each of the four categories:

- Green (minor): walking wounded
- Yellow (delayed): patients with adequate ventilation, perfusion, and ability to follow simple commands but not able to ambulate

- Red (immediate): patients who do not have adequate ventilation, perfusion, or mental status
- Black (deceased/expectant): deceased or with injuries incompatible with life in the emergent environment

Ambulation

First-arriving EMS personnel must commence triage as they arrive on the scene of an incident. When they approach the scene of an MCI, it is not uncommon for them to be overwhelmed by the walking wounded. Because it is important for EMS personnel on the scene not to be distracted by the number of walking wounded who need treatment, they need to designate a location for all walking wounded to congregate so they can continue to conduct primary triage. This will separate the patients who are able to walk from those with critical injuries and/or those who may not be able to ambulate.

For example, when EMS personnel arrive on the scene of a tour bus crash with fifty patients, in order to quickly distinguish the patients who have critical injuries from those who are ambulatory, have the EMS personnel ask all those who can walk to go to a designated location. Someone should be assigned to assist the walking wounded. Failure to do so will allow the walking wounded to return to the triaged areas. This will initially relocate the green patients to one area, allowing for easier management of the remaining victims to triage.

Respirations

Personnel should assess the victim's respirations. If he is not breathing, open the airway and reassess. If the patient is still not breathing, tag him as black (deceased/expectant) and move to the next patient. If the victim is breathing but his respiratory rate is greater than 30, tag him as red (immediate) and move on.

The triage officer does not stop to manage simple airway maintenance. If needed, he will assign someone to manage the airway and move on. If the patient's respiratory rate is less than 30, he moves to the next part of the triage process—perfusion.

Perfusion

EMS personnel need to determine the victim's perfusion status by assessing the capillary refill time. If the patient has no radial pulses or the capillary refill time is greater than 2 seconds, tag him as red (immediate) and move to the next patient. Quickly manage any life-threatening bleeding, if present. If the capillary refill time is less than 2 seconds, move to the next triage process—mental status.

Mental Status

EMS personnel must determine the victim's mental status by assessing his ability to follow simple commands. If the victim is unconscious, or cannot follow simple commands, tag him as red (immediate). If the patient is conscious, can follow simple commands, and meets no other red criteria, tag him as yellow (delayed).

Using the START System

Once personnel have reached a trigger point that defines red criteria for the patient, they tag him as red (immediate) and move on to the next patient. If a victim makes it through the respiration/perfusion/mental status (RPM) assessment with no red criteria findings but is unable to walk, tag him as yellow (delayed).

A mnemonic to remember the START system is "30-2-Can Do." For the adult patient with a respiratory rate less than 30, with capillary refill less than 2 seconds, and who "Can Do" simple commands, if he can walk, he is green (walking wounded), and if he cannot walk, he is yellow (delayed); everyone else is red or dead.

THE JUMPSTART SYSTEM

MCIs can be more stressful when children are involved. This type of MCI can have an emotional impact on personnel that may negatively affect their ability to triage and treat these patients at a time when decision making is critical. The JumpSTART system, developed by Dr. Lou Romig from the Miami (Florida) Children's Hospital, is designed to parallel the adult START triage format and include items that are specific to pediatrics (Romig, 2009). The advantages of using this pediatric triage system to help conduct triage operations during an MCI event are twofold:

1. Using a pediatric system that parallels an existing adult triage system accounts for the physiologic and anatomic differences of pediatric patients, particularly when deciding on a triage category for each patient.
2. It helps manage over-triage of the pediatric patient that might allocate precious resources away from patients who need them more.

These two advantages are designed to help relieve stress so that a more objective decision regarding the care of pediatric patients can be made. The goal of pediatric triage is to allow EMS personnel to ensure that "injured children are triaged by responders with their heads, not their hearts" (Romig, 2011).

The JumpSTART triage system was designed for use in patients between the ages of 1 and 8 years. At younger than 1 year, the patient is likely not ambulatory, and at approximately 8 years of age, pediatric physiology (especially the airway) becomes similar to that of adults. Because of the variation in patient size, if the patient looks like a child, use JumpSTART; if the patient looks like a young adult, use START.

Ambulation

As EMS personnel do in START, identifying and directing all ambulatory patients to the designated green (minor) area for secondary triage and treatment is necessary. Begin assessment of nonambulatory patients as they are found. Nonambulatory patients who are carried by other people (parents, siblings) must be triaged and placed in the correct designated treatment area. Do not attempt to separate children from parents or caregivers unless critical treatment necessitates it.

Respirations

If the patient is breathing spontaneously, go to the next step and determine the respiratory rate. If the patient is apneic or has very irregular breathing, EMS personnel should open the airway using standard positioning techniques. If spontaneous respirations resume after opening the airway, personnel should tag the patient as red (immediate) and move on. If there is no breathing after airway opening, check for peripheral pulse. If no pulse is found, tag the patient as black (deceased/unsalvageable) and move to the next patient. If there is a peripheral pulse, give five mouth-to-barrier ventilations. If apnea persists, tag the patient as black (deceased/unsalvageable) and move on. If breathing resumes, tag the patient as red (immediate) and move to the next patient.

If the patient's respiratory rate is 15 to 45 breaths per minute, move to the perfusion assessment. If respirations are fewer than 15 or more than 45 per minute, then tag the patient as red (immediate) and move to the next patient.

Perfusion

If a peripheral pulse is palpable, proceed to assess the patient's mental status. If no peripheral pulse is present (in the least injured limb), tag the patient as red (immediate) and move to the next patient.

Mental Status

Use the Alert, Verbal, Painful, Unresponsive (AVPU) scale to determine the patient's mental status. If the patient is alert, verbally responsive, or gives an age-appropriate response to pain, tag him as yellow (delayed) and move to the next patient. If the patient is inappropriately responsive to pain or unresponsive, tag him as red (immediate) and move to the next patient.

Other Conditions

JumpSTART takes into account pediatric patients who are not able to walk, children who may be developmentally delayed, children with chronic disabilities, or those who may not have been able to ambulate because of acute injuries that existed prior to the incident.

If the patient meets *any* red criteria, he is tagged as red (immediate). The patient is tagged as yellow (delayed) if significant signs of external injury are present (deep penetrating wounds, severe bleeding, severe burns, amputations, distended tender abdomen). The patient is tagged as green (minor) if there is no significant external injury. Patients tagged as black (deceased/unsalvageable), with the exception of patients suffering from injuries incompatible with life, should be reassessed once all critical interventions for red and yellow patients have been completed.

START/JUMPSTART DIFFERENCES

Specific physiologic differences in the adult and pediatric patients require that the START triage system be modified to incorporate the pediatric patient. (See Figure 2.4.) Some of these differences are as follows:

- *Respirations*—An apneic child is more likely to have a primary respiratory problem than is an adult. Perfusion may be maintained for a short time, and the child may still be salvageable. Depending on the age of the child, a respiratory rate greater than 30 may either under- or over-triage the patient.
- *Perfusion*—Capillary refill may not adequately reflect hemodynamic status in a cooler environment.
- *Mental Status*—Obeying simple commands may not be an appropriate gauge of mental status for younger children.

THE SALT SYSTEM

The Sort, Assess, Lifesaving interventions, Treatment and/or Transport (SALT) triage system was created by a multidisciplinary workgroup and led by researchers at the Medical College of Wisconsin. It incorporates both adult and pediatric patients and is designed to work in any manner of MCI (Medical College of Wisconsin, 2008).

SALT Triage Procedure

The first step in the SALT triage system is Sort. Patients are evaluated using simple voice commands asking them to walk to an area or wave their hands. By the patients following simple commands, or by their inability to do so, paramedics can have a quick idea of the number of potentially critical patients.

The second and third steps—Assess and Lifesaving interventions—begin the assessment and treatment of patients with a focus on life-threatening injuries or conditions, such as major hemorrhage, closed airways, tension pneumothorax, or chemical exposure. The fourth and final step—Treatment and/or Transport—is conducted after providing any life-threatening interventions and color coding

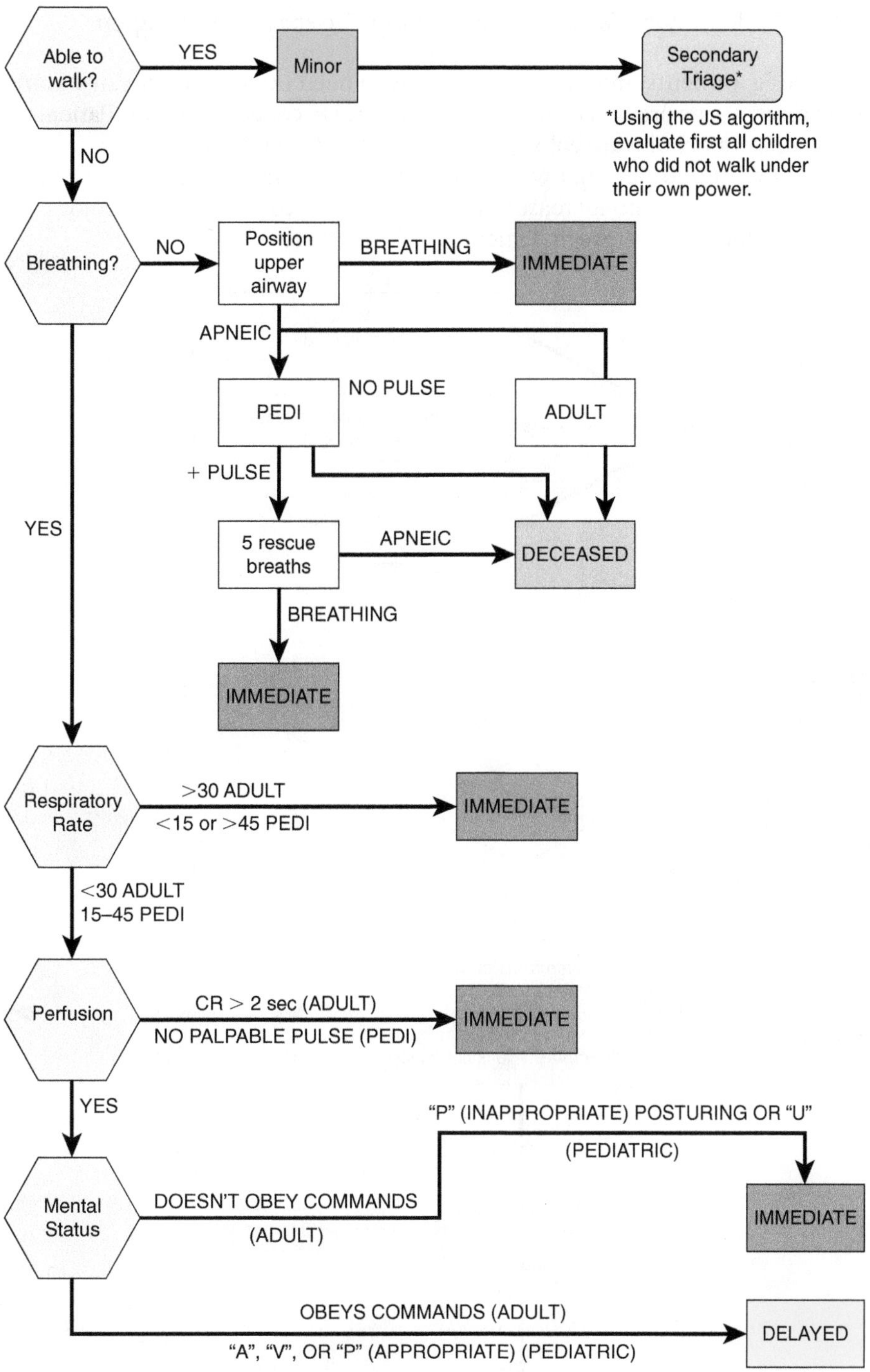

FIGURE 2.4 The START/JumpSTART algorithm can be used for both adult and pediatric triage. *(Source: "START and JumpSTART Algorithm Triage System" in Paramedic Care: Principles & Practice, Volume 7, Operations, 4E by B. E. Bledsoe, R. S. Porter, R. A. Cherry. Copyright © 2013, p. 52. Reprinted and Electronically reproduced by permission of Pearson Education, Inc., Upper Saddle River, New Jersey.)*

of the remaining patients into categories based on the assessments previously made.

Patients with high priority are color coded as red. Minimally injured patients who can tolerate a delay in care with no increased risk of mortality are color coded as green. Patients who need treatment but can wait to receive it are color coded as yellow. Patients considered to be deceased are color coded as black. Patients who are expected to die, even with the resources at hand, are color coded as gray. (See Figure 2.5.)

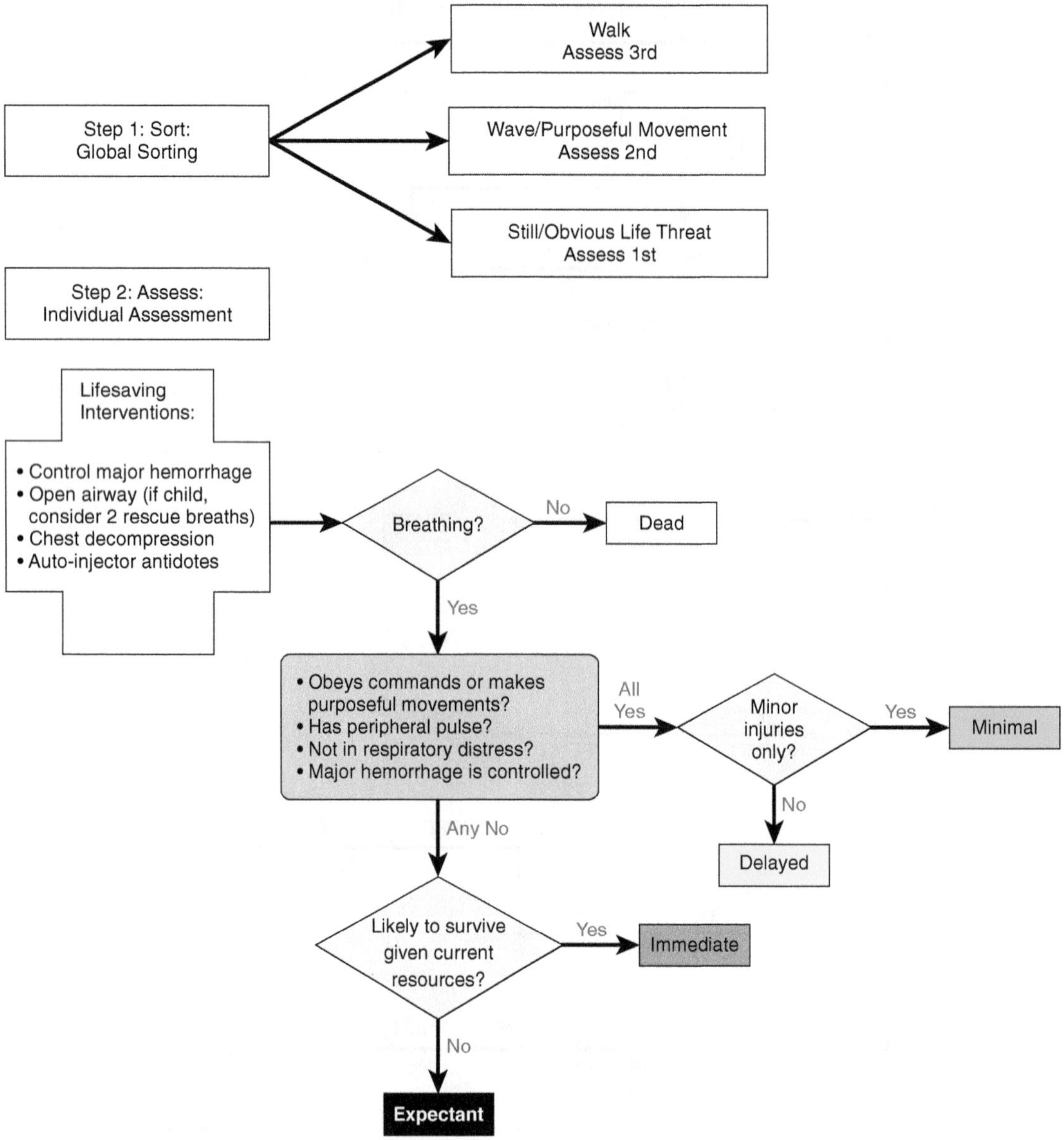

FIGURE 2.5 The SALT algorithm.

DESTINATION DECISIONS

The transport group is responsible for the distribution of patients from the scene of the incident to the receiving facility. Various factors must be taken into consideration when determining the distribution of patients. The number of hospitals in the area will play a major role in this process. If there is only one hospital in the area, choices may be limited. However, regardless of the distance, other hospitals must be considered among the potential destination hospitals.

In 2007, for example, a 56-passenger motor coach with a driver and 52 passengers onboard was traveling on a remote road in southern Utah when it crashed. The bus rolled over an embankment and came to rest on its wheels. The roof was separated from the body and 50 of the 53 occupants were ejected from the bus. Nine of the passengers were fatally injured; 43 passengers and the driver received minor to serious injuries.

The local EMS agency had eight basic life support ambulances. Neighboring EMS agencies sent a variety of transport units to the scene, and units as far away as Colorado responded to the scene. In addition, a 15-passenger van was used to transport the walking wounded. The closest treatment facility was a clinic that was 43 miles away from the crash scene. The more seriously injured patients were transported to a local hospital 75 miles from the crash site; because this hospital had no trauma response capabilities, it was used as the triage hospital to treat and release minor injuries and transfer patients who were in serious condition.

In this scenario, no receiving facilities were within a reasonable range from the incident scene. The patients were distributed to twelve hospitals and one clinic. The nearest trauma center was located 190 miles from the crash site. Air medical was not an option because of weather conditions (National Transportation Safety Board, 2009). This is illustrative of a unique situation; however, it is demonstrative of the fact that when faced with an MCI, the distribution of patients is critical to the success of the patient's outcome. Further, distance should not play a factor, within reason, of the choice of hospitals to transport patients from an MCI.

There is evidence that transporting the patients with minor injuries or the walking wounded to a close hospital, but not the closest hospital, will increase the chance of survival for more critical patients (Bloch, Schwartz, Pinkert, Blumenfeld, Avinoam, et al., 2007). The closest hospitals, if appropriate, should be reserved for the critical patients to reduce the transport time from the scene of the incident.

Transport officers must take all aspects of the distribution into consideration. In addition to the proximity to the incident scene, other considerations, including surge capacity, should be taken into account. Surge is a concern in an MCI. Preplanning and consultation with the hospitals should be part of the process to determine the surge capacity of the hospitals in the region. Specialty patient needs must also be considered in an MCI. If there are burn patients, pediatric patients, or patients with other special considerations who require special treatment, the destination should be considered. Distribution of patients in an MCI is a critical element in the success of managing the incident.

POST-INCIDENT REVIEW

A **post-incident review (PIR)** is an important process for looking at the MCI from a retrospective view. A PIR is not a blame session; rather, it is a session to identify the strengths and weaknesses of the operations of the incident. If a plan is not in place, the PIR is a starting point for establishing a plan for the next

MCI. The PIR establishes the processes and actions that made the incident management run efficiently and effectively. The weak points analysis should identify areas that need improvement.

Any weak points can be addressed by a variety of methods. Training may be the solution to resolve or change and improve the weaknesses. Sometimes the weakness is completely out of the agency's hands and requires another agency to make the change. When this occurs, the change can only be given as a recommendation. For example, the PIR may raise the issue that certain hospitals were not prepared for the number of patients. A change to mediate this can be suggested, but achieving resolution is not the responsibility of the EMS agency.

PIRs are most effective when all players are involved so that everyone has the opportunity to speak openly and discuss the issues that were encountered. PIRs do effect change when they are used in the proper format. A PIR should be held as soon after the MCI as possible. The lead agency from the MCI is generally the sponsor for the PIR and serves as the moderator.

PROVIDING SHELTER AND ORGANIZING EVACUATIONS DURING AN MCI

During times of disaster, it is not uncommon to need shelter of some kind. The **National Response Framework** identifies ESF #6-Mass Care, Emergency Assistance, Housing, and Human Services with the lead coordinator as the Department of Homeland Security/Federal Emergency Management Agency (DHS/FEMA) (FEMA, 2008a, 2008b). Each state has the responsibility to designate the lead agency that will ensure mass care is accomplished. Often, the local emergency management officials will work with the American Red Cross (ARC) for mass care. The determination of need is a joint decision between the emergency operations center and the ARC representative. Shelters are not the property of the ARC but are designated facilities that have been identified by local officials.

Once the determination has been made to open a shelter, the ARC then contacts its local employees and volunteers. The staffing needs are determined by the number of evacuees expected. Once personnel arrive, the startup begins. It is important that plans are made in advance, as shelters need time to set up for the incident.

The ARC stands ready to provide shelter, meals, supplies, and emotional support (American Red Cross, 2011, p. 3). The goal is to provide medical support at all shelters. However, that is not always possible. Even when nursing staff is present, nurses are often limited to providing advanced first aid and administration of OTC medications. Should the patient need more advanced care, then the staff would be directed to utilize local 911 response.

EVACUATING PERSONS WITH SPECIAL NEEDS TO A SHELTER

When evacuees report to shelters, they do not always bring enough medications or perhaps may need specialized care. In these situations, it may fall onto EMS to help relieve the issue at hand. Often this means transporting the evacuees to the local hospital, which may also be overburdened.

Many EMS systems already have in place a system for children discharged with apnea monitors or on home oxygen. By extending this concept, we can identify those persons who require special attention should they be relocated to a shelter. Identifying those **persons with special needs (PSNs)** in advance allows a system to better coordinate efforts to relocate those who may be in harm's way due to impending disasters. For instance, if a person is identified as being dependent on specialized medical equipment that must be powered and has a limited battery backup, a system could relocate this individual well ahead of the impending disaster. This would allow better use of resources during an actual disaster.

Utilizing a collaboration among suppliers, hospitals, and clients, one could develop a program for persons with special needs that, when necessary, helps relocate individuals during times of need, whether a long-term power outage or an impending storm. Should an incident occur, emergency management officials could assist with relocating these individuals. By maintaining lists of PSNs and appropriate shelters, we can better identify the most appropriate type of shelter needed during actual emergencies. The National Response Framework (Federal Emergency Management Agency, 2008a, p. 37) specifically notes that sheltering plans should be prepared for those with special needs and pets.

Should the need for evacuation and shelters be imminent, an evacuation order will be issued. This is where the impact on EMS may begin. It could be as simple as increasing the agency's readiness or assisting the Emergency Operations Center with contacting those previously identified as having special needs. A determination must be made as to which shelter location would be best. Working with emergency management allows EMS to know what types of shelters will be made available during the impending incident.

The shelters may be public (no special needs), public with the ability to handle special needs, nursing care required (nursing homes), and those who need continuous medical care. Such shelters should be identified well in advance of any crisis. Although this is focusing on disasters, a significant disruption of power to a nursing home could prove to be challenging for any EMS system. Having identified shelter options well in advance will make the process of relocation easier.

Once the determination has been made to evacuate, a system must be put in place to handle the relocation of those with special needs. Each system should have a way to store, retrieve, and disseminate the information to those in the field who will carry out the relocation. Most Computer Assisted Dispatch systems can place calls for service as "pending," which allows the information to be readily accessible. The Public Safety Communications Center can forward this information to the PSN dispatcher, a dedicated dispatcher for the event, who then sends it to the PSN or evacuation task force leader.

Best Practice

Ensure that you and your personnel understand how to implement the incident command system. Be sure people understand what role they may play during an incident. Develop cards that outline the basic responsibilities for each job description. A quick review and checklist ensure that tasks are not forgotten.

Understand how to conduct triage and implement drills in sorting patients. This can be as simple as reading pertinent vitals signs to as elaborate as having mock victims who need to be triaged and moved to treatment areas.

Work with your regional hospitals to develop a system for knowing bed availability during a disaster. The Northern Virginia Hospital Alliance was created so that fourteen regional hospitals could communicate and coordinate in times of disasters or major emergencies. This alliance was formed after the events of September 11, 2001.

SETTING UP A TASK FORCE TO ASSIST IN EVACUATIONS

A **task force** (Federal Emergency Management Agency, n.d.) is a combination of single resources assembled for a particular tactical need with common communications and a leader. This group will need the necessary resources to accomplish its goal. These resources include:

- Task force leader
- Advanced life support ambulance
- **Medical ambulance bus**
- Public transportation bus (handicap lift capable preferred)
- School bus (if no other option exists)
- Agency vehicles such as vans

Depending on the size of the response area, several task forces may be necessary. These task forces would pick up and deliver the evacuees to the most appropriate shelter. Once evacuees are delivered to a shelter, the next phase is medical screening by the shelter staff. The ARC has identified that health services workers in disaster situations are to provide health assessments, treatments per protocol, and referrals for care.

ASSIGNMENT OF EMERGENCY MEDICAL SERVICES RESOURCES TO SHELTERS

During the 2009 H1N1 pandemic, some EMS agencies contemplated the potential use of EMS personnel in shelters. This was in response to "what if" shelter health services workers are not available? This brought up questions such as the following:

- If the placement of EMS workers is to occur, how would they operate?
- Are they prepared to handle emergency medical care as primary care providers?
- Does the EMS agency have a protocol that allows for OTC medication administration?

CHAPTER REVIEW

Summary

Under normal circumstances, any system can be taxed due to an increased call volume. When you add in bad weather and multiple simultaneous incidents, things go from bad to worse in a matter of minutes. Understanding a system's capabilities and regional partners will assist in managing the MCI more effectively. Understanding that there is no shame in asking for help early on can make a chaotic scene more manageable. When an MCI with multiple patients is added to a routine day, the ability to manage the scene becomes paramount. When arriving at the scene of an incident, immediately begin scene survey. Initially requesting additional resources will assist in managing the scene of an MCI. Ensuring that responders know how to manage triage, treatment, and transport will make the scene more manageable.

WHAT WOULD YOU DO? REFLECTION

Command and control of the scene are the most critical elements to monitor to ensure a smooth incident scene. Every responder has the obligation to know and understand the principles of triage for the adult and pediatric populations. Reflect back to the case of the car versus school bus. You find yourself in the midst of an emotionally difficult situation.

Your initial actions have established incident command, and triage has begun.

As units begin to arrive, each will receive assignments to help resources be divided appropriately. This would eventually include expanding the treatment transportation sections. A transportation corridor would be set up so that your patients could be taken to the appropriate facilities in the most appropriate fashion.

Review Questions

1. You are asked to do an in-service for monthly training. You are to provide an overview of how the medical branch fits into the incident management system. Provide an overview of the key points you would discuss. Include the functions of the triage, treatment, and transport groups in the medical branch.
2. Why should you conduct a PIR following an MCI?
3. What is considered an MCI in your EMS system?
4. What are the differences between the START and SALT triage processes?
5. What should you consider when determining the transport destination for patients in an MCI?
6. You are part of an MCI. What roles would you establish as part of the ICS?

References

American Red Cross. (2011). "2011 Disaster Relief Program Review." See the organization website.

Bloch, Y. H., D. Schwartz, M. Pinkert, A. Blumenfeld, S. Avinoam, et al. (2007). "Distribution of Casualties in a Mass-Casualty Incident with Three Local Hospitals in the Periphery of a Densely Populated Area: Lessons Learned from the Medical Management of a Terrorist Attack." *Prehospital and Disaster Medicine 22*(3), 186–192.

Dible, J. H. (1959). "D. J. Larrey: A Surgeon of the Revolution, Consultate, and Empire." *Medical History 3*(2), 100–117.

Federal Emergency Management Agency. (n.d.). "Glossary of Terms: Task Force." See the organization website.

Federal Emergency Management Agency. (2008a). "National Response Framework." See the organization website.

Federal Emergency Management Agency. (2008b). "Emergency Support Function #6—Mass Care, Emergency Assistance, Housing, and Human Services Annex." See the organization website.

Infoplease. (2007). *San Francisco Earthquake of 1906: Census Facts.* Information Please Database, Pearson Education. See the organization website.

Lerner, E. B., R. B. Schwartz, P. L. Coule, and R. G. Pirrallo. (2010). "Use of SALT Triage in a Simulated Mass-Casualty Incident." *Prehospital Emergency Car 14*(1), 21–25.

Medical College of Wisconsin. (2008). "National Guideline for Mass Casualty Triage Proposed." See the Newswise website.

National Transportation Safety Board. (2009, April). "Single-Vehicle Accident, Motorcoach Run-Off-the-Road and Rollover, U.S. Route 163, Mexican Hat, Utah, January 6, 2008." Highway Accident Report, NTSB/HAR-09/01/ PB2009-916201. Washington, DC: Author.

Pullum, J. D., and K. D. Kaull. (2001, January). Simple Triage and Rapid Treatment (START) Distance Learning Program.

Romig, L. E. (2011). "The *JumpSTART* Pediatric MCI Triage Tool." Team Life Support, Inc. See the Jump START triage website.

Wiseman, D. B., R. Ellenbogen, and C.I. Shaffrey. (2002). "Triage for the Neurosurgeon." *Neurosurgical Focus 12*(3), E5.

Key Terms

mass casualty incident (MCI) An event in which there are more patients than resources immediately available. This can vary in geographic regions depending on the availability local resources.

medical ambulance bus A specially designed medical bus to accommodate a large amount of patients for transport. These vehicles are designed to hold litters and administer oxygen with medically trained providers on board.

National Response Framework A national guide or framework for an all-hazards approach to mitigating crisis situations.

persons with special needs (PSNs) Patients or victims who require additional services in order to maintain their quality of life.

post-incident review (PIR) An important process for looking at the MCI from a retrospective view. This is utilized to identify the strengths and weaknesses of the operations of any incident.

primary triage The first phase of immediately identifying those critically injured patients so as to formulate an action plan to treat and transport patients from the scene of the incident.

secondary triage The process in which patients receive another assessment to identify if their condition has changed. It is done when the patient is moved from one location to another.

task force a group of people who deal with a specific problem.

triage Based on the French word meaning "to sort out", this is the process of identifying the status of patients during an MCI.

3 CHAPTER

Mass Gatherings and Special Events

Eric Powell

Objectives

After reading this chapter, the student should be able to:

3.1 Analyze and plan for unique EMS aspects of scheduled events that involve mass gatherings (planned and unplanned).

3.2 Identify the planning considerations for EMS operations during a variety of scheduled events involving mass gatherings.

3.3 Identify the factors that are used to determine the level of medical protection provided during mass gatherings.

3.4 Discuss the role of the EMS provider during a variety of scheduled events involving mass gatherings.

3.5 Discuss the value of the EMS provider's personal safety awareness at mass gatherings and special events (planned and unplanned).

Key Terms

complexity analysis
event
fusion centers
incident
incident action plans (IAPs)
incident command post (ICP)
operational period
planning meeting
situational awareness
size-up
SMART (objectives)
surveillance
tactics meeting

WHAT WOULD YOU DO?

Five months ago, you were promoted to the position of EMS division chief for your fire-rescue department. It is Monday morning, and you find out that you have been tasked to provide EMS support at a local high school playoff game. It is expected that 12,000 people will attend and that the possibility exists for a 15,000 to 16,000 participants overflow. Your municipality has eight stations with six advanced life support (ALS) paramedic-level ambulances in service 24 hours a day. All eight of your first-due engine companies are ALS paramedic first-response capable. You have been covering the local high school regular season football games for the last 15 years and have a good understanding of this type of service provision. The responsibility of planning for this event is yours, and you have 12 days to pull this project together. In addition, you have a new county manager who is tasked with cutting the budget of various county departments and has staffers currently performing a "top-to-bottom" review of your EMS system.

Questions

1. What preexisting resources and materials at your fire-rescue department could help you with planning for and executing this task?
2. With which, if any, other agencies/entities do you expect to coordinate and plan for this event coverage?
3. For what contingencies should you plan? How could those contingencies be mitigated?

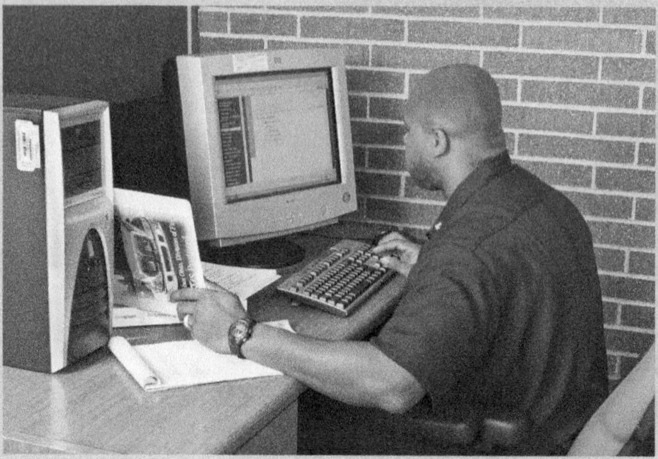

FIGURE 3.1 Staffing a special event can be difficult for an EMS supervisor if he is not prepared.

INTRODUCTION

Mass gatherings and special events take many forms. These events range from standing by at a local high school football game to being detailed to the Super Bowl, World Series, or a Lollapalooza-type concert. These situations can be unplanned as well. Consider the 2011 Occupy Wall Street protests across the United States, which caused consternation for many public safety entities as their movement gained national momentum. Natural disasters can also bring forward conditions in which mass gatherings can occur on short notice, such as at food and water distribution points. Preplanning for any of these events is critical to the safety of personnel working these events.

In the past, EMS has not had a seat at the table with respect to many disaster management or fire service–related planning events. In the most recent report of the Institute of Medicine of the National Academies (2007), entitled "Emergency Medical Services at the Crossroads: Future of Emergency Care," the lack of EMS participation within the disaster planning construct is well-explained:

> EMS and trauma systems have to a large extent been overlooked in disaster preparedness planning at both the state and federal levels. This is due in part to the fact that EMS is often regarded as a subset of fire response, though the medical role that would be undertaken by EMS personnel in the event of a major emergency is distinct from the role of fire suppression teams. (*Source: Excerpt from Emergency Medical Services at the Crossroads: Future of Emergency Care by the Committee on the Future of Emergency Care in the United States Health System, Board on Health Care Services and Institute of Medicine. Published by The National Academies Press, © 2007, p. 196.*)

This chapter focuses on EMS special operations; however, it is noted that many of the special operations roles occur within the context of disaster preparedness planning. EMS planning with regard to mass gatherings and special events fits within what the Institute of Medicine (IOM) was trying to convey. In fact, the IOM report is widely regarded as the new "White Paper." The National Fire Academy (NFA) realized this fact and has broadened its course offerings to include specialized EMS courses, ranging from management to incident management to special operations.

EMS planners and policy makers should review the difference between incidents and events before they begin the main subject material for mass gatherings and special events. There is a distinct difference between the two situations, and the EMS manager will have to employ specific skill sets to meet the challenges brought forward from them. No event or incident is ever the same.

An **incident** is an unexpected occurrence that happens in connection with something else. These situations are defined by their no-notice characteristics. An example of an incident would be the Boston Marathon improvised explosive device (IED) bombings of April 2013. The NFA, (n.d.) provides the following factors that affect incident planning:

- Time criticality
- Unstable, changing situation
- Potential rapid expansion of incident and response
- Difficult communications
- Incomplete information
- Lack of experience managing expanding incidents

An **event** is a planned activity. The EMS manager typically has some time to plan for and meet the mission for these events. An example of an event would be the Macy's Day Parade held in New York City each Thanksgiving Day. The National Fire Academy (n.d.) also provides the following factors that affect event planning:

- Type of event
- Location, size, expected duration, history, and potential
- Number of agencies involved
- Single or multiple jurisdiction
- Command staff needs
- Kind, type, number of resources required
- Projected aviation operations
- Staging areas required
- Other facilities required
- Kind and type of logistical support needs
- Financial considerations
- Know limitations or restrictions
- Available communications (p. 7–3)

MASS GATHERINGS

Mass gatherings can occur through planned or unplanned events. For the EMS manager tasked to cover these events, the best countermeasures are the proper use of the incident command system and well-thought out planning methods. When performed properly, a well-planned and executed mass gathering operation with few problems can be one of the best public relations actions that can be accomplished by the department.

As with any event, planned or unplanned, the incident commander will perform a **size-up**. The size-up allows for analysis of five variables about an incident and is done in order to conceptualize the incident objectives. These variables are:

- Nature and magnitude of the incident
- Hazards and safety concerns
  - Hazards facing response personnel and the public
  - Evacuation and warnings
  - Injuries and casualties
  - Need to secure and isolate the area
- Initial priorities and immediate resource requirements
- Location of **incident command post** and staging area
- Entrance and exit routes of responders (National Fire Academy, n.d., p. 7–6)

The incident commander will also need to have **situational awareness**. The NFA (n.d.) states that situational awareness involves:

- Identifying problems or potential problems
- Recognizing the need for action
- Not ignoring information discrepancies; rather, you must analyze discrepancies before proceeding
- Seeking and providing information before acting
- Continuing to collect information about the incident and assignments made
- Assessing your own task performance
- Identifying deviations from the expected
- Communicating your situational awareness to all team members (p. 7–7)

The NFA (n.d.) also addresses **complexity analysis** as a combination of involved factors that affect the probability of control of an incident. Many factors determine the complexity of an incident, including:

- Effects on life, property, and the economy
- Community and responder safety
- Potential hazardous materials
- Weather and other environmental influences
- Likelihood of cascading events
- Potential crime scene (including terrorism)
- Political sensitivity, external influences, and media relations
- Area involved and jurisdictional boundaries
- Availability of resources (p. 7–7)

PLANNED EVENTS

The EMS personnel role in a planned event may involve one practitioner to dozens, depending on the event. The EMS manager who takes time to consider the variables of a planned event and establishes reasonable contingencies will be postured for success. The three most common planned events that the EMS manager may handle are sporting events, marathons, and concerts. (See Figure 3.2.)

Sporting Events

Sporting events are some of the best planned events for which to develop foundational **incident action plans (IAPs)** as they share characteristics to some degree. During these events typically people are very tightly packed and have differing interests with respect to competitive groups. The possibility of violence is definitely a contingency for which to plan.

Marathons

Marathons will require multiple care-related venues along a predetermined route. Typically,

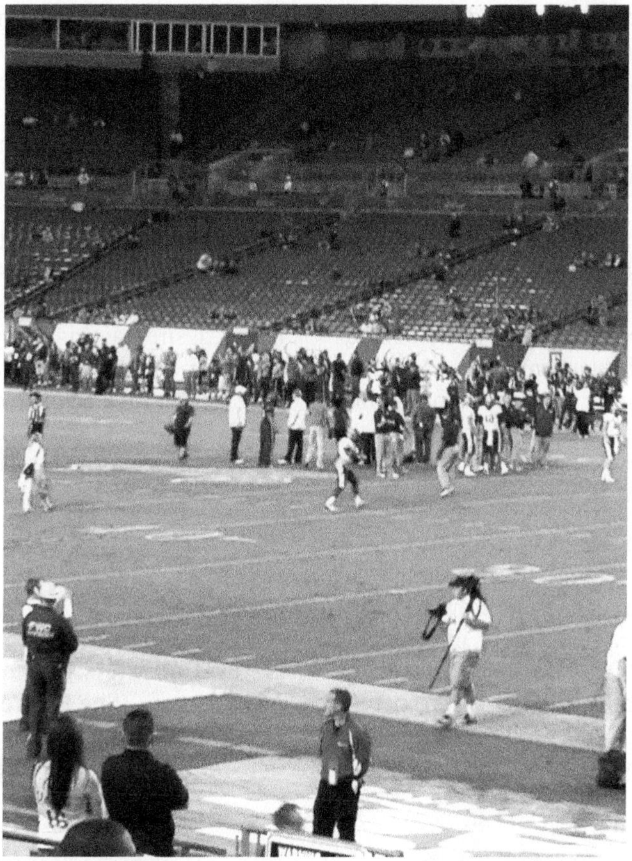

FIGURE 3.2 The three most common planned events that the EMS manager may handle are sporting events, marathons, and concerts. *Source: Courtesy of Jeffrey T. Lindsey, Ph.D.*

participating athletes, when training appropriately, will have few relative problems. These may include physical fatigue/exhaustion, dehydration, and orthopaedic injuries.

Concerts

Concerts can be as routine as a weekday afternoon family concert in the park to a heavy metal battle-of-the-bands concert in a municipality's major music venue. The goal of the EMS planner in this situation would be to know what type of crowd to expect. This will help determine if you should increase supplies or equipment such as Narcan or AEDs. Again, creating positive relationships with local law enforcement can be helpful.

Protests

Protests can be planned events. There may be a small window for the EMS special operations manager to meet the challenge of this type of event. A strategy to assist in mitigating untoward events is for the manager to communicate with the protest organizer(s) about assisting in providing EMS care. The goal of covering this type of situation is providing efficient and effective care and protecting EMS personnel working the event.

UNPLANNED EVENTS

Unplanned events will provide the EMS manager with substantive challenges to overcome and mitigate. Little- or no-notice events will tax operations quickly. The EMS manager will have to gain situational awareness as soon as possible as well as working right away to catch up on resource and logistical needs. A critical variable in unplanned events is the possibility of untoward/dangerous crowd behaviors.

Political Protests

Political protests, in particular, can be volatile and polarizing, with counter-groups engaging each other. EMS special event crews must be concerned with their own safety, interact and collaborate with law enforcement, and be informed about the group and its specific issues. By knowing the specific issues of the protests, EMS crews can better interact with the protesters in an appropriate and professional fashion. This does not mean that the EMS personnel advocate what the protesters do; rather, it means that the EMS personnel working the situation remain neutral and have the best intelligence possible to remain safe. EMS crews must be cognizant that some political protesters bring videography equipment and attorneys to these events. The goals of the protesters might be for self-protection; others might desire gaining entry into litigation via a real or perceived untoward event, such as a civil rights violation by public safety entities. If the EMS crews are well informed, practice appropriate patient advocacy, and carry themselves professionally, there is little risk of an unwanted situation. Civil disorder can be an unwanted variable in these types of events.

Natural Disasters

Natural disasters create new challenges for public safety. (See Figure 3.3.) The worst-case scenario in this situation would be civil disorder that cannot be mitigated by the police or

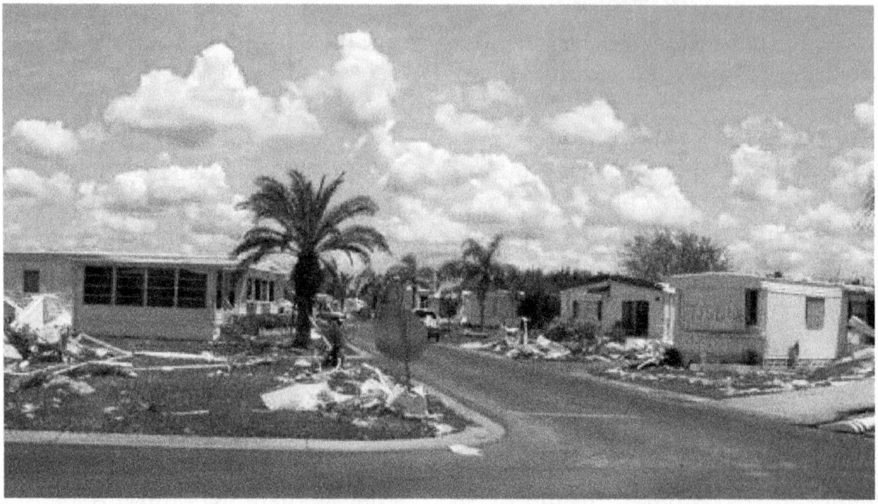

FIGURE 3.3 Natural disasters can create complex incident situations that require planning for a large-scale event. *Source: Courtesy of Jeffrey T. Lindsey, Ph.D.*

the military, forcing EMS to be significantly limited in its role of providing care. In this situation, mass gatherings could occur at shelters, food/water distribution points, and evacuation routes. Positive relationships with law enforcement as well as an active presence at state and regional intelligence **fusion centers** will increase the chances of a successful EMS mission within the context of a natural disaster (U.S. Department of Homeland Security, 2012).

Civil Disorder Situations

As in natural disaster and political protest situations, civil disorder can lead to participants behaving very violently. The first consideration in this type of event is the safety of the public safety personnel working the incident/event. Civil disorder ranges from riots after a hockey game, such as in Vancouver in 2011, to the various incidents that transpired after the police beating of Rodney King in Los Angeles. The violence at these situations is indiscriminate. Even though the EMS mission is to care for everyone no matter the situation, violent actors do not discriminate when it comes to attacks on EMS personnel. Personal safety in this situation cannot be emphasized enough.

INITIAL ACTIONS

As is common with most public safety situations, there are three main objectives. The NFA (n.d.) addresses those objectives via the following priorities:

- *First priority: Life safety*—Determine if life is at immediate risk. This includes responders and the public.
- *Second priority: Incident stabilization*—What should be done to keep the situation from becoming worse?
- *Third priority: Property conservation*—What can be done to protect or minimize damage to public and private property? Are there any environmental issues that need to be addressed? (p. 7–4).

EMS personnel will integrate easily into the first two priorities. Their mission does not traditionally include the third priority of property conservation as is commonplace for the fire service. EMS personnel can be valuable with respect to the potentially toxic environment as they can provide observation and **surveillance** during an event.

INITIAL RESPONSE ACTIONS

The initial response phase for EMS to an incident follows National Incident Management System (NIMS) methodology. The NFA (n.d.) indicates the following:

- Assume Command and establish Incident Command Post (ICP).
- Establish immediate Incident Objectives, strategies, and tactics. The size-up should provide information about what needs to be done first to prevent loss of life or injury and to stabilize the situation. For small incidents, the initial IAP may be verbal and may cover the entire incident. For larger, more complex incidents, the initial IAP may cover the first operational period. A written IAP then will be developed.
- Determine if there are enough resources of the right kind and type on scene or ordered. The incident objectives will drive resource requirements. What resources are required to accomplish the immediate incident objectives? If the right kind and type of resources are not on scene, the incident commander (IC) must order them immediately.
- Establish the initial organization that maintains span-of-control. At this point, the IC should ask, "What organization will be required to execute the IAP and achieve the objectives?" He should establish that organization, always

keeping in mind safety and span-of-control concerns. The span-of-control range of three to seven is to ensure safe and efficient use of resources. (p. 7–4).

Table 3.1 illustrates the various command and general staff positions. It also provides a description of each the responsibilities for these positions.

SMART OBJECTIVES

SMART (objectives) is an acronym for specific, measurable, action oriented, realistic, and time sensitive:

- *Specific*—The objective needs to provide a clear-cut description of the task.
- *Measurable*—Write the objective so you can measure the progress of the task.
- *Action oriented*—All objectives should include a verb.
- *Realistic*—The objective needs to be able to be achieved.
- *Time sensitive*— Set a specific amount of time to accomplish the task. (*Source: Excerpt from "All Hazards Incidents: Setting Objectives and Strategies" by Larry Miller in Fire Engineering 165(2), February 2012, pp. 75. Used by permission of Pennwell Corporation.*)

After completing the size-up and developing SMART incident objectives, a briefing will occur for the command staff. You will need to use the incident command system (ICS) Incident Briefing Form (Form ICS 201).

TABLE 3.1 Command and General Staff Planning Responsibilities

Incident Commander	Provides overall Incident Objectives and strategy Establishes procedures for incident resource ordering Establishes procedures for resource activation, mobilization, and employment Approves completed IAP by signature
Safety Officer	Reviews hazards associated with the incident and proposed tactical assignments Assists in developing safe tactics Develop(s) safety messages
Operations Section Chief	Assists in identifying strategies Determines tactics to achieve Command objectives Determines work assignments and resource requirements
Planning Section Chief	Provides incident and resource status reports Develops contingency plans Manages the planning process Produces the IAP
Logistics Section Chief	Ensures that resource ordering procedures are communicated to appropriate agency ordering points Develops a transportation system to support operational needs Ensures that the Logistics Section can support the IAP Completes assigned portions of the written IAP Places orders for resources
Finance/Administration Section Chief	Provides cost implications of Incident Objectives, as required Ensures that the IAP is within the financial limits established by the IC Evaluates facilities, transportation assets, and other contracted services to determine if any special contract arrangements are needed

Source: NFA (n.d.), p. 7–12.

OPERATIONAL PERIOD FACTORS

The **operational period** is a set period of time for an incident—for example, it can be 6, 8, 12, or 24 hours. The amount of time can vary due to a number of different factors, including the following.

- Safety conditions—Safety of responders, victims, and others is always the first priority on any response
- Condition of resources—Planning must be done far enough in advance to ensure that additional resources needed for the next operational period are available
- The length of time necessary or available to achieve the tactical assignments
- Availability of fresh resources
- Future involvement of additional jurisdictions or agencies
- Environmental conditions—Factors such as the amount of daylight remaining and weather and wind conditions can affect decisions about the length of the operational period. (pp. 7–10)

Typically the IC sets the operational period. The IC rarely makes this decision unilaterally; it is best done with counsel from the command staff. The operational periods can change from day to day based on what incident objectives are covered or by any of the preceding factors.

TACTICS MEETING

The **tactics meeting** is done in order to review tactics created by the operations section chief. There are three main parts to this meeting:

- Determining how the selected strategy will be accomplished in order to achieve the incident objectives
- Assigning resources to implement the tactics
- Identifying methods for monitoring tactics and resources to determine if adjustments are required (e.g., different tactics, different resources, or new strategy)

The operations section chief, safety officer, planning section chief, logistics section chief, and resources unit leader attend the tactics meeting. The meeting is led by the operations section chief. The Operational Planning Worksheet (ICS 215) and Safety Analysis (ICS 215A) forms are used to document the tactics meeting. For less complex incidents, the tactics meeting may be an informal gathering of the key players (NFA, n.d., p. 7–13).

PLANNING MEETING

The **planning meeting** allows for the command and general staff to analyze what the operations section chief has brought forward with respect to his operational plan. The ICS 215 and 215A forms are a substantial part of this meeting. As the NFA (n.d.) explains:

> The Planning Section Chief leads the meeting following a fixed agenda to ensure that the meeting is efficient, while allowing each organizational element represented to assess and acknowledge the plan. The Operations Section Chief delineates the amount and type of resources he or she will need to accomplish the plan. The Planning Section's Resources Unit will have to work with the Logistics Section to fulfill the resource needs." (p. 7–19)

INCIDENT ACTION PLAN

After the planning meeting, the incident action plan (IAP) is prepared. It is recommended that an IAP be created in a few generalized situations:

- First, consider when two or more jurisdictions are involved in the response. Mutual or automatic aid agreements need to be in place. Care should be taken to differentiate and confirm tactics between the two jurisdictions.
- Second, if the incident continues into another operational period, personnel, incident command changeover, and other logistical considerations may be of importance. If General

Staff sections are staffed, this indicates a substantial incident and that numerous organizational elements have been activated.

- Third, if a hazardous materials incident is involved or if agency policy dictates that an IAP is to be used, use it. (NFA, n.d., p. 7–21)

The IAP is not a singular form; rather it is a set of standardized forms and other documents that explain what the incident commander and operations section chief are directing in order to accomplish tasks during an operational period. The necessary forms and other documents are as follows:

- IAP cover sheet (not an ICS form)
- ICS 202, Incident Objectives
- ICS 203, Organization Assignment List
- ICS 204, Division or Group Assignment List
- ICS 205, Incident Communications Plan
- ICS 206, Medical Plan
- Safety messages, maps, forecasts (not ICS forms) (NFA, n.d., p. 7–22)

The ICS 206, Medical Plan Form, is of particular interest to EMS planners at a mass gathering and/or special event. This form provides for integration of EMS operations within the plan, as does the implementation of a medical branch within the ICS system. The form provides information on incident medical care locations, EMS and EMS-related transportation systems, hospitals, and medical emergency procedures. This form is typically created by the medical unit leader and reviewed by the safety officer.

The ICS 214, Unit Log, is important as it is a record of unit activities and is the basic reference document for information in an after-action report. It is initiated and maintained by command and general staff members, field command, and unit leaders. Anything important should be logged in an ICS 214. This form can be of immeasurable value when personnel are logging in information that can be utilized later in an after-action report or as a guide to revise procedures or guidelines.

EMS PLANNING

The NFA recommends three broad-based initial considerations for EMS planners. These considerations are as follows:

1. Develop and implement a plan that will maintain the present level of EMS in the community and provide the same level of service for the scores of citizens and visitors who will be attending the event.
2. Build on previous experience.
3. Perform a hazard analysis for each venue and other designated locations. (NFA, n.d., pp. 7–35)

A community-oriented approach, coupled with an attitude of advocacy, will help successfully execute the mission. If the EMS manager cannot provide an adequate and effective level of service for the community while covering a mass gathering or special event, he will be excoriated by citizens. In addition, the local governance will seize a political opportunity and denigrate the EMS system and its personnel. Unfair criticism typically is never corrected by the media or by word of mouth. The EMS manager must plan effectively and anticipate the possibility of contingencies, especially for their jurisdiction.

Prior special events planning and an agency's coverage experience will be of exceptional value to the planning process. As EMS professionals, learning from mistakes is of tremendous benefit. The value of an immediate debrief will offer revisions for the next event.

The hazard mitigation program for EMS is similar to the preplanning process performed by the fire service. Haddow and Haddow (2009) indicate that a hazard mitigation process is a four-step method:

1. Establish a community partnership that involves all members of the community in developing a community-based hazard mitigation plan.
2. Identify the community risks (i.e., floods, hurricanes, earthquakes, etc.).

3. Identify potential mitigation actions to address these risks and develop a prioritized plan.
4. Generate the funding, political, and public support needed to implement the plan. (*Source: Excerpt from Disaster Communications in a Changing Media World by K. S. Haddow and G. D. Haddow. Published by Elsevier, © 2009, p. 70.*)

Planning efforts within the context of mass gathering and special events can begin with building a foundation of an EMS-related hazard mitigation program, one that is not often found in EMS systems across the country.

PARTICIPATING GROUPS

Groups that will participate in planned and unplanned gatherings/events vary from peaceful vigils with overlapping safety oversight to those people intent on civil disorder and disobedience. The EMS manager must gather information as to what group is expected in any planned/unplanned events. This information allows the EMS manager to better care for the participants and keep EMS personnel as safe as possible.

Gathering information and properly analyzing it can be the foundation of a rudimentary EMS intelligence function. Knowing the composition of a participating/attending group is similar to knowing your audience as a speaker or teacher. For example, fostering a positive relationship with key individuals involved with protest events can provide for smoother patient/group interactions, transfer out of the event to medical care, and improve safety for your personnel. In addition, an EMS organizational dynamic that recognizes the value of cultural sensitivity and respect will be of considerable value when considering group dynamics and perspective. This situation typically is more of a problem for law enforcement than for EMS; however, it is an evolving situation for EMS.

SCHEDULED EVENTS

Scheduled events are going to occur with regularity, and we can learn a great deal from each event, even those that are not problematic. The opportunity to collect data and anecdotal experience will be of exceptional value. As a planner, take time to be attentive to a continuous quality improvement process, make notes, and ask the crew for feedback after events in order to be more efficient in the operations phase. When interacting with stakeholders during the planning process, make sure to indoctrinate them to schedule as far in advance as possible.

Scheduled special events for EMS may be the only time that most citizens have contact with EMS. Look upon these events as great public relations opportunities. The EMS crews covering these events must be educated about their importance and the criticality of professional and positive interpersonal interactions for the event. In addition, creating and maintaining consistent relationships with those people and institutions that request EMS service at special events cannot be overstated. Not only can EMS professionals receive positive feedback from the public they serve, but they also can observe and seize opportunities for future EMS public education prospects. These events can certainly be win-win situations for EMS service when approached correctly and with some creativity.

UNSCHEDULED EVENTS

EMS services have a great deal of experience with day-to-day operations and single-incident, single-resource events. That particular experience is valuable when it comes to the unplanned event that produces a mass gathering. One of the variables that the EMS manager has control over is knowledge of resources and the understanding of variables that can impact a mass gathering and/or special event. (See Figure 3.4.) Identifying EMS resource needs is a great place for the EMS planner to start.

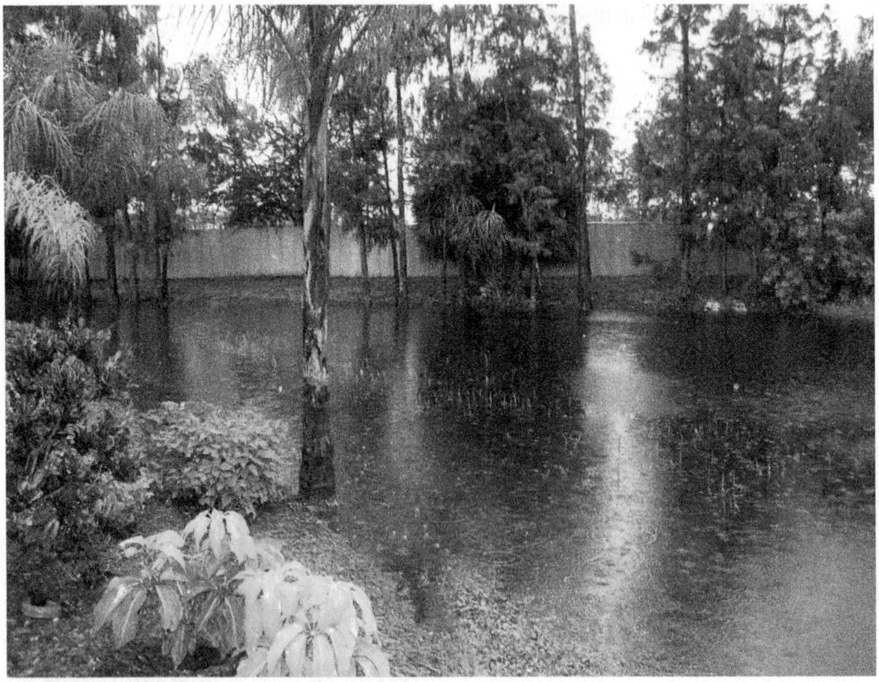

FIGURE 3.4 One of the variables that the EMS manager has control over is knowledge of resources and the understanding of variables that can impact a mass gathering and/or special event. *Source: Photo courtesy of Jeffrey T. Lindsey, Ph.D.*

There are four main considerations for identifying EMS resource needs:

- Anticipated call volume
- Event factors
- Human and environmental factors
- Type of operation (NFA, n.d., pp. 7–26)

In a major incident, call volume has two aspects: baseline volume and anticipated requests over baseline. The goal is to meet the needs of the event while maintaining a level of service. Some standards recommend a minimum of 3.5 advanced life support units per 50,000 people. It is important to determine if the service is operating at resource levels that meet the baseline request volume or if there is any room for expanded needs. If resource levels only meet baseline volume, there must be plans for immediate requests for assistance through mutual aid and regional response assistance requests (NFA, n.d., 7–26).

VARIABLES INVOLVED IN EMS PLANNING

The EMS manager, when planning for an event or when thrown into an unplanned situation, has a significant number of variables to consider. (See Figure 3.5.) This section takes into account a few of the most important to consider.

WEATHER CONSIDERATIONS

Maintaining relationships with local weather media outlets and/or the National Weather

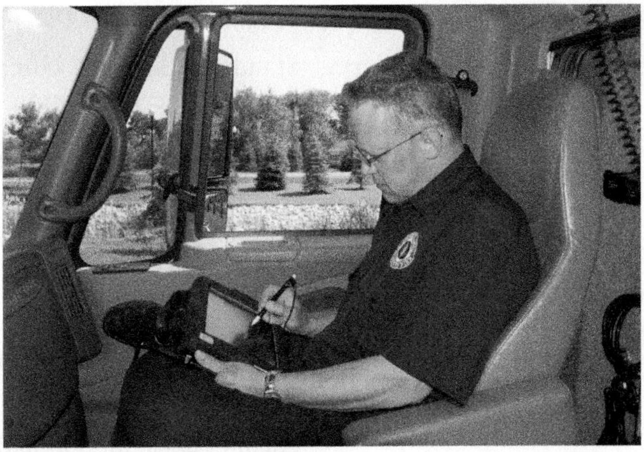

FIGURE 3.5 The EMS manager, when planning for an event or when thrown into an unplanned situation, has a significant number of variables to consider.

Service can be a great help for EMS when planning for mass gatherings (whether planned or unplanned). For some events, EMS may be able to pass along weather-related information to assist in mitigating illnesses or injuries for a planned or unplanned event.

High heat and humidity during events call for increased water consumption as well as cooling measures. Cooling fans or tents may be a part of the EMS planner's strategy in such a situation along with water distribution facilities. This can also be an opportunity for positive public interactions by providing sunscreen and/or counseling for sunburns. Major concerns would be heat exhaustion and heat stroke. Surveillance of weather by EMS personnel covering an event or on standby for a mass gathering is of particular value.

Cold weather calls for warming equipment (warming fans or blowers). Blankets or other layered coverings can be utilized as well. Caloric intake for humans is actually increased in cold weather. The availability of hot foods can be of assistance in mitigating cold illness/injuries. Again, surveillance by EMS personnel in a cold weather event in a mass gathering or special event can catch problems before they develop.

In addition, severe weather during a special event or mass gathering can create a mass casualty incident if proper consideration is not given to the threat. For instance, lightning can strike 5 to 10 miles ahead of the storm. Winds generated by a thunderstorm can exceed 70 miles per hour, and hail can cause considerable injuries for an individual caught outside without shelter. Cancelling or postponing an event

Side Bar

Types of Illnesses and Injuries That Could Occur to Spectators or Participants

- Dehydration
- Exacerbation of cardiac and COPD histories
- Exacerbation of diabetes history
- Exposure to insects (causing anaphylaxis or disease-carrying vectors)
- Medication interaction issues
- Excessive alcohol intake
- Intentional and unintentional prescription and illicit drug overdoses

Side Bar

Injuries That Could Occur at Mass Gatherings and Special Events

- Assaults (all-inclusive, including sexual)
- Musculoskeletal injuries
- Soft-tissue injuries
- Neurological injuries
- Blunt and penetrating injuries

due to severe weather is much more preferable to the alternative.

SIZE OF EVENT

The size of the event affects resource management directly. There are many variables to consider with respect to the event size. The chief considerations are personnel and logistics. As the EMS manager, understanding the need to scale back or call forward assets is best done prior to the event. Experience will guide the EMS manager in subsequent events on how to staff an event when the size is known. Remember, the EMS manager will bear the brunt of the responsibility and accountability if the prudent variables are not planned for fully and properly.

MEDICAL PROTOCOLS

Standard EMS protocols and operating guidelines are the foundation for mass gatherings and special events. Many EMS systems have specific annexes within the protocol manual that address these events. Having a medical director staff mass gatherings and special events is a value-added option, but it is not the case in most situations.

ALCOHOL CONSUMPTION AND ILLICIT DRUG USE

Alcohol consumption and illicit drug use will increase call volume. Alcohol consumption can precipitate many adverse events such as violence, compounding the problems expected and experienced at a mass gathering. Sometimes the problem does not present itself until people begin leaving an event, exacerbating instances of driving while impaired. Illicit drug use can also create problems (typically violence and overdose). The intelligence function within the incident command system can be of use in this situation. In addition, if an event is held near a body of water, this can complicate issues substantially. EMS planning considerations for this type of event would include lifeguards and watercraft equipment requests and allocations. Expect noncompliance with

Best Practice

St. Anthony's Hospital Event Medicine Team

St. Anthony's Hospital in St. Petersburg, Florida, has an Event Medicine Team staffed by EMS professionals. The group is comprised primarily of experienced paramedics and emergency medical technicians who work regular EMS and fire service jobs in the area. The group has handled events such as the Tampa Bay Rays major league baseball team, the Mahaffey Theater, and the St. Petersburg Grand Prix Race. Other events such as the Little League World Series, the PGA Tampa Bay Championship, major league baseball spring training, and triathlons are the norm. The Event Medicine team is well experienced with event planning and considers prudent contingencies when faced with an increased workload.

swimming restrictions in events involving alcohol consumption near bodies of water.

CALLING IN PERSONNEL FOR UNSCHEDULED EVENT

Standard operating guidelines that address personnel recall should be in place. If an agency does not have a recall policy, creating one is a good place to start. Writing a standard operating guideline (SOG) related to personnel recall involves writing about accepted human resources principles. This is not a task that an EMS planner can do alone. When creating the SOG it is important to receive feedback from command staff, human resources, chief executive officer, attorney, and so on.

READILY ACCESSIBLE SUPPLIES

Making sure that supplies are readily accessible might be as easy as using a utility pickup truck to tow a mass-casualty trailer full of supplies to the mass gathering/special event site. Do not underestimate the value of distributing supplies in a reasoned manner to crews; give them equipment applicable to the event and their role during that event. In addition, listen to feedback regarding supply utilization during the operational period and adjust supply distribution accordingly. If the event requires changing supply distribution points, do not hesitate to do so unless it affects provider safety in an adverse way.

COMMUNICATIONS SYSTEM

The EMS radio communications system must be able to handle a rapid increase in volume. When evaluating many untoward events in EMS operations and disaster management situations, the greatest failures often lie in communications problems. Many emergency management offices have equipment such as the ACU-1000 that can cross-connect up to twenty-four radio channels simultaneously. The issue of communications interoperability is of critical importance within the mass gatherings and special events venue. The EMS special operations manager who prioritizes this variable will be much more effective in most any complex response.

AGREEMENTS WITH OUTSIDE AGENCIES FOR MUTUAL AID

Setting up agreements with outside agencies for mutual aid is best completed when a mass gathering or special event is not pending. Having extra ambulances or a strike team or two available is of exceptional importance in a mass gathering or special event that does not go so well. Insurance issues are a very important variable here. The ability to work out insurance and liability issues is of critical importance and requires municipality/county/private institution legal communication and agreement.

TRAINING OF PERSONNEL

The training of EMS personnel in the incident command system is of particular importance. The EMS planner should make sure that all personnel are ICS 100, 200, 700, and 800 compliant. Crews should also be trained in ICS 300, and all EMS command staff should be trained in ICS 400. Any time that a training evolution can use an ICS construct, it should be integrated for practice. Traditionally, EMS has not utilized the ICS system as fire service and law enforcement agencies have in the past. Training that involves mass gatherings/special events and vulnerable populations, such as children, the elderly, and the handicapped, should be pursued aggressively by the EMS planner.

EASY ACCESS AND EGRESS FOR TRANSPORTING UNITS

Consideration of access and egress should be made in the planning process, carried through to the creation of the IAP, and maintained throughout the operational periods. Coordination with law enforcement and other critical public safety agencies is a good idea. Vigilance during the operational phase to make sure that ingress and egress routes are kept clear should be tasked to personnel who can observe these areas without impacting their primary job tasks.

PROVISION FOR PRIVACY

When establishing the provider–patient relationship, it is still incumbent on the provider to use due diligence and provide privacy measures when performing assessments, diagnostics, and/or treatment modalities.

PROTECTION FROM THE ELEMENTS

Setting up an area where there is protection from the elements is a very important provision of service and may require some type of vendor agreement (most certainly time spent creating relationships). Children, pregnant women, the elderly, and other special needs populations may require this type of refuge.

Do not forget about protection of medical and ancillary personnel from the elements as well. The shelter should be large enough to accommodate medical personnel and anticipated patients.

WATER

There are several different expert guides to assist medical and relief workers in planning for water distribution in planned and unplanned mass gathering and special events. For example, the U.S. Agency for International Development (USAID) provides the following information:

- Drinking—3 to 4 liters per day
- Cooking and cleanup—2 to 3 liters per day
- Hygiene—6 to 7 liters per day
- Washing of clothes—4 to 6 liters per day
- Total water needs, per person, per day—15 to 20 liters (Coppola, 2011, p. 320)

UNIT RESOURCES

Other established mathematical formulae can assist the EMS planner in his task. When the EMS planner begins to work through resource requests and total management, the NFA (n.d.) indicates following this criteria:

- Historical review of the events in the past
- Venue and event management
- Other EMS agencies with similar events
- Additional factors
    - Add 33% call volume for the consumption of alcohol
    - Add an additional 33% for the presence of illicit/illegal drugs
    - Consider special factors (e.g., elderly, handicapped). (p. 7–28)

The NFA (n.d., p. 7–28) also brought forward a formula called the Belgian Ambulance Methodology. This formula is used when planning for EMS unit resource requirements. The formula is as follows:

$$X = Nt/Tn$$

Where,

X = number of ambulances required
N = number of persons requiring transport
t = round-trip travel time to hospital, including time to return to service (in hours)
T = total time available for operations (in hours)
n = number of persons to be transported per ambulance

The following example shows how the formula is used to estimate resource needs:

Using the Belgian Ambulance Methodology

Situation: Evacuation of a hospital prior to a storm.

Hospital census: 120 patients (N = 120)

Round trip travel time: 1 hour (t = 1)

Must be accomplished in 6 hours ($T = 6$)
Will be transported 1 per ambulance ($n = 1$)

$$X = Nt/Tn$$
$$X = (120 \times 1)/(6 \times 1)$$
$$X = 20 \text{ ambulances (4 five-ambulance strike teams)}$$

EQUIPMENT AND SUPPLIES

Depending on the geographic location, and rural versus urban environment, the basic list of equipment and supplies needed when responding to a mass gathering or special event will vary. The following items are listed in no particular order and are quite broad in their scope, yet they provide a good starting point when checking to see if an agency has what is needed.

Tents

These will vary in size considerably. In the planning phase, make sure the EMS providers know how to set up the tents.

Treatment Supplies

Common EMS unit supplies are a good starting point when planning for mass gatherings and special events. Having basic supplies that are easily carried by person, by cart, or by small vehicle is optimal. Staging treatment supplies and other equipment securely within the operational area is a good idea as well.

Extra Equipment

Extra equipment could range from extra cots, stretchers, blankets, and pillows to fuel, diesel exhaust fluid, generators, rope, twine, duct tape, personal food and water, index cards and markers. The list can be extended based on needs and experience.

Identification Vests

These vests can be labeled as to task (e.g., Staging, Triage, Paramedic, EMT, etc.). When working on a highway/road, remember that vests are mandated by OSHA. Many public safety providers are killed on United States roadways every year.

Additional Radios

The main issue is knowledge of working frequencies, recharging, and accountability. Make sure to keep a log of who has what. Access to and accountability for radios should be strictly tracked and managed.

ALL-TERRAIN VEHICLES/MINI-AMBULANCES/WHEELED CONVEYANCES

These helpful transport vehicles can range from bicycles; to golf carts; to six-wheeled, all-terrain vehicles with a standard wheeled EMS stretcher. They can be self powered, battery powered, or fuel powered. In a large-scale mass gathering or special event, they can be of considerable help with response, moving personnel and equipment, and assisting with surveillance.

FINANCIAL CONSIDERATIONS

Some events are cost recoverable from federal or state funding specifically set aside for natural and/or manmade disasters. However, many events will be routine and covered by the agency's budget. The funding set aside for mass gatherings and special events can vary greatly across the United States. Some events can have a cost-recovery component attached to them. These can be planned for as well as negotiated prior to the event.

MEDIA

The media's relationship with public safety can be a double-edged sword. Although many public safety agencies, such as EMS, can maintain a positive relationship with the media, it should never be forgotten that a mistake or untoward event can create a rather contentious situation between the two institutions. Cahill (2003) privdes good information on the media with regard to the disaster management/humanitarian relief context when he writes,

> The mass media can do the following:
> - Raise consciousness about health issues
> - Help place health on the public agenda
> - Convey simple information
> - Change behavior if other enabling factors such as the following are present:
>   - Existing motivation
>   - Supportive circumstances
>   - Advocating simple one-off behavior change
>
> The mass media cannot:
> - Convey complex information
> - Teach skills
> - Shift people's attitudes or beliefs
> - Change behavior in the absence of enabling factors. (*Source: "Points on Mass Media" from Emergency Relief Operations, 2003, p. 105–106. Used by permission of Fordham University Press.*)

Cahill (2003) brings up some important points for the EMS planner. During an event, the media should be handled by the public information officer (PIO). However, if the EMS planner knows on the front end that the media can convey simple information, prepackaged messages can be developed by the EMS planner for the PIO. It is important to know that the media cannot teach skills or convey complex information; make sure to keep it simple.

CHAPTER REVIEW

Summary

There are many different considerations and variables that the EMS planner must analyze and synthesize for mass gatherings and special events. The incident command system should be the foundation for all EMS planners, and that should be advocated as EMS has not been a traditional end-user of the process. In addition, EMS should also take a proactive role in emergency management and its concepts. Incident action plans (IAPs) should be completed for every mass gathering and special event, and these plans should be logged and analyzed to better meet the mission for subsequent events. Experience is the value in that situation. Performing hazard analyses is also a good practice in which EMS should become proficient. Special events are a great way for EMS to enjoy a positive public relations/public education venue when done correctly. In addition, the most important factor in EMS involvement in mass gatherings and special events is personal safety.

WHAT WOULD YOU? Reflection

As the EMS division chief for your department, your job is made much easier as you have been providing this service for many years. Having IAPs (incident action plans) to review from the past games will be invaluable as you have kept data on attendance, number of EMS calls/contacts during the standby, types of calls/contacts during the standby, preexisting public safety contacts (e.g., law enforcement, other EMS agencies, school system key contacts, custodial contacts), preexisting ingress/egress routes, hospital contacts, and so on. Remember that IAPs are fluid and require the EMS special operations manager to be able to change and revise them on short notice.

Having a close relationship with the school system key contacts and law enforcement will be critical for this next special event. Keeping the command staff in the loop early as to your projected needs also will be very important. Expect to include the school board, high school sports representatives, athletic trainers, law enforcement, school security, the fire service (i.e., fire marshal and EMS first response), local hospital emergency departments, EMS medical director, and quite possibly the local/regional fusion center.

You may plan for twice the amount of personnel for this event with a contingency for an additional unit if needed. Briefing the on-duty personnel at the other stations will be important to continue the flow of information. Safety of the personnel will be of particular importance for this event. Write an IAP for this event as you would for any other. You may want to set up a medical branch ICS system for this event, even if for practice.

The EMS special operations manager is well advised to make sure that all EMS providers within the system are compliant with ICS 100, 200, 700, and 800. The resource for these courses may be found at the FEMA website.

Review Questions

1. What is the difference between an incident and an event?
2. What are the five characteristics of developing incident objectives per the SMART methodology?
3. What is surveillance, and why is it an important strategy for EMS?
4. Using the Belgian Ambulance Methodology formula, what would be the requirements for a sporting event mass gathering that your fusion center considers could be target for a terrorist bombing? The potential for injuries is 200 people of various ages. The goal is to transport all patients within the Golden Hour. You estimate that the round-trip travel time is 30 minutes. You can transport two patients per ambulance. What are your resource requirements?
5. Which is completed first: the incident action plan or the planning meeting?
6. What are the requirements for water, per person, per day? What is the breakdown for each type of use (i.e., drinking, bathing, etc.)?
7. What is the function of an intelligence fusion center?
8. What four elements does a well-written incident action plan (IAP) provide?
9. Investigate your own EMS budget or interview an EMS director and investigate what type of funding is tasked for mass gatherings or special events (inclusive of disaster events). What did you find?

References

Cahill, K. M. (2003). *Emergency Relief Operations.* New York: The Center for International Health and Cooperation, Fordham University Press.

Clements, B. W. (2009). *Disasters and Public Health: Planning and Response.* Boston, MA: Butterworth-Heinemann.

Coppola, D. P. (2011). *Introduction to International Disaster Management.* Boston, MA: Butterworth-Heinemann.

Haddow, G. D., and K. D. Haddow. (2009). *Disaster Communications in a Changing Media World.* Boston, MA: Butterworth-Heinemann.

Institute of Medicine of the National Academies. (2007). "EMS at the Crossroads: Future of Emergency Care." Washington, DC: The National Academies Press.

Miller, I. (2012, February). "All Hazards Incidents: Setting Objectives and Strategies." *Fire Engineering 165*(2), p. 75.

National Fire Academy. (n.d.). "EMS Special Operations Curriculum." Emmitsburg, MD: Author.

U.S. Department of Homeland Security. (2012). *State and Major Urban Area Fusion Centers.* See the organization website.

Key Terms

complexity analysis A combination of involved factors that affect the probability of control of an incident.

event A planned activity.

fusion center(s) A set point for the receipt, analysis, gathering, and sharing of threat-related information between the federal, state, and local governments and private sector partners.

incident An unexpected occurrence that happens in connection with something else.

incident action plans (IAPs) Formally documents incident goals (known as control objectives in NIMS), operational period objectives, and the response strategy defined by incident command during response planning.

incident command post (ICP) The field location at which the primary tactical level, on scene incident command functions are performed.

operational period A set period of time specified for an incident (e.g., 6 hours, 8 hours, 12 hours, etc.).

planning meeting A meeting held as needed throughout the duration of an incident, to select specific strategies and tactics for incident control operations, and for service and support planning.

situational awareness The idea of understanding what is happening at an incident, and the measures that are needed to mitigate the incident.

size-up The steps taken when first arriving on scene to help set up the immediate incident objectives.

SMART objectives An acronym used in incident planning to describe five characteristics to create an effective plan. These are *smart, measurable, action oriented, realistic,* and *time sensitive.*

surveillance The collection and analysis of health-related data to assist in preventing a serious adverse clinical event.

tactics meeting The time set to review the tactics developed by the operations section chief.

Tactical Response

4 CHAPTER

Sam Bradley

Objectives

After reading this chapter, the student should be able to:

4.1 Explain modern dangers to fire, EMS, and law enforcement personnel and the justification for increased interoperability.
4.2 Define the role of SWAT teams.
4.3 Justify the need for tactical paramedics as an integral part of the SWAT team.
4.4 Explain responsibilities of the tactical paramedic on a special weapons and tactics unit.
4.5 Explain considerations for EMS involvement with a SWAT team.
4.6 Discuss advantages and challenges of EMS involvement as TEMS paramedics.
4.7 Discuss costs associated with supporting TEMS paramedics.
4.8 Discuss TEMS paramedic protocols and equipment.
4.9 Explain TEMS paramedic initial and ongoing training needs.

Key Terms

barricaded subjects
counter-sniper operations
diving or marine operations
dignitary protection
hemostatic agents
interoperability
medical intelligence
medical team officer
medical threat assessments
special weapons and tactical (SWAT) team
tactical medicine
tactical emergency medical support (TEMS)
tactical tourniquets

WHAT WOULD YOU DO?

You are in the middle of your morning administrative chores when the dispatcher announces there's a train derailment. Although most of the trains that go through your district haul freight, this one happens to be a high-volume, high-speed commuter train. You start for the scene. First reports state there are about a hundred people in three cars who need to be triaged. You call for support from your company's operation in adjacent counties.

You go to the command post and become part of the unified command with fire and law enforcement. Due to the number of patients, the relatively small number of response personnel, and the requirement for three branches of the operation, resources are limited. Your supervisors are given key incident command system (ICS) roles in triage, treatment, and transport.

Although the incident is ultimately considered a success, one of the complaints in the review was that your ambulance company supervisors had no idea what they were doing in terms of understanding their ICS role. They had to be assisted and corrected a number of times by fire personnel who were engaged in fire suppression and extrication.

The only ICS training your supervisors received were the minimum required classes, which were completed online. When the time came time to transfer this knowledge to a real world incident, they were not prepared.

Questions

1. As an EMS manager, what has your company done to prepare EMS employees for interacting in the ICS system on a large incident?
2. Does your agency train with fire and law enforcement to prepare for large patient incidents?
3. What kind of relationship has been established with public safety agencies to promote safety for all responders?

INTRODUCTION

With budget cuts reducing the number of law enforcement personnel, the risk to EMS goes higher. With intentional acts of terrorism, EMS personnel can become targets, as seen in the 1993 World Trade Center attack, the bombing of the Alfred P. Murrah Federal Building in Oklahoma City, any number of school shooting incidents, and, most notably, the 2011 attacks on the World Trade Center and the Pentagon. There are also dangers from multiple patient incidents secondary to transportation accidents, and the aftermath of natural disasters.

One consideration about **tactical emergency medical support (TEMS)** is its diversity. Urban police operations with EMS units and hospitals in close proximity are very different from rural areas without such support and are subject to long transport times. The complexity of a TEMS program should be founded on an agency's ability to mitigate and stabilize hemorrhage. A TEMS program should be tailored to the needs of the specific law enforcement operation.

What about the issues EMS providers deal with every day?

- Hysterical family members or bystanders who can become verbally or physically assaultive
- Increased prevalence of handguns due to a perceived need for added security

- Additional stress from an economy in recession—losing jobs and homes, lost pensions, and businesses closing—causing people to act desperately
- Domestic abuse situations, assaults, or acts of violence that include weapons
- An increased number of mentally ill patients and the need for disturbed or violent people to seek care in emergency rooms due to the closure of mental health care facilities
- Mentally ill patients released from facilities with the hope (not always fulfilled) of compliance with medications
- Increased gang activity, with drug use and abuse. (With the increased numbers of drug abusers, the likelihood of hospitals, pharmacies, clinics, and even ambulances becoming targets for desperate drug seekers is higher.)
- Potentially unsafe environments like bad neighborhoods or poorly lit parking lots (Often, there is no immediate means of obtaining backup. This is made worse by low staffing numbers and limited or inadequate communication equipment.)
- Lack of staff training for recognizing and managing assaultive and escalating hostile behavior

From the police side, "line-of-duty deaths jumped by 37% in 2010, according to the report by the National Law Enforcement Officers Memorial Fund. . . . and 2011 added another 13% to this tragic number". (*Source: Excerpt from "Complacency Kills" by M. Kahlberg in Law Enforcement Today, January 2012.*)

Side Bar

The National Law Enforcement Officers Memorial Fund website states, "A total of 1,799 law enforcement officers died in the line of duty during the past 10 years, an average of one death every 53 hours or 164 per year. There were 163 law enforcement officers killed in 2011. On average, over the last decade, there have been 53,469 assaults against law enforcement each year, resulting in 15,833 injuries."

(Source: From "Law Enforcement Facts: Key Data about the Profession" from The National Law Enforcement Officers Memorial Fund.)

Active shooter situations, **barricaded subjects**, and hostage situations are not uncommon for police, and lessons learned from recent incidents made it all too clear that they were sometimes unprepared or underarmed.

A good example was the shootout in front of a Bank of America building between North Hollywood Police and two heavily armed bank robbers in 1997. Before the robbers were eventually killed, 2,000 rounds of ammunition were fired and eleven police officers and seven civilians were injured. The police were armed with pistols or shotguns, but the robbers had fully automatic AK-47 and M16 rifles capable of penetrating body armor. The military-grade body armor they wore prevented the police officers' bullets from harming them initially. Only the **special weapons and tactical (SWAT) team** had rifles powerful enough to penetrate the body armor.

One controversy occurred over the fact that the Los Angeles Police Department would not allow medical personnel to treat one of the injured robbers. The department claimed to have been following a current procedure, which stated that ambulance personnel were not allowed to enter a hot zone in a hostile situation. Understanding the need for **interoperability** with law enforcement, the "tactical paramedic" role has become of increasing interest. Many law enforcement agencies have integrated specialized EMTs, paramedics, and sometimes physicians into their tactical teams. The fact that EMS was tactically separate from law enforcement operations sometimes resulted in a delay of care.

If tactical medical personnel had been present during this event, or events like the Columbine High School shooting in 1999, or the killing of four police officers in Oakland in 2009, there might have been a different outcome. Personnel may have been able to reach injured officers sooner and could have provided medical care to injured civilians in areas where untrained ambulance personnel could not go.

TACTICAL LAW ENFORCEMENT TEAMS

Tactical law enforcement teams may be known as special weapons and tactics teams, special response teams, emergency services units, or emergency tactical response teams. They may be full time or on call. They may be local police, sheriff's department personnel, or federal officers.

Law enforcement is a hazardous profession for anyone who chooses to uphold the law. Some situations call for a higher level of training, specialized skills, and an interest and ability to operate in austere and unsecure environments. These men and women are dedicated and committed to the extent that this may be their singular focus in life. They are prepared to handle the most difficult and dangerous of situations, knowing the possibility of injury or death is high. They need to maintain optimum fitness both physically and mentally. Given that life or death could depend on a quick decision or perfection of a skill, the need for training is constant.

TYPES OF SWAT MISSIONS

Teams are called out to situations that involve unconventional hazards and require specialize skills. Types of incidents include the following:

- Hostage incidents
- Barricaded suspects
- Suicidal subjects
- High-risk warrant service and arrests
- Gang and drug mitigation
- Dignitary protection
- Situations with the likelihood of armed resistance

Specialty teams may also engage in any of the following:

- **Counter-sniper operations**
- Explosives mitigation
- **Diving or marine operations**
- Air operations or search-and-rescue operations
- Terrorism mitigation

Criminals and terrorists are more resolute, heavily armed, and violent than ever before, and there is no indication that this will change any time soon. Law enforcement tactics and tactical medical techniques need to constantly evolve to treat and evacuate the wounded, the sick, and the injured as well as address and eliminate threats. (See Figure 4.1.)

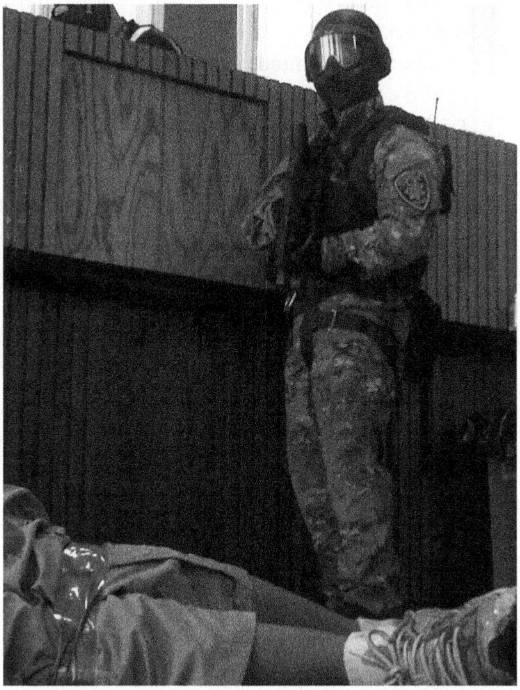

FIGURE 4.1 In this situation, a SWAT officer is holding a suspect. *Source: © Sam Bradley, Urban Shield, 2011.*

TACTICAL PARAMEDICS AS A NEW STANDARD

With the current climate of economic unrest, justification is greater for deployment of tactical law enforcement teams. In the document "Tactical Medicine and Tactical Casualty Care," the California Commission on Peace Officer Standards and Training (POST, 2013) states, "Operational tactical medical support programs provide a necessary and significant linkage between law enforcement personnel and EMS services during dangerous or sustained operations." With more deployment comes more risk. Ensuring the health and safety of a tactical team is a command responsibility and requires skills and personnel maintenance as well as medical support. Having tactical paramedics qualified, trained, and skilled in law enforcement operations is becoming an accepted and necessary standard.

Tactical and SWAT teams are not currently required to have a **tactical medicine** program, but in 2005 POST recommended that medical programs be incorporated into a tactical law enforcement program. The recommendation states that if a tactical medical program is adopted, the personnel will be trained as "Tactical EMTs," "Tactical Paramedics," or "Tactical Physicians" and will complete an approved tactical medicine class.

According to the POST website, tactical medicine has evolved in recent years due to better-trained personnel who assist at incidents that involve potentially violent outcomes. Tactical medics are used to provide immediate care to the tactical officers and to any other victims at the scene, which result in better outcomes for all involved (POST, 2013). (See Figure 4.2.)

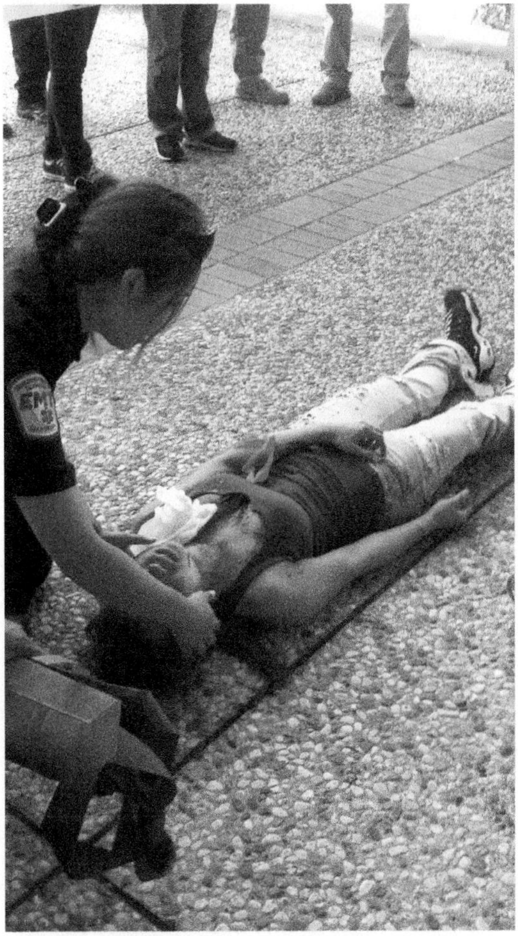

FIGURE 4.2 ■ EMS may assist an injured patient after an explosion during a tactical event. *Source: © Sam Bradley, Urban Shield, 2011.*

The POST Operational Guideline for SWAT was derived from California Penal Code Section 13514.1, which created a standard that provided information, education, and training to those who function in the tactical environment (POST, 2013).

Since then, POST has collaborated with the California Emergency Medical Services Authority (EMSA) and "completed development of guidelines to provide baseline development and implementation of operational programs developed as required and described in the SWAT Guidelines." The "POST/EMSA Tactical Medicine Operational Programs and

Side Bar

Tactical Medicine

The delivery of medical services for law enforcement special operations, states, "The tactical incident response environment presents unique challenges to law enforcement personnel and for the personnel providing emergency medical care and support services in that environment. Tactical medical care providers must have a clear understanding of, and consideration for, law enforcement response, tactics, and the mission-specific objectives of a tactical operation when planning for and providing medical support" (POST, 2013).

Standardized Training Recommendations" (California POST in Collaboration with Emergency Medical Services Authority, 2009) is meant to serve as a companion document to the SWAT guidelines and describes the critical role that tactical medicine planning and threat assessment play in the overall contingency planning as part of the SWAT operational plan.

THE ROLE OF A TACTICAL PARAMEDIC

A tactical paramedic, or **medical team officer**, is considered part of a tactical medical or TEMS team. The term *tactical paramedic* is used here for clarity, but the majority of SWAT teams rely on EMT-Bs to support their operations. Paramedics provide additional capabilities but are not always available to teams. The term *tactical paramedic* is used even though the scope of practice of the practitioner may vary. Tactical paramedics support law enforcement personnel and are considered a necessary component of the team.

Even though paramedics may use their ALS skills, this is not everyday EMS. A prehospital-based paramedic may have the same level of dedication, professionalism, and commitment as his law enforcement counterparts, but a tactical operation requires a very different mind-set and skills set.

To operate in a tactical environment, paramedics must develop skills in situational awareness and performing **medical intelligence** assessments. Paramedic training assumes that a paramedic will be managing patients injured during an event that has already taken place and is now deemed safe. Tactical paramedics are involved in the situation before and during the mission. Their focus is to consider, and potentially mitigate, hazards necessary to minimize the morbidity and mortality of personnel working in a tactical operation. They prevent casualties when at all possible, treat casualties when they occur, and complete the mission. A basic medical intelligence assessment would be similar to surveying the scene for hazards, while also looking much deeper into the potential for problems and how best to mitigate them.

After the January 2011 shooting of U.S. Representative Gabrielle Giffords, it was recognized that immediate treatment and transport is what makes the difference in saving someone's life that has sustained a serious life-threatening injury. Regardless, of whether it is an urban environment or rural environment, time is of the utmost critical element for a patient. During such situations, law enforcement is faced with the issue of gaining control over the situation and cannot provide the immediate treatment needed for the victim (Kastre and Kleinman, 2012). If paramedics were trained as a part of a tactical team, they would be where and when they were needed, rather than standing by and waiting for the area to be cleaned.

The tactical paramedic may also have a role outside of a mission that would support team

Best Practice

The California Model

The State of California Emergency Medical Services Authority (EMSA) and the California Commission on Peace Officer's Standards and Training (POST) created tactical medicine guidelines designed to provide baseline development and implementation standards for tactical medicine programs, as described in the 2005 SWAT Guidelines. EMSA sets minimum statewide medical standards for initial tactical medicine training. These guidelines are for the development of public safety agency programs in California and are contained in the 77-page document entitled "Tactical Medicine: Operational Programs and Standardized Training Recommendations" (California POST in Collaboration with Emergency Medical Services Authority, 2009). This document recommends seven components that should be included in a comprehensive Tactical Medicine Operational Program:

- Medical Oversight
- Medical Contingency Planning
- Operational Support/Tactical Emergency Support (TEMS)
- Quality Improvement
- Team Health Management
- Training and Education

The State of California has approved a 2-week, 80-hour comprehensive tactical medicine course, which covers the core content of tactical medicine. It utilizes didactic education, hands-on training, scenario-based teaching, and firearms instruction. The program is broken into modules.

Tactical Medicine Course Module A is open to medical people actively involved in providing emergency medical support for military and law enforcement special operations teams or those looking to establish a new team. Course Module B provides additional intensive training and skills in tactics and advanced medical care. A newer Module C covers topics not developed in Module A or Module B and satisfies some CE and CME requirements. This module can be used as refresher training, additional training, or to provide new skill sets.

Another unique thing about California was the establishment of an annual SWAT training exercise, Urban Shield. This comprehensive full-scale regional preparedness exercise was started by the Alameda County Sheriff's Office in 2007 and provides opportunity for SWAT and tactical response teams to exercise in real-world scenarios.

Urban Shield is a full-scale exercise designed to "assess and validate the speed, effectiveness and efficiency of capabilities, as well as test the adequacy of regional policies, plans, procedures and protocols. This training provides first responders, homeland security officials, emergency management officials, private and non-governmental partners, and other personnel with the knowledge, skills, and abilities needed to perform key tasks required in large-scale disasters". (*Source: Excerpt from "The Urban Shield Exercise" in Articles: Urban Shield the Event a. Published by Urban Shield, © 2014.*)

For the 2011 event, twenty-nine individual events were set up in several counties in the Bay Area. These scenarios are very realistic and very relevant. Teams compete against other regional teams as well as with teams from across the country and internationally. In 2011, challengers included teams from Jordan, Bahrain, and the State of Israel. Originally focused on SWAT teams, the event has expanded to include Explosive Ordinance Disposal Team (EOD; otherwise known as bomb squads), fire, Urban Search and Rescue (USAR), Hazmat, and EMS.

The value of Urban Shield is that it allows each agency to evaluate its own tactical capabilities, while training together with EMS, Fire, and EOD strengthens capabilities to manage large-scale events utilizing the National Incident Management System (NIMS) concepts.

health and readiness. This may include maintaining medical histories, immunization records, and health status information for team members. This information is confidential, of course, so he would assure that only those with a need to know would have access to this information.

The tactical paramedic may conduct **medical threat assessments** specific to the mission outcome. He may help develop physical fitness and stress reduction training. He should be knowledgeable about the medical effects of conditions found on a typical mission: stress, sleep deprivation, nutritional replacement and hydration, and environmental impact. These issues could be addressed in training prior to an event and monitored during an event.

The tactical paramedic would serve as a health information resource for the team as well as a liaison and advocate for how an injured or ill officer would be managed in the health care system. This would involve creating positive relationships and sometimes establishing agreements with health care facilities.

The tactical paramedic could be a resource in terms of interacting with and providing training for local EMS, fire, and transport entities so they would learn how to appropriately interact when assuming care of an ill or injured officer. Another role for a tactical paramedic could be responsibility for police dogs that become injured or ill. He could learn basic supportive care that would stabilize an animal until it could be transferred to a veterinarian. There is also potential for TEMS paramedics to manage problems that occur with the public as well as officers during more routine, but potentially dangerous, events like warrant services.

CONSIDERATIONS FOR CREATING OR PROVIDING ASSISTANCE FOR A TACTICAL MEDICAL TEAM

The typical model of a tactical team/EMS relationship is where paramedics wait with their ambulance and are called in only when needed. These "standby" agreements are becoming more obsolete as cases are being made for failure to provide appropriate and expedient care. The deaths resulting from the Columbine shootings provide an example of how law enforcement procedures have changed and medical response needs have been reconsidered.

DIFFERENT MODELS

Areas such as Pinellas County, Florida, have gone in a different direction. Once paramedics agree to train to become tactical paramedics and meet the requirements, they engage in the same rigid training as SWAT officers. A repercussion of this kind of model is that it raises the frequency of responses for EMS on tactical incidents and may require rethinking on the operational side as well as more districtwide training for the other emergency service providers.

Another example of how the models are changing are that hazmat response teams, who typically manage spills and releases, now find themselves working with law enforcement when a hazardous material incident might be part of a weapons of mass destruction (WMD) event. This requires EMS and hazmat-trained professionals to work with law enforcement specialty teams to enter into questionable situations and perform rescues.

Hazmat incidents pose different challenges and require methodical analysis and planning. This is where tactical cops need to enter the EMS world and become familiar with air monitoring equipment and appropriate personal protective equipment (PPE) for this kind of incident.

ADVANTAGES OF A TEMS UNIT

Police, fire, and EMS all have knowledge and training that can be mutually beneficial. For instance, SWAT officers can learn forcible entry techniques and victim extrication methods from fire. In general, all involved agencies need a better understanding of each other's roles to interact positively and effectively at incidents. Cross-training would strengthen this relationship. Better cooperation leads to better communication, which leads to better safety for all personnel.

Side Bar

TEMS: A Better Option?

Why is having a TEMS team a better option than an ambulance standing by somewhere? It's a matter of speed, knowledge, and having the right equipment to mitigate a traumatic injury that can kill in minutes. Paramedics not only need to be trained in the medical procedures to handle life-threatening bleeding, but they also must have the training and PPE to go into a hot zone and extricate a fallen officer. When specialty paramedics are not trained and available to treat and evacuate a victim, then other SWAT officers must, which takes them out of the battle. (See Figure 4.3.)

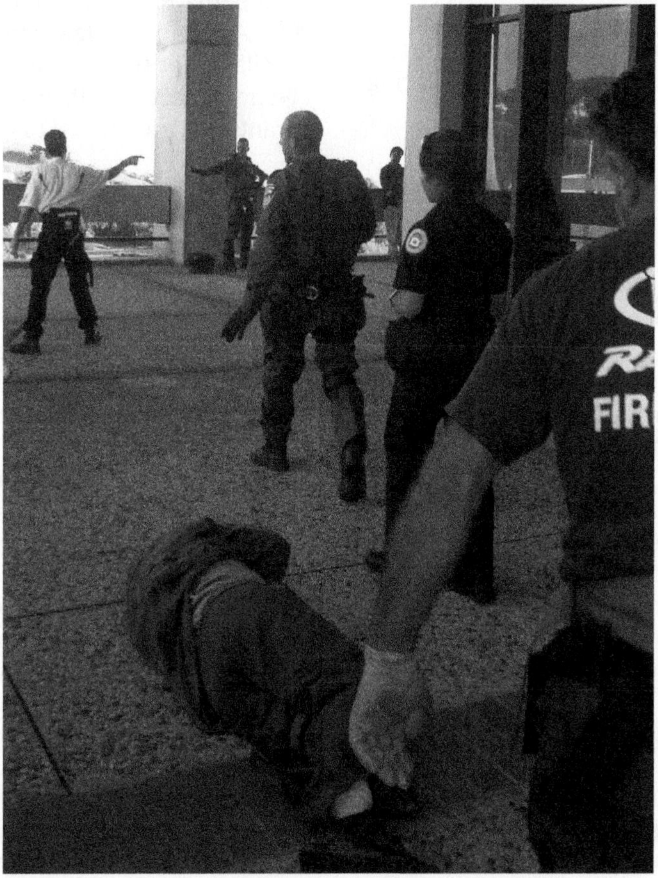

FIGURE 4.3 EMS may interact with SWAT during various situations. *Source: © Sam Bradley, Urban Shield, 2011.*

Training in a tactical environment logically gives a paramedic better situational awareness and critical thinking skills. They are more likely to develop better skills in terms of preplanning an incident and handling calls with difficult skills requirements. Information learned from cross-training also could translate into training for other members of the primary agency or department.

CHALLENGES OF A TEMS UNIT

No program is without challenges, nor are they free. Tactical medical programs can incur heavy expenses for training and equipment, but grant funding is available. A high-risk program like this also involves liability. These are matters to be studied when considering a program.

Funding

There are costs involved in selecting tactical paramedics since candidate requirements are stringent. The first large expense is seen with initial training. Not only is the fee for a 2-week course high, but the employee will also have to be paid for his time and his agency will have to pay to backfill his position. Ongoing training is another necessary and regular expenditure.

Once tactical paramedics are trained, they will need PPE similar to that of law enforcement, including ballistic (bulletproof) vests and Kevlar helmets. In some cases, law enforcement may pay for this equipment with the proceeds of confiscated property from drug arrests or seized assets.

Funding an EMS TEMS component of a team usually requires each agency to pay its own personnel for engaging in SWAT missions. This allows the sharing of costs and makes it simpler to manage overtime and liability issues. On the other hand, there is a cost savings in eliminating the need for an emergency vehicle to sit standby for an event.

How to Get Funding

If an opportunity exists for public support, the team should engage the media to promote the team. When the public understands what the program does as well as the specific role of TEMS medical personnel, people will be more inclined to support funds requested. If the team goes to the voters for a bond issue or a parcel tax, having promoted the team as community friendly benefits the entire program.

One way of accomplishing this is through public visibility. Create a display for local preparedness fairs. Go to big-box stores and set up a table to provide informational materials and perhaps offer free blood pressure checks.

A number of law enforcement grants are available for training and supplies, such as the National Tactical Officers Association (NTOA) grants that are offered to its members.

LIABILITY

A major issue regarding tactical paramedics is whether or not they should be trained to shoot and/or carry firearms. Generally, EMS professionals want the public to understand that they do not bear arms, but some wonder if tactical paramedics should be part of a special category that is allowed to do so.

Originally, roles within a tactical team were clearly defined: Law enforcement handles police matters, and paramedics handle medical and trauma issues. Over time, however, the role of the tactical paramedic has evolved, and needs are now based on the area served, team specialty, and types of deployment typically seen. Paramedics train with the team and are already familiar with the tools that the team uses. Considering the low percentage of time paramedics are needed for patient care, it seems an efficient decision to use them for other assignments during the operation. Some teams find it appropriate to integrate tactical paramedics into other tactical roles on the team. Police officers trained as paramedics, or paramedics with law enforcement training, could operate in dual roles.

In many cases, administrators on both sides value the progressive scope of these emerging roles. One theory is that they become more useful to the team. They can function as SWAT members until they are needed as paramedics. They may have more limited and less dangerous duties, such as covering a perimeter, deploying distraction devices, or assisting with breaching. Another side of the argument is that some believe it is better to have team members assigned to one particular job, which allows them to gain the experience necessary to do it effectively. Specialization ensures that an individual will not be overwhelmed during stressful events or have specific skills diluted.

Some teams prefer their tactical paramedics to be unarmed and want them to focus only on providing medical support. They have concern that placing additional tactical responsibilities on them runs the risk of the paramedic not being available to treat someone in a timely manner. If the paramedic is armed and tasked with cover for the team, would it compromise the safety of other officers if the paramedic had to race to the aid of a downed officer? Other questions arise about situations in which the paramedic shoots and injures or kills someone. Would that affect his ability to provide the best care for someone who just shot at him or someone he just shot?

Another option is to arm tactical paramedics with less-than-lethal weapons, such as beanbag guns, or rubber-bullet guns. This would provide them protection without the training and liability of a lethal weapon.

Whether a team requires that paramedics be armed or unarmed would depend on the needs of the unit, the mission, and the resources available. A key issue regarding whether tactical paramedics are armed is whether or not they are sworn to duty. If not sworn, then the tactical paramedic should not (and cannot) engage in law enforcement tasks. If armed, the only reason for a non–law enforcement officer to have a weapon is for self-defense. Law enforcement as well as the EMS agency would have to agree. Law enforcement would need to ensure appropriate training and proficiency. Were the tactical paramedic to shoot a civilian, it is unlikely he would have the same legal protections, access to counsel, and psychological support as law enforcement, unless established in policy.

CREATION OF A TEMS UNIT

A needs assessment would be required to determine the necessity for a TEMS unit to meet the specific medical needs of a SWAT/tactical team. Medical oversight and medical direction would need to be provided, which would require coordination with the local EMS agency. A program medical director would need to take responsibility for the program and define patient care protocols and procedures for medical support during tactical operations. Before partnering with the police, the fire department or EMS agency must ensure that this expanding role would not take resources away from fundamental fire missions or negatively affect day-to-day ambulance operations.

The "law enforcement first" option can be time consuming and expensive as obtaining a paramedic license requires 1,000+ hours of classroom studies, clinical practice, and an internship. Paramedic classes are focused on fire and ambulance personnel, not law enforcement. A police department would also have to factor in the potential cost of overtime for covering an officer during training. Another issue is required ancillary certifications, such as ACLS, and the time and cost of continuing education and cyclical relicensure.

The advantage to this option is that the paramedic is armed and fully trained and functional as a law enforcement officer. In reality, though, most city police departments do not receive the volume of SWAT-type calls necessary to maintain the medical proficiency of a tactical paramedic, which makes it logical for paramedics to fill this role.

The "paramedic first" option would require law enforcement to draw from local EMS personnel. This requires an attitude of cooperation and interoperability among agencies and provides benefit to both in terms of sharing training and resources. EMTs and paramedics appreciate the opportunity and challenge of learning new skills. With this option, EMS personnel would be required to apply, submit to a background check and physical exam, possibly an agility requirement, and then training to learn law enforcement basics. Initial and ongoing training requires top physical shape. Personnel thus trained will need to manage obstacles to reach the officer, move quickly while carrying medical gear, and be able to tolerate PPE such as gas masks.

Where law enforcement is inherently more dangerous, prehospital medicine can be fairly routine and is rarely dangerous. In the former, paramedics would have to function under stress and less-than-ideal conditions; skills they may be quite proficient in will become more difficult to perform in a hot-zone scenario.

Once accepted on the team, tactical paramedics would be required to train regularly with tactical law enforcement team members to build relationships and trust as well as to understand the operational side of a SWAT-type operation. There is little doubt that police and EMS agencies working together will result in lower mortality and morbidity to police officers as well as civilians. (See Figure 4.4.)

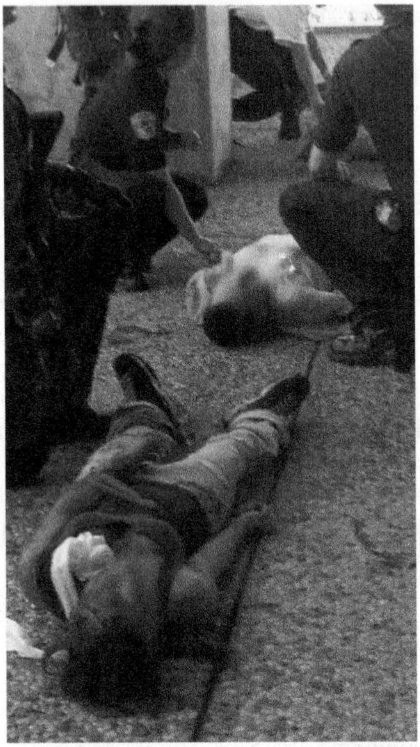

FIGURE 4.4 ■ Sometimes EMS will assist a SWAT event. *Source: © Sam Bradley, Urban Shield, 2011.*

TACTICAL PARAMEDIC PROTOCOLS AND EQUIPMENT

Tactical medicine is not a matter of transferring prehospital training or equipment into a law enforcement venue. The most obvious difference is time. The paramedic does not have the luxury of time to apply direct pressure for several minutes, start an IV, or even apply a splint when under fire. The main goal of the tactical paramedic is quick, decisive action and immediate control of severe bleeding, then getting himself and his patient to safety. Much has been learned from recent conflicts overseas. Innovative military needs have driven the creation of new tourniquets and bleeding control substances appropriate for urban high-threat environments.

Tactical paramedics do not carry large medical bags like they would on an EMS vehicle. Supplies are kept in vests pockets, backpacks, pouches, or small kits. They may have to travel quickly and can find themselves in confined spaces. They may have to carry their gear for many hours. Equipment may be adjusted based on the mission. An active shooter, hostage scenario, or barricaded suspect call may have different requirements than a high-risk warrant or **dignitary protection** assignment.

Even though specialized trauma treatments and equipment are filtering into prehospital care, their best use is in tactical medical situations. These include tools such as **tactical tourniquets**, tactical compression dressings, and **hemostatic agents**. (See Figure 4.5.)

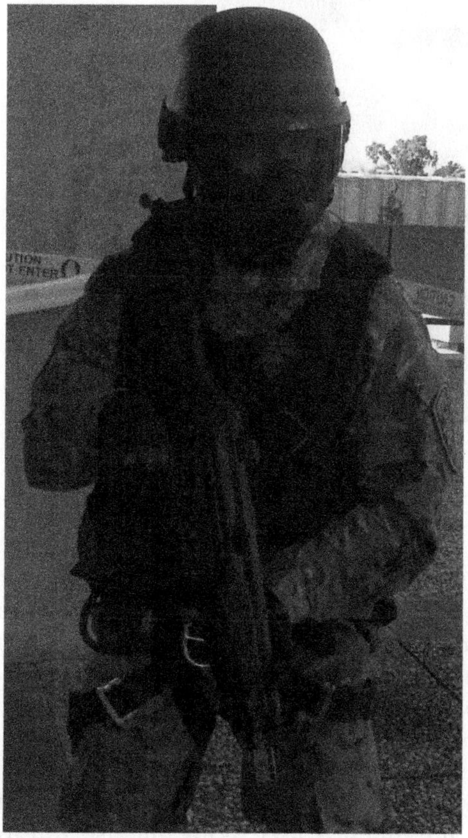

FIGURE 4.5 ■ A fully equipped SWAT officer.
Source: © Sam Bradley, Urban Shield, 2011.

TRAINING

A number of companies offer tactical paramedic training, but it is still an emerging field, and curricula have not been standardized nationally. The Committee for Tactical Emergency Casualty Care (C-TECC), modeled after the Committee for Tactical Combat Casualty Care (CoTCCC), is comprised of a broad range of experts in high-threat medicine from across the United States. Subject matter experts come from emergency medicine, emergency medical services, police, fire, and military special operations.

C-TECC was tasked to study and transition military medical lessons learned from the battlefield to civilian crisis response in order to reduce preventable causes of death in first responders and the civilian population. Based on the principles of Tactical Combat Casualty Care (TCCC), the TECC guidelines are a set of best practice recommendations for casualty management during high-threat civilian tactical-and-rescue operations. This may well form the basis for a national standardized tactical medical curriculum. (See Figure 4.6.)

PRIMARY TRAINING

Tactical training should be extensive and comprehensive to meet the needs of the high-stress tactical environment. Whether the responder's primary career is law enforcement or EMS, training requires an understanding of both police and emergency medical roles.

Paramedics signing up for tactical duty must be in prime shape and ready for basic training. They will learn about the role of the tactical paramedic, tactical triage, legal and liability issues, mission-specific equipment needs, police defense and control tactics, firearms training, and the psychology of managing stress as well as understanding the psyches and behavior of their police

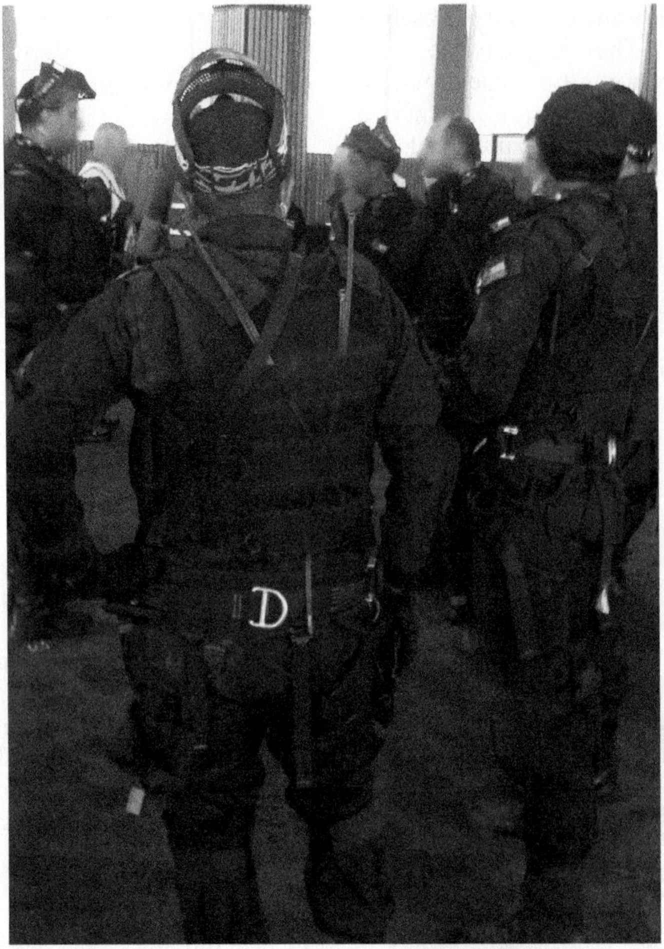

FIGURE 4.6 ■ It is common to debrief after a SWAT event. *Source: © Sam Bradley, Urban Shield, 2011.*

counterparts, gangs, and the suspects with whom they interact.

ONGOING TRAINING

Regular practice is important for any job that requires quick thinking and high-end skills. Simulated scenarios addressing types of responses that are rare, such as acts of terrorism, keep the team sharp for such events. Simulations also raise awareness that terrorists will look for opportunities to strike, especially when they feel public safety personnel are feeling complacent. Training reinforces the need to be vigilant for the signs of potential terrorism, not just during operations but also when encountering familiar, everyday scenes. The tactical paramedic who takes part in training will not only stay sharp on infrequently used skills but also will foster tighter relationships with team members. (See Figure 4.7.)

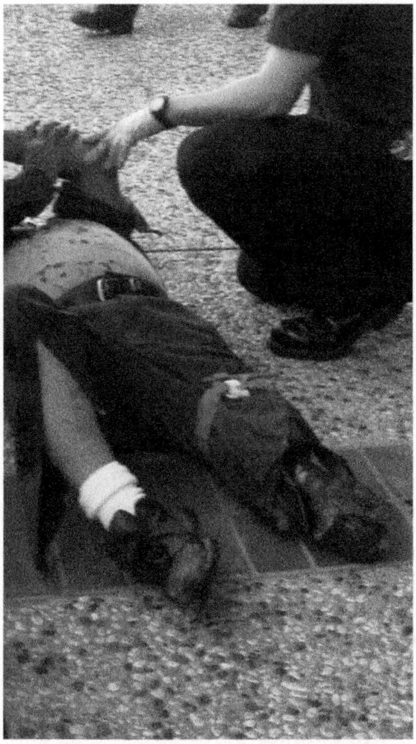

FIGURE 4.7 A "patient" prepped with moulage for a SWAT training event. *Source: © Sam Bradley, Urban Shield, 2011.*

CHOOSING A TACTICAL MEDICINE TRAINING PROGRAM

Since tactical training includes knowledge of police tactics and is conducted by and for law enforcement personnel, acceptance into primary training programs is dependent on careful screening. Most programs require the applicant to be a paramedic and work within the public safety arena of police, fire, or EMS. They also consider candidates from the military, or people working within a division of the U.S. Department of Homeland Security.

Specifics to consider when researching a tactical medical training provider include the following:

The Education Provider

- How long has the program been in existence?
- Is the program certified by a state agency, which may also provide law enforcement training approval?
- Is the program certified by a state emergency medical services authority, which provides approval and oversight for tactical paramedics?
- Does the U.S. Department of Homeland Security approve the program for domestic preparedness?
- Does the program offer continuing education (CE) for EMT/paramedics or continuing medical education (CME) for physicians?
- Is the course long enough to provide the in-depth didactic and practical training required?

Faculty

- Are the instructors sworn law-enforcement officers, non–law enforcement personnel, or a combination of both?
- What background and experience do the instructors have?
- Are instructors active on a tactical team?
- Are physician instructors board certified in emergency medicine or trauma surgery?
- Are TCCC certifications or trauma certifications, such as ITLS or PHTLS, required?

Instructional Techniques

- Is firearms instruction done with real or simulated weapons?
- Is the course curriculum relevant to your needs?
- Is the course heavy with reality-based scenarios or mostly didactic?

Funding

- Can the program qualify for Homeland Security or other grant funding?

The best way to determine if a program meets your needs is to check out the program's website, contact graduates of the program, and/or use social media and tactical medical websites to get feedback on the course.

One example of available training is the Tactical Combat Casualty Care (TCCC) course, which is considered "the military counterpart to the PHTLS course" and is "designed for military medics, corpsmen, and pararescuemen who are preparing to deploy in support of combat operations." TCCC guidelines center on the goals of treating the casualty, preventing additional casualties, and completing the mission. The 48-hour course covers tactical combat casualty care principles and prepares the student to use medical care skills in hostile and austere conditions (National Association of Emergency Medical Technicians, 2013).

CHAPTER REVIEW

Summary

The idea of EMTs and paramedics becoming tactical medical providers on a SWAT team is quickly becoming a standard. It is a reflection of a time when careers in public safety and law enforcement have become more dangerous. There is a need for fire, EMS, and law enforcement to work together for the benefit and safety of all involved.

It is important to emphasize, however, that the desire for TEMS support of law enforcement teams must originate from within the law enforcement organization. It would not work for EMS to train to a TEMS standard, then offer services to law enforcement. TEMS personnel support the health of the law enforcement team, provide immediate care if an injury occurs, and serve as a liaison to EMS. The agreement of a fire department or EMS agency to provide personnel for training and assignment with a law enforcement tactical team needs careful consideration in terms of cost, liability, and the benefit to involved agencies.

Candidates' qualifications may include physical conditioning, medical experience, ability to work under great stress, and ability to adapt skills to a tactical environment. The tactical paramedic will also need to commit to training time with the SWAT or tactical team to keep skills fresh. This can be a challenging, rewarding, and beneficial role for a medical provider who wants to make a bigger difference.

WHAT WOULD YOU DO? Reflection

Tactical paramedics are trained to interact with and follow the command of the special operations team to which they are assigned. Most EMS providers have limited interaction with other agencies on a day-to-day basis and work within familiar roles. In a multiple patient incident, everything changes.

This case study illustrates the need to get out of the mind-set of "our" versus "their" role responsibilities. In an MCI, personnel from EMS, fire, and law enforcement may be asked to function in roles that are usually delegated to someone in another agency. Although fire typically assumes ICS roles, EMS personnel may be assigned to roles in medical operations, triage, treatment, staging, or transportation.

EMS employees should be prepared to go out of their comfort zone and function in these roles. Preparation requires more than just taking an online course in basic ICS. If the opportunity arises to take part in a tabletop or functional exercise, it would be beneficial for EMS to engage. The management of an MCI is very different from smaller, more common incidents that do not require multiple agencies to mitigate.

One of the biggest issues in a large incident is that of responder safety. Responders may be running on adrenaline, facing new challenges, or serving in roles that are unfamiliar. The larger number of responders makes accountability more difficult and even more important. By preplanning and rehearsing an MCI, critical questions can be answered and potential safety issues mitigated.

EMS supervisors must be prepared to take on an ICS role if needed. Taking part in ICS training and engaging in MCI exercises with other agencies would ensure that everyone was prepared for the next big one.

Review Questions

1. What are some of the modern dangers to fire, EMS, and law enforcement that justify the need for increased interoperability?
2. What is the role of SWAT teams?
3. Why is there a more visible need for tactical paramedics to engage as part of the SWAT team?
4. What are some of the responsibilities of the tactical paramedic on a special weapons and tactics unit?
5. What are some of the things to be considered if an EMS department or agency wishes to involve personnel with a SWAT team?
6. What are some of the advantages and challenges of EMS involvement as TEMS paramedics?
7. What cost factors are associated with supporting TEMS paramedics?
8. What types of equipment would a TEMS paramedic require?
9. What are some of the TEMS paramedic initial and ongoing training requirements?

References

Bolton, B. (2010). "California's Medical Reserve Corp Unites Build for the Future." EMS Dispatch. See the organization website.

Burke, T. (2006). "The Tactical Paramedic: Not Just for SWAT Ops. *EMS World Magazine*. See the organization website.

California Commission on Peace Officer Training and Standards. (2013). "Tactical Medicine and Tactical Casualty Care." See the California Emergency Medical Services Authority website.

California POST in collaboration with California Emergency Services Authority. (2009). "Tactical Medicine: Operational Programs and Standard Training Recommendations." Sacramento, CA: California Commission on Peace Officer Standards and Training (POST).

Callaway, D., R. Smith, G. Shapiro, J. Cain, S. McKay, and R. L. Mabry. (2011). "TECC Evolution and Application of TCCC Guidelines to Civilian High Threat Medicine." *Journal of Special Operations Medicine 11*(2), pp. 95–100.

Central Officers. (2012, March 18). "1997 North Hollywood Shootout Remembered." See the organization website.

Coalition for Tactical Medicine. (2011). "CTM Receives Continued Support from Combat Medical Systems CMS. See the PRLog website.

Dinnage, R. (2004). "New Kentucky Team Is a Model for Medical and Tactical Unit." *Firehouse.* See the organization website.

Evans, B. (2009). "The Time for Tactical Medics Has Arrived." *Fire Chief.* See the organization website.

Heiskell, L., and R. Carmona. (1994). "Tactical Emergency Medical Services: An Emerging Subspecialty of Emergency Medicine." *Annals of Emergency Medicine 23*(4), pp. 778–785.

Johnson, J. (2011, December 29). "Line of Duty Police Officer Deaths Increase By 13% In 2011." *The Inquistr*. See the organization website.

Kahlberg, M. (n.d.). "Complacency Kills." Law Enforcement Today. See the Law Enforcement Today wesbite.

Kastre, T., and D. Kleinman. (2012, May 2). "Tactical EMS Saved Lives after Giffords Shooting." *Journal of Emergency Medical Services*. See the organization website.

Moreau, G. (2012, October 1). "Tactical Medics: Armed vs. Unarmed." See the Eclipse Tactical Medicine website.

National Association of Emergency Medical Technician. (2013). "TCCC Guidelines and Curriculum." Clinton, MS: National Association of Emergency Medical Technicians.

National Law Enforcement Officers Memorial Fund. (n.d.) "Law Enforcement Facts: Key Data about the Profession." See the organization website.

Public Safety Wireless Network (PSWN) Program. (n.d.). "Public Safety and Wireless Communications Interoperability: Critical Issues Facing Public Safety Communications." See Connecticut Department of Emergency Services & Public Protection website.

Urban Shield. (2013). "Urban Shield the Event." See the organization website.

Vayer, J., and R. Schwartz. (2003). "Developing a Tactical Emergency Medical Support Program." *Advanced Emergency Nursing Journal 25*(4), pp. 282–293.

Key Terms

barricaded subjects Criminal suspects who are holding ground in a physical location, are refusing to submit to police requests to surrender, and are in possession of, or have access to, weapons.

counter-sniper operations Tactics used by a sniper to mitigate damage or disable another sniper.

diving or marine operations SWAT teams that specialize in marine or maritime operations.

dignity protection Tactical assignment to mitigate the threat of violence against an important person.

hemostatic agents Material that assists in stopping bleeding and promoting clotting; applied to or mixed into a trauma dressing.

interoperability The ability of different organizations to work together to promote efficiency, effectiveness and safety in an operation.

medical intelligence Gathering of medical information about conditions, suspects, and other data that may have an impact on a tactical operation.

medical team officer A role performed by a tactical provider that would include gathering and monitoring information to ensure the health of tactical team members.

medical threat assessments Identification of threats that can have negative consequences to the physiologic and psychologic health of a tactical team.

special weapons and tactical (SWAT) teams Specialized units of law enforcement that focus on mitigating high-risk incidents such as barricaded suspect, hostage rescue, incidents with high-powered firearms, drug enforcement, high-risk warrants, and dignitary protection.

tactical medicine Emergency medical services support to the SWAT team provided by specially trained medical providers.

tactical emergency medical support A group of people providing medical support in a tactical law enforcement environment.

tactical tourniquets A device used in a tactical setting to control hemorrhage from bleeding.

CHAPTER 5

Pandemics

RANDY KEARNS

Objectives

After reading this chapter, the student should be able to:

5.1 Define *communicable disease* and *infectious disease*, and discuss where the terms differ.

5.2 Discuss and define the different infectious disease material: virus, bacteria, fungi, and parasite.

5.3 Define and differentiate a pandemic and an epidemic.

5.4 Discuss the impact pandemics have made in world population in the last thousand years.

5.5 Describe key developments in managing a pandemic.

5.6 Discuss the basic principles of communicable disease.

5.7 Describe the key components of Universal Precautions for the health care workforce.

5.8 Discuss response and medical management strategies for a pandemic event.

5.9 Describe the impact a potential pandemic would have in the health care workforce.

Key Terms

anthrax
antibiotics
antivirals
bacterium
Black Death/Plague
cholera
communicable disease
epidemic
fungi
hepatitis
Human Immunodeficiency Virus (HIV)
influenza
influenza-like illness (ILI)
novel virus
outbreak
pandemic
parasite
polio
quarantine
Severe Acute Respiratory Syndrome (SARS)
smallpox

surge capacity
tularemia
Universal Precautions
viral hemorrhagic fever (VHF)
World Health Organization (WHO)

WHAT WOULD YOU DO?

Over the past several weeks, news reports have indicated an unusually high number of cases of the "flu" being reported in many countries around the world. As the weeks unfold, a consistent story emerges, including an unusually high infection rate with similar symptoms to **influenza-like illness (ILI)** (Flick et al., 2013). Patients who had received the flu vaccine were being infected with a frequency similar to those who had not been inoculated with it. The Centers for Disease Control and Prevention (CDC) are reporting that they have identified a novel virus and the initial flu vaccine distributed did not reflect this virus strain. Health officials over the past 2 months are reporting similar outbreaks in major cities throughout the world.

This morning, your local public health department notified your EMS organization that the state surveillance system has not indicated an atypical outbreak in your jurisdiction. However, more than a hundred patients, none of whom had a fever, showed up this morning for the department's free clinic. Furthermore, most have reported seeing the previous afternoon or evening newscast featuring how hard hit certain communities were in several of the cities where the outbreaks are reported.

Shortly after 15:00, you receive a 9-1-1 call to a home for a patient reporting difficulty breathing, fever, and chills. During your response, communications also relays that the patient had attended a conference in Los Angeles and had returned by commercial airline earlier this week. Is the patient's travel history significant? Your partner reminds you, "I have a newborn at home. If this is what I think it is, I'm not going near the patient."

Questions

1. What are your strategies for managing this patient? Do you motivate your partner to stay engaged with the call? If yes, how do you do this?
2. Does this scenario include the elements of a potential pandemic?
3. Are the patients who presented to the public health clinic this morning indicative of a new outbreak or what some would describe as the "worried well"?

INTRODUCTION

Infectious diseases are caused by pathogenic microorganisms, such as viruses, bacteria, parasites, or fungi. Diseases can be spread, directly or indirectly, from one person to another. Zoonotic diseases are infectious diseases of animals that can cause disease when transmitted to humans (World Health Organization, 2013). When an infectious disease is easily spread from one human to another, it is more accurately described as a **communicable disease**.

Another somewhat commonly used term is *tropical diseases*. However, this term describes all diseases that occur principally in the tropics. This includes those countries that lie between the latitudes of the Tropic of Cancer and the Tropic of Capricorn. While most such diseases are communicable, the term can be confusing since tropical diseases also include diseases that are not communicable, are genetic disorders, and are caused by nutritional deficiencies and environmental conditions encountered within the tropics (Zumla and Ustianowski, 2012).

When a communicable disease is recognized to be spreading at rates that are unusually high or atypical in nature in a given location, it is often described as an **outbreak**. There is no consensus about how to specifically pinpoint when an outbreak begins or ends. However, the term *outbreak* is more commonly used before either epidemic or pandemic is used to describe the nature of a communicable disease being spread to others in a given location.

A **pandemic** is a global disease impacting a population that has little or no immunity and for which there is no vaccine. An **epidemic** can occur in a small confined area such as a community, state, or country, and a vaccine may or may not be available. Generally, a communicable disease is described as an epidemic if it has not reached globally and not affected a significant number of people. The broader the reach internationally, and the greater the numbers impacted with no known means of vaccination, the more likely the epidemic is described as a pandemic.

THE ROLE PANDEMICS HAVE IN EMS OPERATIONS

It is statistically unlikely that your response area will be the first or one of the first to see patients demonstrating symptoms that become or are later associated with a pandemic outbreak. Nevertheless, illness and airborne and blood-borne diseases always pose a risk to the EMS provider; personal protective equipment (PPE) should be used to protect the responder. Understanding the simple principles of communicable disease and how it is spread both in the general population and to the EMS provider are essential for self-protection. These practices include activities such as cleaning the surface areas of the ambulance and medical equipment after transports, use of PPE, and frequent hand washing. It is essential to know how to clinically manage a patient, but it is equally important to understand and minimize the risk of communicable disease.

The variety of environments that EMS providers see patients in can harbor microorganisms that are more likely to be found in a distinct subset of the patients who either do not or cannot practice good personal hygiene. For some poor hygiene is a choice, and for others it is a limitation based simply on access and affordability. Regardless, there is ample evidence of EMS providers contracting a communicable disease from patients. These situations remind us to remain vigilant to protect ourselves, relying on **Universal Precautions** and being aware of these threats. A report by Harris and Nicolai (2010) showed that EMS providers in Canada did not consistently use universal precautions. Given the similarities in overall operations between Canada and many other countries, it is reasonable to believe that this threat also looms large for EMS providers internationally.

The everyday threats that EMS providers face include communicable diseases. However, the greatest threat is the emergence of a communicable disease that spreads quickly throughout the human population with little or no known means of self-protection. This threat becomes the basis for a pandemic. The primary threat of a pandemic today rests with the emergence of a **novel virus**. When a new and atypical virus is identified, it is described as a novel virus. A novel virus is considered dangerous until better understood and measures to manage it are identified. Having a basic understanding of the more common viruses is crucial to developing a strategy to manage the care of patients, to remain healthy, and to keep an EMS agency functional during an outbreak.

VIRUSES

A virus is a tiny organism that multiplies within cells and causes diseases such as influenza, measles, mumps, rabies, and hepatitis. A virus is not affected by **antibiotics**. Other viruses, such as those that cause yellow fever and West Nile virus, rely on transmission through mosquito bites (insect vector).

One of the more recently identified viruses is the **Human Immunodeficiency Virus (HIV)**, which attacks the human autoimmune system. HIV can lead to Acquired Immune Deficiency Syndrome (AIDS). According to the International HIV/AIDS charity formerly known as the AIDS Education and Research Trust (today referred to as AVERT), an estimated 34 million people live with HIV/AIDS worldwide as of 2010 (AVERT, 2013). AIDS is the world's greatest ongoing pandemic.

Hepatitis is a virus that is both commonly found in the United States and remains a threat to EMS personnel. Currently, there are five known variants of the hepatitis virus, identified as hepatitis A, B, C, D, and E. Hepatitis A and E are associated with ingestion of contaminated food or water. Hepatitis B, C, and D are associated with infected blood or bodily fluids. There is a known and recommended vaccination for hepatitis B. Patients with hepatitis may display a jaundiced appearance (yellowing of the skin and sclera of the eyes) and may report experiencing fatigue, malaise, dark urine, nausea, vomiting, and/or abdominal pain.

For all viral infections, the commonly noted signs and symptoms include fever and associated fatigue. Management is focused on comfort care and symptom management, including both respiratory support and fluid management to prevent dehydration. PPE and hygiene practices such as frequent hand washing and thorough cleaning of patient compartment surfaces remain essential means of personal safety.

Viruses pose the greatest pandemic risk today due to their ability to evolve. Their rapid evolution creates a difficult environment for science to remain current with effective vaccination and treatments, such as antivirals. **Antivirals** are developed to target either a specific virus or, in certain instances, to have a more broad application for viruses that are similar in nature. For an array of reasons, antivirals are more difficult to create and difficult to optimally modify as the virus mutates. Furthermore, although a broader array of antibiotics has been developed to combat bacterial infections, antivirals have thus far been difficult to develop on the same scale and variety as antibiotics.

BACTERIA

A **bacterium** is a one-celled organism that exists throughout the environment. (The plural of *bacterium* is *bacteria.*) Some bacteria are harmful and cause disease. Several of the more notable communicable diseases include cholera, Legionellosis (Legionnaires' disease), pneumococcal disease (leads to pneumonia), meningococcal disease (bacterial meningitis), methicillin-resistant Staphylococcus aureus (MRSA), Staphylococcus infection (Staph infection), typhus (typhus fever), spotted fever, tetanus, pulmonary tuberculosis (TB), and salmonella.

The most common method of treating a bacterial infection is to use an antibiotic. The first antibiotic was penicillin (Centers for Disease Control and Prevention, 2013i). Today, an array of antibiotics ranges from targeted use for a specific strain of bacteria to broad-spectrum antibiotics. Although there are multiple reasons why we have more antibiotics available to us today, one key point is that the nature of the bacterium is such that it does not evolve or mutate as frequently as a virus.

Tularemia, also bacterial in nature, is a communicable disease that generally is spread by tick or mosquito bites, or direct contact with infected animals, or inhalation of contaminated dust particles. Although there are many ways to contact tularemia, person-to-person contact has not been identified as one of those methods. Due to the nature of how tularemia is spread (it is easily aerosolized), it has been weaponized by several countries including the United States. Vaccines for prevention of tularemia are not commercially available.

Most agree that the world's second and greatest pandemic, the **Black Death/Great Plague** from 1347 to 1351, which killed 60 percent of the European population, had a bacterial source: the bacterium *Yersinia pestis*. There are three known varieties of the Great Plague: bubonic plague, septicemic plague, and pneumonic plague (Centers for Disease Control and Prevention, 2013d). The Plague has not been eradicated and occasionally is diagnosed in North America. Nevertheless, it is scarce and more likely to be seen in the western states of North America. Although EMS providers may face an individual with bacterial infection, it is less likely that a bacterial source will be as contagious as the Plague. Nor is it as likely to lead to a pandemic event as is a viral source. Bacterial infections pose a risk to EMS providers providing care for the individual, but this risk can be mitigated with traditional PPE and other protective measures.

Anthrax is also a bacterial-based communicable disease. The Anthrax bacterium is generally associated with hoofed animals. Those populations most likely to be at risk include farm workers and those who work with animal pelts/hides. The Anthrax bacterium can be inhaled as a spore, ingested through eating Anthrax-tainted meat, or through cutaneous contact where there is a break in the skin.

Anthrax bacteria were associated with domestic terrorism actions in the months following the 9/11 attacks (referred to as the Anthrax or 10/12 attack, based on when the first Anthrax-contaminated letter was found) (Kournikakis, Martinez, McCleery, Shadomy, and Ramos, et al., 2011; Zink, 2011). The Anthrax used with this specific attack was genetically enhanced to substantially increase mortality and morbidity. The particular deoxyribonucleic acid (DNA) composition of the Anthrax used in these attacks was traced to a U.S. weapons lab at Fort Detrick, Maryland. Although no arrest was ever made, the person of interest identified by the Federal Bureau of Investigation (FBI) committed suicide after an extensive search was conducted of his personal property and he was notified of charges pending by the FBI. The FBI closed the case in 2010.

Refer to Table 5.1 for a summary of viruses and bacteria.

PARASITES

A **parasite** is an organism whose life is co-dependent on a living host that is typically a mammal. A parasite gets its food from or at

TABLE 5.1 ■ Fact Sheet of Viruses and Bacteria

Distinctions	*Virus*	*Bacteria*
Management	Vaccines/Antivirals	Antibiotics
Size	Small	Large
Cellular	No cells	Unicellular
Reproduction	Invades host cell, takes over the cell causing it to make copies of the viral DNA/RNA	Fission
Living Attributes*	Non-living*	Living*

**The "living determination" is based on ability to reproduce outside of a host. Viruses do not have a nucleus and require a host. Bacteria are single-cell organisms that can metabolize food and can replicate without a host.*

the expense of the host. Some parasites can cause the host to become ill. Several of the more significant and well-known parasitic infestations include African sleeping sickness, bedbugs, body lice, pubic lice (commonly referred to as crabs), hookworm, intestinal roundworm, malaria, and mites (scabies). Most parasites can be managed with good hygiene practices. Nevertheless, if ample hosts are available for the parasite to live and thrive, many parasites have active and rapid reproductive cycles that, without measures to abate the spread, can lead to widespread infestation.

EMS providers may be charged with managing a patient with a parasitic infestation, but it is unlikely that a parasitic source will lead to a pandemic event. Sickness secondary to a parasitic infection poses a risk to EMS providers providing care for the individual; this risk can be mitigated with traditional PPE and other personal protective measures. However, managing a patient with a parasitic infestation is one of the more common situations from which responders can become infected during regular daily duties.

FUNGI

Fungi interact with humans in both beneficial and deadly manners. A number of fungi are native and common to a given environment and live in the soil and plants. Fungal infections include opportunistic infections such as cryptococcosis (frequently seen in patients with AIDS), hospital-acquired infections such as candidemia, and community-acquired infections such as coccidioidomycosis or valley fever.

EMS providers may face an individual with a fungal infection, but it is unlikely a fungal source will lead to a pandemic event. Fungal infections do pose a risk to EMS providers providing care for the individual; again, this risk can be mitigated with traditional PPE measures.

INFLUENZA VIRUS

The most common communicable disease that kills thousands each year is the **influenza** virus. The influenza virus is frequently described based on the two distinct proteins of the virus and their varieties. These proteins are hemagglutinin and Neuraminidase. The most common influenza virus proteins are known as hemagglutinin 1 and neuraminidase 1, or H1N1. All known influenza viruses have zoonotic origins, such as avian (bird) and swine (pig).

Influenza is seasonal in temperate regions of the world. There is year-round influenza activity in tropical climates, such as the equatorial portion of Africa and Southeast Asia. Often cited is an article from the *Journal of the American Medical Association*, which reports that approximately 200,000 hospitalizations are related to influenza complications each year with 36,000 deaths (Thompson, Shay, Weintraub, et al., 2003). However, the CDC reports that there is great variability. The mortality from 1979 to 2010 ranged from approximately 3,000 to approximately 49,000, which underscores the variability and unpredictability of morbidity and mortality associated with influenza (Centers for Disease Control and Prevention, 1995, 2013n).

The most common influenza virus is the H1N1. Each year it goes through various changes (also referred to as reassortment) throughout the flu season. Other strains of influenza virus are caused by distinctly different versions of either the hemagglutinin or the neuraminidase or both. Prior to 2009, the last pandemic declared by the **World Health Organization (WHO)** was the 1968 H3N2 Hong Kong flu. This novel virus was first identified in an outbreak in Hong Kong, thus its name. That same year, the most common flu virus remained H1N1, and it was being contracted around the world. Nevertheless, with no vaccine and limited human immunity developed to ward off the novel virus, it was the H3N2 outbreak in Hong Kong that posed the greatest threat.

One example of a recently identified zoonotic source of influenza that has thus far produced a high mortality rate is H5N1. The first four deaths directly attributed to H5N1 were in China and Vietnam in 2003 (Morbidity and Mortality Weekly Report, 2004). H5N1 is a particularly deadly virus; some estimates are as high as 75 percent mortality rate (Trampuz, Prabhu, Smith, and Baddour, 2004). It is known as the avian influenza virus, H5N1, or (more commonly) the "bird flu." It has been seen in Asia, Europe, and Africa on a limited basis, thus far. At this time, with few exceptions, it is only passed from the zoonotic host (a bird such as a chicken) to a human. It has not yet become highly contagious, but it poses enormous risk if it does.

As any flu virus mutates, so does the autoimmune response of the human body. National and international health organizations, such as the CDC and the WHO, rely on simple and sophisticated surveillance systems around the world to track known and identify new typical, atypical, and novel viruses. When an unusually virulent strain of H1N1 emerged in 2009, the WHO declared a pandemic in June 2009. Both the CDC and the WHO were actively engaged, working with partners in the private pharmaceutical industry. A vaccine targeting this particular variety of the virus was produced and made available in the months that followed. However, this did not occur before thousands had died and the virus had made its way around much of the industrialized world, leading to one of the world's most recent pandemics. The 2009 pandemic was the first pandemic declared by the WHO since what was known as the Hong Kong flu of 1968 (Du et al., 2009).

During 2009, there were two distinct strains of H1N1. The anticipated H1N1 strain

Side Bar

What Is a Pandemic?

- Pandemics are sporadic and unpredictable.
- They spread from person to person and cause human illness.
- Most of the population is susceptible.

Three conditions must be met for a pandemic to start. To better understand these three condition, influenza will be used for the following example:

- For influenza, a new influenza virus subtype must emerge for which there is little or no human immunity.
- It must infect humans and causes illness.
- It must spread easily and sustainably (continue without interruption) among humans.

emerged as it typically does and was similar to what was anticipated by the WHO and CDC. Vaccination programs were in place, and the vaccine had been produced in sufficient quantities to meet public needs. However, a novel strain was reported in Mexico in the spring of 2009 that produced flu-like symptoms. After further examination, it was determined that the virus was not the same H1N1 that had been anticipated for the flu season. This particular strain was highly infectious and easily spread from human to human. By April, it was in the United States and had appeared in Asia and Europe (Cohen and Enserink, 2009). Scientists at both the WHO and CDC worked quickly to identify the virus and develop a vaccine. Vaccine was rushed to production and became available by mid-October, but not before the virus became a worldwide pandemic event (Dawood, Jain, Finelli, Shaw, Lindstrom, et al., 2009).

The greatest fear was that this novel strain of H1N1 would infect someone infected with H5N1 and that the two strains of flu infecting the same patient would allow the viruses within the same host (the patient) to mutate into a supervirus (WHO Informal Network, 2009). The thought of combining the mortality and morbidity percentages seen with H5N1 patients with this novel strain of H1N1 flu that was easily passed from person to person could lead to a catastrophic health event not seen since the 1918 Spanish flu outbreak.

COMMUNICABLE DISEASES: THIRD WORLD EXPERIENCES

Communicable diseases—whether indigenous or now commonly found—are more often present in harsh environments and where clean water or hygienic measures are limited. Given the ease and frequency of international and intercontinental travel of people, goods, and products, the likelihood of managing a patient with an atypical communicable disease is more a threat today than it once was. Significant efforts are undertaken to screen, monitor, and include surveillance activities necessary to keep these threats at bay. Nevertheless, it is important to discuss several of the more notable communicable diseases and their potential impact.

Cholera is one of the more common communicable diseases associated with a lack of access to ample amounts of potable water for both consumption and food preparation. Cholera is caused by a bacterium that, once ingested (and infected by the bacteria), will result in patients reporting frequent and painful watery diarrhea that continues for an extended period. Dehydration is a common complication and must be a key consideration, along with an antibiotic, in management.

The most frightening viruses are classified as a **viral hemorrhagic fever (VHF)**. Yellow fever (YF) is one of the less lethal VHFs, but it is one that has been seen in Western civilization (Jentes, Poumerol, Gershman, Hill, Lemarchand, et al., 2011). A vaccination is available for YF. For persons traveling from the United States or most of the countries where Western-style medicine is practiced to areas where YF is a threat, vaccination is highly recommended.

Two of the more notable VHF viruses include Marburg and Ebola. Both are similar in signs and symptoms. Little is known about them, and there is no known vaccination or cure. Signs and symptoms of VHF include elevated temperature with any or all of the following: bloody emesis, blood-tinged sputum, blood-tinged tears, and blotchy areas on either or both the torso and extremities, along with rapid decline in health. Management includes comfort care. There is little evidence of antiviral medication effectiveness at this time. Mortality rates for patients with Marburg or Ebola can be as high as 80 percent (Allaranga, Kone,

Formenty, Libama, Boumandouki, et al., 2010; Balter, 2000; Leroy, Baize, and Gonzalez, 2011).

COMMUNICABLE DISEASE IN THE MOVIES

Hollywood has given the world several pandemic-themed films, such as *Outbreak* and *Contagion.* Although neither is a documentary or based on actual scenarios, the general premise of how interconnected the world population has become, and how a novel virus could readily spread worldwide in a short period of time, is a plausible situation. Regardless, aside from the entertainment factor, both movies serve as a reminder to the general public of the clear and present danger a pandemic could present if the communicable disease is particularly virulent.

HISTORIC EPIDEMICS AND PANDEMICS

Civilization has been struck by pandemics throughout recorded history (Echenberg, 2002; Lagace-Wiens, Rubinstein, and Gumel, 2010; Murray, Lopez, Chin, Feehan, and Hill, 2006). The two greatest influences on sudden changes in regional or world population over the past 3,000 years have included war and pandemic (Barry and Gualde, 2008; Perrone and Tumpey, 2007). Trends correlated with war and violent deaths do impact world population (Obermeyer, Murray, and Gakidou, 2008) but not to the extent of pandemic.

BLACK DEATH/FOURTEENTH-CENTURY PANDEMIC

The greatest morbidity and mortality rates from a pandemic are typically known as the Black Death of 1347 or the Fourteenth-Century Pandemic (Tsiamis, Poulakou-Rebelakou, Tsakris, and Petridou, 2011). The Black Death was mostly bubonic plague and pneumonic plague. Between 1346 and 1365, the infectious disease spread over much of the Europe, Eastern Asia, and Northern Africa. It is estimated that more than 40 percent of the world population (60 percent of the European population) died during the 20 years of the epidemic (Beran, 2008). The epidemic ended only after millions had died, with most of the survivors having developed immunity to the disease (Haensch, Bianucci, Signoli, Rajerison, Schultz, et al., 2010).

SMALLPOX

A virus that made its way through history, leaving staggering death tolls, was **smallpox**. Today, smallpox is considered eradicated, following aggressive worldwide vaccination programs. Nevertheless, the lack of immunity to smallpox and other communicable diseases brought to the Americas by European explorers in the sixteenth and seventeenth centuries was responsible for the deaths of up to 80 percent of the indigenous population. Some scholars suggest that the number was closer to 90 percent in the hardest hit areas (Aufderheide, Rodriguez-Martin, and Langsjoen, 1998). Regardless, smallpox was the principal communicable disease that decimated the indigenous populations of the Americas.

Effects of the smallpox virus were identified on mummified remains in Egypt (Hopkins, 1980). It is believed that the virus has infected the human population for more than 12,000 years (Perrin, Noly, Mourer, and Schmitt, 1994). Particularly lethal in children, it has been estimated that the death rate was as high as 80 percent in Europe in the eighteenth century, with an estimated 400,000 dying each year from the disease (Riedel, 2005).

A similar virus that is zoonotic in nature and found primarily in Central Africa and West Africa is monkeypox. Monkeypox is typically seen in primates and rodents, but there have been cases of human monkeypox identified in Africa (Bayer-Garner, 2005). Based on the limited number of cases seen and documented, monkeypox in humans is less lethal. It is believed that the smallpox vaccine provides sufficient protection to monkeypox. However, since smallpox being declared eradicated, smallpox vaccinations have stopped in most civilian populations. An outbreak of monkeypox was linked to an exotic pet store owner in Chicago in 2003, sickening dozens but resulting in no fatalities.

POLIO

The pandemic virus that posed a significant threat to the U.S. population from approximately 1840 to 1955 years ago was poliomyelitis (**polio**) (Centers for Disease Control and Prevention, 2013o). Polio, a viral disease, remained a major public health threat until a vaccine was developed in the 1950s. Today, it is largely eradicated in the Western world through vaccination programs. Polio in the United States is rare today, but outbreaks continue in countries where the vaccine is either not available or not widely distributed for use.

Polio is transmitted from person to person contact with blood or body fluids (more specifically, respiratory mucus or fecal material). Polio can manifest in any of three ways: subclinical, nonparalytic, and paralytic; thus, polio has been and can be a devastating virus. There is no known cure for Polio, but symptom management and comfort care have improved quality-of-life outcomes for those infected. The best management is prevention through vaccination.

SPANISH FLU

Spanish flu is the most recent pandemic with significant worldwide loss of life. It is estimated that between 5 percent and 20 percent of the world population (approximately 20 million to 50 million) died of the flu (National Vaccine Program Office, n.d.). More Americans died of the influenza pandemic of 1918–1919 than during all of World War I. Further complicating the outbreak was the disproportionate mortality rate of teens and young adults in their twenties. This flu was seen in three distinct waves before subsiding in 1919. Although never confirmed, it was believed that the robust autoimmune response found in teen and younger adult patients may have contributed to the vulnerability and the subsequent higher mortality rates for this age group.

UNKNOWN COMMUNICABLE DISEASES

Emerging diseases continue to be a great unknown we face in health care. When a group of infected patients emerges with an unknown source but the preponderance of evidence suggests that all the patients have the same infection, it is typically referred to as a "syndrome" until its source can be determined. The syndrome label allows researchers to focus on building a body of work to both stop the spread of the communicable disease and treat those who have been infected.

The most recent syndrome to emerge with consequences that threatened the general population and impacted the health care systems of western civilizations was identified as the **Severe Acute Respiratory Syndrome (SARS)** (Cheng, Chan, To, and Yuen, 2013). It appeared over a span of less than 12 months from

November 2002 until the summer of 2003. As indicated by its name, the syndrome had dramatic respiratory system impact. Antibiotic treatment was ineffective. SARS faded away almost as fast as it had emerged. However, during its brief lifespan, it killed hundreds, including health care workers in Canada and Asia who seemingly had taken traditional Universal Precautions. In one Canadian hospital alone, 25 percent who entered the room of a SARS-infected patient became infected (Xing, Hejblum, Leung, and Valleron, 2010). For the general population, death rates ranged from 9 percent to 12 percent of those diagnosed, but they were more than 50 percent in the 65 years and older population (Ofner-Agostini, Wallington, Henry, Low, McDonald, et al., 2008).

Potential explanations were offered that include a novel virus of unknown etiology with avian, swine, or bovine origin to the more bizarre, which included a bioweapon that escaped a military lab. Today, we know that it was a novel virus, identified as a coronavirus, and it is thus recorded in the literature as SARS-CoV (Thiel, 2007).

BIOWEAPONS, COMMUNICABLE DISEASES, AND PANDEMICS

A number of countries today either operate or have operated labs for the purpose of developing weapons using biological agents (Jacobs, 2004). Countries that operate bioweapon labs do so for one or two specific reasons. The first is developing more potent or atypical strains of a given biological agent, in effect developing biological weapons. The second is to understand how naturally occurring communicable disease can be spread and how to develop medical countermeasures to combat an attack using a biological weapon.

Biological agents used as weapons can decimate both a military and civilian population, without causing widespread death. Death, it can be argued, is much easier to deal with than sickness, given the conclusiveness and immediacy of loss and body disposal. In comparison, sickness, particularly widespread sickness, impacts not only the person who is sick as it can cause a great burden for those left to provide ongoing care for the ill and injured (Schreiber, Yoeli, Paz, Barbash, Varssano, et al., 2004).

In war, it is a paradox to use a biological agent that has the potential to set off a pandemic with a communicable disease that has been genetically altered. On one hand, the bioweapon could cause widespread sickness or kill many of the enemy. However, without strict vaccination and adherence to avoid cross-contamination, the release of a potent bioweapon could also lead to widespread sickness or kill many of those who released the biological agent. Furthermore, the more novel and contagious the biological agent, the greater the likelihood it could use the returning soldiers as a vector and spread to the civilian population.

Thus, the challenge of using a biological agent is to do so without infecting the military troops or civilian population of the attacking country. Bioweapons can be seen as a deterrent to attack because they create a position of mutually assured destruction. Given that bioweapons can be developed and created with less sophistication and financial investment than required for nuclear weapons, bioweapons are one way to shift the balance of military power.

The more likely threat of bioweapon use comes from terrorist organizations. In Oregon in 1984, 751 people became ill after eating from salad bars that had been intentionally contaminated with salmonella (Jacobs, 2004; Scripps Howard News Service, 2007). The intent was to make local residents sick and prevent them from voting. With those supporting a local fringe candidate knowing of the plot and staying away from those restaurants, the intention was to swing the election. However, the outcome desired by the terrorist did not produce the intended result. Nevertheless, it did make people sick and reminded us how vulnerable we are to purposeful contamination using a biological agent.

EMS AND PANDEMICS TODAY

Pandemics have a long history of creating social chaos and disruption as well as morbidity and mortality rates that are unlike anything we have seen in our lifetime. A challenge faced by EMS today pertaining to pandemics includes the potential for responders being infected before a vaccine can be developed, mass produced, and distributed to EMS employees and volunteers as the first wave moves quickly across the country. The U.S. Department of Transportation developed the "EMS Pandemic Influenza Guidelines for Statewide Adaption" (National Highway Traffic Safety Administration, 2007). Key points in the guide include the following:

- EMS Planning
- Role of EMS in Influenza Surveillance and Mitigation
- Maintaining Continuity of EMS Operations During Influenza Pandemic
- Legal Authority
- Clinical Standards and Treatment Protocols
- EMS Workforce Protection

The guide is slightly dated but provides a good structure for discussing EMS operations and pandemic preparedness. Key aspects include planning and preparation for an EMS system. For clinical personnel, the planning activity increases awareness, improves understanding regarding the real risks, and can serve as a means of allaying unfounded fears.

EMS can play a vital role in conducting surveillance to aid in identifying an outbreak. Patients presenting with an ILI in cluster, or spikes in calls with similar chief complaints, can produce vital information early in an outbreak. This is most successful when tracked in a computer-aided dispatch (CAD) system that is linked to either regional or state public health surveillance systems that can recognize and trend atypical volumes of similar symptoms. Surveillance can take on all forms of linking data. Ginsberg, Mohebbi, Patel, Brammer, Smolinski, et al. (2009) have discussed the use of search-engine queries to trend symptom searches. Combined with geocoding to identify the location where the queries are taking place, such queries can provide researchers with another edge in monitoring an outbreak at its onset as the general population turns to the Internet to ask about symptoms.

Best Practice

Preparing for a Pandemic

The three common means of contracting a communicable disease include inhalation, ingestion, and absorption. Best practices include how to best care for your patient while keeping you healthy. Think in terms of how a communicable disease is transmitted, and ensure that the necessary protection steps have been taken for yourself, fellow EMS providers, other responders, the patient, and the public.

Personal Protection Equipment, Vaccine, and Hygiene

- *Gloves*—Use properly fitting gloves and have spare exam gloves with you at all times. If you have multiple patients, change gloves between patients.
- *Mask/eye protection*—Follow organizational standards, but for any potential interaction with either a patient who has an infectious disease, or where the nature of the response is unknown, eye and inhalation protection must include the use of glasses with side splash shields and a properly fitting mask. Eye protection can include glasses, a shield, goggles, or another means of shielding the eyes while providing the EMS provider with sufficient transparency to accurately evaluate the patient. Most organizations follow Occupational Safety and Hazards Administration (OSHA) Standard 1910.134 (OSHA, 2010), or a state standard that may be more specific or strict and is based on the federal standard. For many organizations, a mask complies with National Institute for Occupational Safety and Health (NIOSH) Approved N95 Particulate Filtering Facepiece Respirators (Centers for Disease Control and Prevention, 2013p). The 2011 data from NIOSH identify seven types of particulate filtering facemasks, but those more useful in the health care profession are based on ease of use, storage, and access to the product.
- Traditional barrier-type masks do not offer the same protection and will not comply with the OSHA 1910.134 standard, but they may offer some limited protection if nothing else is available during a pandemic with a medical disaster unfolding.
- Another step that has been practiced (but lacks scientific data to confirm its value) where transmission of the communicable disease is airborne includes placing an oxygen mask on the patient at an appropriate flow in part to aid in the oxygenation of the patient and in part to serve as a means of capturing all or a portion of the patient's aerosolized exhalation.
- *Vaccine*—Follow your organization's policies and procedures, which generally include receiving vaccines for the seasonal flu, hepatitis B, and tetanus along with a screening for tuberculosis. These may or may not be included in your vaccination and screening profile for your organization's records, but some may include your vaccine history for measles, rubella (also known as German measles), and mumps. This could also include noncivilian vaccines or international travel vaccine history such as for yellow fever, anthrax, smallpox, tularemia, and other communicable diseases not commonly found in the United States today.
- *Personal Hygiene*—You should report for duty with a clean body and a clean uniform. In addition to wearing gloves, wash your hands after each patient contact and between patients to avoid cross-contamination. Keep a small bottle of hand sanitizer with you at all times and use it any time soap and water are not immediately available. Sneeze into the bend of your arm. During known outbreaks, practice social distancing. The best way to manage communicable disease is to prevent it. It starts with you, the EMS professional, and cleanliness.
- *Ambulance or Response Vehicle Cleanliness*—During your initial duties on the ambulance or response vehicle, and after each patient, be sure the interior surfaces of the ambulance patient compartment are clean. This includes reusable items that will touch a patient, such as the head of a stethoscope. Also, clean and maintain cleanliness of items within the truck where contamination can be overlooked and transmitted to other patients or to EMS personnel; this includes door handles, seat belt buckles, steering wheels, and so on.

GENERAL EMS PATIENT ASSESSMENT AND MANAGEMENT STRATEGIES

For the EMS provider, the key aspect of managing a patient with a communicable disease starts with identifying if the patient has the signs and symptoms associated with a communicable disease. A fever is the most common sign and symptom associated with a communicable disease. Generally, the fever is accompanied by perspiration and chills as well as aches and pains. Until determined otherwise, the patient is assumed to have a communicable disease when presenting with a fever of unknown origin.

Patient management is generally limited to comfort care and symptom management. Patients in acute distress secondary to a communicable disease may include oxygen, airway and respiratory support, and fluid management for dehydration. Nevertheless, throughout the provision of care, Universal Precautions are emphasized for the EMS provider.

Two common patient management strategies used are **quarantine** and the development of field hospitals for **surge capacity**. Quarantine is used to isolate the infected from those who are well (Markel, Lipman, Navarro, Sloan, Michalsen, et al., 2007). The intent is to reduce the spread of the disease. Quarantine is difficult to manage under ideal circumstances and is mostly considered a solution that cannot be achieved today in most Western countries (Markel, Stern, and Cetron, 2008). Laws and procedures continue to exist to permit restricted access and movement when a public health emergency is declared, but restricting freedom of movement is difficult in contemporary society. The better approach is known as social distancing. This approach has two views: one from those infected and one from those who are well. Either may practice social distancing with the intent to not infect others or to not be infected by others through direct contact or droplet contamination. Social distancing is a common principle of continuity of ongoing operations plan (COOP).

Surge capacity strategies include adaptation of space such as churches and gymnasiums in order to create large field hospitals. The outbreak spread very quickly and dozens became hundreds that became thousands in less than a month, quickly overwhelming the health care system. In the aftermath of the 9/11 attacks, a better definition has emerged to describe surge capacity. Stratifying what we know as surge capacity with respect to staff, space, and supplies aids those involved in planning for and responding to the disaster. It is a quick size-up of the state of disaster response (Hick, Barbera, and Kelen, 2009).

EMS SYSTEM SUSTAINABILITY DURING A PANDEMIC

EMS is a vital service that must be supported and maintained during a pandemic event. As such, this includes developing and potentially activating a continuity of ongoing operations plan (COOP). COOP is essential to an EMS system surviving during a pandemic. For additional education regarding COOP, refer to the Federal Emergency Management Agency (FEMA) Independent Study programs IS 546.12: Continuity of Operations Awareness Course; IS 547.a: Introduction to Continuity of Operations; and IS 548: Continuity of Operations (COOP) Program Manager (FEMA EMI, 2009a, 2009b, 2009c). (See the sidebar on "Key Concepts of COOP Planning.")

One often overlooked aspect of COOP planning is devolution planning. Do you have a plan to close the service and transfer the responsibility to another agency? In many cases, this is not an option. Sometimes, taking

Side Bar

Key Concepts of COOP Planning

The three FEMA independent study courses offer great insight into COOP. The key concepts of COOP planning that are applicable to the EMS profession include the following:

1. The plan to keep employees healthy *must* also include keeping families of employees healthy. Who is prioritized to receive vaccinations? Can you vaccinate your own personnel? How quickly will vaccines be available? Will you require all of your employees to be vaccinated?
2. Absenteeism may run high with both those who are sick and those who refuse to report for duty based on the risk of exposure.
3. A pandemic may also interrupt other infrastructure, such as the supply chain (medical supplies, PPE supplies, etc.), vehicle repair, vehicle fuel, electricity, water supply, and garbage collection.
4. System processes must allow for a decentralized approach where office-based employees can operate from other locations (including home, if needed).
5. Organizational systems must facilitate the ongoing operation with a decentralized approach.
6. Organizational considerations must be sorted. Concentration should be focused on essential functions, with prioritization of those you may struggle to maintain.
7. What services can you suspend during a pandemic?
8. How will the pandemic impact your ability to rely on other agencies that routinely support your activities (e.g., fire department or volunteer first responders, mutual aid agencies)?
9. Do you have an order-of-succession plan? If so, is it three deep?
10. Maintain a work-well environment. Sick employees or those exhibiting signs/symptoms of sickness *must* go home!
11. Do you have or have you considered a policy to restrict travel either on duty or off duty if certain communities are known to be high risk for exposure?
12. Have you consulted with human resources about these potential policy decisions and, where applicable, with the union representative? Get people on board with what could be needed long before it is needed.
13. Develop a general guide for the staff to include reinforcing simple strategies such as a staff notification plan, a communication plan (keep the lines open and flowing), social distancing, closing noncritical common areas, and refocusing on hygienic practices from hand washing to cleaning patient care reusable items.

a committee of employees through the steps of closing the service and transferring the responsibility reminds all involved how essential the service is and to what extent and extreme it should be carried to protect this vital service. Nevertheless, there are times—such as when a hospital was struck by a tornado in Joplin, Missouri, in 2011—when devolution is a possibility. The hospital continued to operate in a temporary structure, but at greatly reduced capacity and capability. Regardless, for pandemic preparedness the focus should be on how to safely continue to operate the service while keeping employees, patients, and employees' families safe. All three of these areas must be addressed in the planning and preparedness process.

THE FUTURE

Over the past 10+ years, three events have shaped the future for pandemic preparedness in the United States. They include the anthrax letters in 2001, the threat of avian influenza

(H5N1) in 2005, and the H1N1 influenza pandemic in 2009. Although none of these situations was as dramatic as the 1918–1919 pandemic or the Black Death of 1347, the potential for a public health catastrophe has been and remains significant. Pandemic preparedness is an important aspect of all hazards preparedness and planning for the health and medical function of disaster planning.

Future leaders must be able to quickly adjust to changing landscapes to include advocating for vaccination distribution for EMS as an equal partner with other health care providers. EMS continues to evolve in the overall health care profession. When the next pandemic occurs, EMS preparedness efforts will be reflected at each agency's level of preparedness.

CHAPTER REVIEW

Summary

The next pandemic may or may not be more virulent than that of the 2009 pandemic influenza. Nevertheless, the consensus range for the 2009 pandemic influenza is 151,700 to 575,400 deaths. The wide range in variability is due to accounting for adjustments for age, as well as the variety of sources, and in some cases the need to create estimates where data from some countries did not exist. This is clearly not the 5 million to 20 million deaths seen in the 1918–1919 pandemic Spanish flu outbreak, nor is it as virulent.

The next pandemic may be years from now. Then again, the novel or atypical virus that emerges to start a pandemic may have already claimed the first few lives in some little-known community. Based on historical and recent experiences, we do not know when it will happen, but we do know it will happen.

Communicable disease is something the EMS provider will not usually see with the same degree of frequency, but particularly during the peak of an outbreak it may rise to the most frequent reason for EMS alarms. Regardless, making sure that each EMS provider uses basic PPE on every call and having a plan in place if an outbreak occurs will make EMS providers better prepared to deal with potential outbreaks, epidemics, or pandemics.

WHAT WOULD YOU DO? Reflection

Each year, EMS clinicians manage literally millions of patients with a communicable disease. As with any patient for whom you have reason to suspect his illness may be linked to a communicable disease, PPE is essential in these cases. The evidence suggests, and you must presume, that this is a patient with, perhaps, a novel virus. Nevertheless, you have to encourage and keep your EMS partner engaged. Some respond best based on duty and obligation; others respond to encouragement or greatest good; still others respond to logic, regardless, to ensure the best patient outcome and mitigate exposure for the clinicians. All responders must stay engaged and focused on the patient at hand.

Although certainly not conclusive, it is reasonable to believe that this case could be linked to the pandemic outbreak. The signs and symptoms (facts of the situation) are the facts that should be conveyed to the receiving hospital during your radio encode prior to arrival as well as to the receiving clinician. The balance is to ensure that they have the information you have and are taking reasonable precautions and concerned without creating undue panic.

Most likely they are "worried well." An unfortunate impact from the 24/7 news cycle is a saturation of tragic and troubling news. Informing a population without instilling fear and panic is a difficult balance that both news and weather forecasters deal with frequently.

Review Questions

1. What is the difference between communicable disease and infectious disease?
2. What is the difference between a viral infection and a bacterial infection? How are these types of infections managed?
3. What fungal and parasitic conditions have been seen in your ambulance or could be seen in your jurisdiction?
4. What is the difference between an epidemic and a pandemic?
5. What is COOP, and does it have a role in EMS system planning for pandemic preparedness?
6. Discuss the Universal Precautions that make the most difference during an outbreak of patients with ILI.
7. How can surveillance strategies diminish the impact of a pandemic?
8. Discuss response and medical management strategies for a pandemic.

References

A.D.A.M. Medical Encyclopedia. (2013). "Cholera." PubMed Health. See the MedlinePlus medical encyclopedia website.

A.D.A.M. Medical Encyclopedia. (2013). "Meningitis." PubMed Health. (See the MedlinePlus medical encyclopedia website.)

A.D.A.M. Medical Encyclopedia. (2013). "MRSA." PubMed See the MedlinePlus medical encyclopedia website.

A.D.A.M. Medical Encyclopedia. (2013). "Salmonella enterocolitis." PubMed Health. See the MedlinePlus medical encyclopedia website.

A.D.A.M. Medical Encyclopedia. (2013). "Spotted Fever." PubMed Health. See the MedlinePlus medical encyclopedia website.

A.D.A.M. Medical Encyclopedia. (2013). "Tetanus." PubMed Health. See the MedlinePlus medical encyclopedia website.

A.D.A.M. Medical Encyclopedia. (2013). "Tularemia." PubMed Health. See the MedlinePlus medical encyclopedia website.

A.D.A.M. Medical Encyclopedia. (2013). "Typhus." PubMed Health. See the MedlinePlus medical encyclopedia website.

A.D.A.M. Medical Encyclopedia. (2013). "Penicillin." PubMed Health. See the MedlinePlus medical encyclopedia website.

AIDS Education and Research Trust (AVERT). (2013). "Worldwide HIV & AIDS Statistics: Global HIV and AIDS Estimates, 2011." See the organization website.

Allaranga, Y., M. L. Kone, P. Formenty, F. Libama, P. Boumandouki, et al. (2010). "Lessons Learned During Active Epidemiological Surveillance of Ebola and Marburg Viral Hemorrhagic Fever Epidemics in Africa." *East African Journal of Public Health* 7(1), 30–36.

Aufderheide, A. C., C. Rodriguez-Martin, and O. Langsjoen. (1998). *The Cambridge Encyclopedia of Human Paleopathology*. Cambridge (UK) and New York: Cambridge University Press.

Balter, M. (2000). "Emerging Diseases. On the Trail of Ebola and Marburg Viruses." *Science 290*(5493), 923–925.

Barry, S., and N. Gualde. (2008). "The Black Death in Christian and Muslim Occident, 1347–1353." *Canadian Bulletin of Medical History 25*(2), 461–498.

Bayer-Garner, I. B. (2005). "Monkeypox Virus: Histologic, Immunohistochemical and Electron-Microscopic Findings." *Journal of Cutaneous Pathology 32*(1), 28–34. doi: 10.1111/j.0303-6987.2005.00254.x.

Beran, G. W. (2008). "Disease and Destiny-Mystery and Mastery." *Preventive Veterinary Medicine 86*(3–4), 198–207. doi: 10.1016/j.prevetmed.2008.05.001.

Centers for Disease Control and Prevention. (1995, July 21). "Pneumonia and Influenza Death Rates—United States, 1979–1994." *Morbidity and Mortality Weekly Report 44*(28), pp. 535–537.

Centers for Disease Control and Prevention. (2013a). "Emergency Preparedness and Response: Smallpox." Author. See the organization website.

Centers for Disease Control and Prevention. (2013b). "Reconstruction of the 1918 Influenza Pandemic Virus." Author. See the organization website.

Centers for Disease Control and Prevention. (2013c). "Anthrax." Author. See the organization website.

Centers for Disease Control and Prevention. (2013d). "Cholera." Author. See the organization website.

Centers for Disease Control and Prevention. (2013e). "Parasites - Bed Bugs." Author. See the organization website.

Centers for Disease Control and Prevention. (2013f). "Parasites - Body Lice." Author. See the organization website.

Centers for Disease Control and Prevention. (2013g). "Parasites Hookworm." See the organization website.

Centers for Disease Control and Prevention. (2013h). "Parasites Intestinal Roundworms." Author. See the organization website.

Centers for Disease Control and Prevention. (2013i). "Parasites - Malaria." Author. See the organization website.

Centers for Disease Control and Prevention. (2013j). "Parasites - Pubic "Crab" Lice." Author. See the organization website.

Centers for Disease Control and Prevention. (2013k). "Parasites - Scabies." Author. See the organization website.

Centers for Disease Control and Prevention. (2013l). "Parasites Sleeping Sickness." Author. See the organization website.

Centers for Disease Control and Prevention. (2013m). "Polio." Author. See the organization website.

Centers for Disease Control and Prevention. (2013n). "Viral Hepatitis." Author. See the organization website.

Centers for Disease Control and Prevention. (2013o). "Estimating Seasonal Influenza-Associated Deaths in the United States: CDC Study Confirms Variability of Flu." See the organization website.

Centers for Disease Control and Prevention. (2013p). "The National Personal Protective Technology Laboratory (NPPTL)." Author. See the organization website.

Centers for Disease Control and Prevention. (2013q). "Disease Listing." Author. See the organization website.

Centers for Disease Control and Prevention. (2013r). "VaccinesGov Glossary." Author. See the organization website.

Cheng, V. C., J. F. Chan, K. K. To, and K. Y. Yuen. (2013). "Clinical Management and Infection Control of SARS: Lessons Learned." *Antiviral Research*. doi: 10.1016/j.antiviral.2013.08.016.

Cohen, J., and M. Enserink. (2009). "Infectious Diseases. As Swine Flu Circles Globe, Scientists Grapple with Basic Questions." *Science 324*(5927), 572–573. doi: 10.1126/science.324_572.

Dawood, F. S., S. Jain, L. Finelli, M. W. Shaw, S. Lindstrom, et al. (2009). "Emergence of a Novel Swine-Origin Influenza A (H1N1) Virus in Humans." *New England Journal of Medicine 360*(25), 2605–2615. doi: 10.1056/NEJMoa0903810.

Du, N., X. X. Yang, Y. Lan, L. Y. Wen, X. D. Li, et al. (2009). "Review on the etiological property of 1968 Hong Kong flu virus (H3N2)." *Bing Du Xue Bao 25* (Suppl:17–20).

Echenberg, M. (2002). "Pestis Redux: The Initial Years of the Third Bubonic Plague Pandemic, 1894–1901." *Journal of World History 13*(2), 429–449.

FEMA EMI. (2009a). "IS-546.A: Continuity of Operations Awareness Course." Emergency Management Institute (ed.). (See the organization website.)

FEMA EMI. (2009b). "IS-547.A: Introduction to Continuity of Operations." Emergency Management Institute (ed.). See the organization website.

FEMA EMI. (2009c). "IS-548: Continuity of Operations (COOP) Program Manager." Emergency Management Institute (ed.). See the organization website.

Flick, H., M. Drescher, J. Prattes, K. Tovilo, H. H. Kessler, et al. (2013, August 4). "Predictors of H1N1 Influenza in the Emergency Department: Proposition for a Modified H1N1 Case Definition." *Clinical Microbiology and Infection*. doi: 10.1111/1469-0691.12352

Ginsberg, J., M. H. Mohebbi, R. S. Patel, L. Brammer, M. S. Smolinski, et al. (2009). "Detecting Influenza Epidemics Using Search Engine Query Data." *Nature 457*(7232), 1012–1014. doi: 10.1038/nature07634.

Haensch, S., R. Bianucci, M. Signoli, M. Rajerison, M. Schultz, et al. (2010). "Distinct Clones of Yersinia pestis Caused the Black Death." *PLoS Pathogens 6*(10). doi: 10.1371/journal.ppat.1001134.

Harris, S. A., and L. A. Nicolai. (2010). "Occupational Exposures in Emergency Medical Service Providers and Knowledge of and Compliance with Universal Precautions." *American Journal of Infection Control 38*(2), 86–94. doi: 10.1016/j.ajic.2009.05.012.

Hick, J. L., J. A. Barbera, and G. D. Kelen. (2009). "Refining Surge Capacity: Conventional, Contingency, and Crisis Capacity." *Disaster Medicine and Public Health Preparedness 3* (2 Suppl), S59–S67. doi: 10.1097/DMP.0b013e31819f1ae2.

Hopkins, D. R. (1980, May). "Ramses V, Earliest Known Victim?" *World Health* 22(1).

Jacobs, M. K. (2004). "The History of Biologic Warfare and Bioterrorism." *Dermatologic Clinics 22*(3), 231–246. doi: 10.1016/j.det.2004.03.008.

Jentes, E. S., G. Poumerol, M. D. Gershman, D. R. Hill, J. Lemarchand, et al. (2011). "The Revised Global Yellow Fever Risk Map and Recommendations for Vaccination, 2010: Consensus of the Informal WHO Working Group on Geographic Risk for Yellow Fever." *The Lancet Infectious Diseases 11*(8), 622–632. doi: 10.1016/s1473-3099(11)70147-5.

Kournikakis, B., K. F. Martinez, R. E. McCleery, S. V. Shadomy, and G. Ramos. (2011). "Anthrax Letters in an Open Office Environment: Effects of Selected CDC Response Guidelines on Personal Exposure and Building Contamination." *Journal of Occupational and Environmental Hygiene 8*(2), 113–122. doi: 10.1080/15459624.2011.547454.

Lagace-Wiens, P. R., E. Rubinstein, and A. Gumel. (2010). "Influenza Epidemiology—Past, Present, and Future." *Critical Care Medicine 38*(4 Suppl), e1–e9. doi: 10.1097/CCM.0b013e3181cbaf34.

Leroy, E., S. Baize, and J. P. Gonzalez. (2011). "Ebola and Marburg Hemorrhagic Fever Viruses: Update on Filoviruses]." *Médecine Tropicale: Revue du Corps de Santé Colonial 71*(2), 111–121.

Markel, H., H. B. Lipman, J. A. Navarro, A. Sloan, J. R. Michalsen, et al. (2007). "Nonpharmaceutical Interventions Implemented by U.S. Cities During the 1918–1919 Influenza Pandemic." *Journal of the American Medical Association 298*(6), 644–654. doi: 10.1001/jama.298.6.644.

Markel, H., A. M. Stern, and M. S. Cetron. (2008). "Theodore E. Woodward Award: Non-pharmaceutical Interventions Employed by Major American Cities During the 1918–19 Influenza Pandemic." *Transactions of the American Clinical and Climatological Association 119*, 129–138, discussion 138–142.

Morbidity and Mortality Weekly Report. (2004). "Outbreaks of Avian Influenza A (H5N1) in

Asia and Interim Recommendations for Evaluation and Reporting of Suspected Cases—United States, 2004." Morbidity and Mortality Weekly Report *53*(5), 97–100.

Murray, C. J., A. D. Lopez, B. Chin, D. Feehan, and K. H. Hill. (2006). "Estimation of Potential Global Pandemic Influenza Mortality on the Basis of Vital Registry Data from the 1918–20 Pandemic: A Quantitative Analysis." *Lancet 368*(9554), 2211–2218. doi: 10.1016/s0140-6736(06)69895-4.

National Vaccine Program Office. (n.d.). "Glossary of Terms." Author. See the organization website.

National Highway Traffic Safety Administration. (2007). "EMS Pandemic Influenza Guidelines for Statewide Adoption." (Washington, DC: National Highway Traffic Safety Administration.)

Obermeyer, Z., C. J. Murray, and E. Gakidou. (2008). "Fifty Years of Violent War Deaths from Vietnam to Bosnia: Analysis of Data from the World Health Survey Programme." *BMJ 336* (7659), 1482–1486. doi: 10.1136/bmj.a137.

Ofner-Agostini, M., T. Wallington, B. Henry, D. Low, L. C. McDonald, et al. (2008). "Investigation of the Second Wave (Phase 2) of Severe Acute Respiratory Syndrome (SARS) in Toronto, Canada. What Happened?" *Canada Communicable Disease Report 34*(2), 1–11.

OSHA. (2010). "Regulations (Standards – 29 CFR): 1910.134." Author. See the organization website.

Perrin, C., V. Noly, R. Mourer, and D. Schmitt. (1994). "Preservation of Cutaneous Structures of Egyptian Mummies: An Ultrastructural Study." *Annales de dermatologie et de vénéréologie 121*(6–7), 470–475.

Perrone, L. A., and T. M. Tumpey. (2007). "Reconstruction of the 1918 Pandemic Influenza Virus: How Revealing the Molecular Secrets of the Virus Responsible for the Worst Pandemic in Recorded History Can Guide Our Response to Future Influenza Pandemics." *Infectious Disorders Drug Targets 7*(4), 294–303.

Riedel, S. (2005). "Edward Jenner and the History of Smallpox and Vaccination." *Proceedings (Baylor University. Medical Center) 18*(1), 21–25.

Schreiber, S., N. Yoeli, G. Paz, G. I. Barbash, D. Varssano, et al. (2004). "Hospital Preparedness for Possible Nonconventional Casualties: An Israeli Experience." *General Hospital Psychiatry 26*(5), 359–366. doi: 10.1016/j.genhosppsych.2004.05.003.

Scripps Howard News Service. (2007, January 28). "Health Experts Fear Bioterror Attack." *Grand Rapids Press*, p. G1.

Thiel, Volker. (2007). *Coronaviruses: Molecular and Cellular Biology*. Norfolk, UK: Caister Academic Press.

Thompson, W. W., D. K. Shay, E. Weintraub, et al. (2003). "Mortality Associated with Influenza and Respiratory Syncytial Virus in the United States." *Journal of the American Medical Association 289*(2), 179–186. doi: 10.1001/jama.289.2.179.

Trampuz, A., R. M. Prabhu, T. F. Smith, and L. M. Baddour. (2004). "Avian Influenza: A New Pandemic Threat?" *Mayo Clinic Proceedings 79*(4), 523–530, quiz 530. doi: 10.4065/79.4.523.

Tsiamis, C., E. Poulakou-Rebelakou, A. Tsakris, and E. Petridou. (2011). "Epidemic Waves of the Black Death in the Byzantine Empire (1347–1453 AD)." *Le infezioni in Medicina: Rivista Periodica di Eziologia, Epidemiologia, Diagnostica, Clinica e Terapia delle Patologie Infettive 19*(3), 194–201.

WHO Informal Network. (2009). "Studies Needed to Address Public Health Challenges of the 2009 H1N1 Influenza Pandemic: Insights from Modeling." *PLoS Currents 1*(Rrn1135). doi: 10.1371/currents.RRN1135.

World Health Organization. (2013). "Infectious Diseases." Author. See the organization website.

Xing, W., G. Hejblum, G. M. Leung, and A. J. Valleron. (2010). "Anatomy of the Epidemiological Literature on the 2003 SARS Outbreaks in Hong Kong and Toronto: A Time-Stratified Review." *PLoS Medicine 7*(5), e1000272. doi: 10.1371/journal.pmed.1000272.

Zink, T. K. (2011). "Anthrax Attacks: Lessons Learned on the 10th Anniversary of the Anthrax Attacks." *Disaster Medicine and Public Health Preparedness 5*(3), 173–174. doi: 10.1001/dmp.2011.71.

Zumla, A., and A. Ustianowski. (2012). "Tropical Diseases: Definition, Geographic Distribution, Transmission, and Classification." *Infectious Disease Clinics of North America 26*(2), 195–205. doi: 10.1016/j.idc.2012.02.007.

Key Terms

anthrax An infectious disease due to a bacterium called *Bacillus anthracis*. Infection in humans most often involves the skin, gastrointestinal tract, or lungs.

antibiotics Types of medication used to damage or destroy bacteria, thus allowing the body to ward off an infection.

antivirals A broad application that is developed to target either a specific virus or in certain instances.

bacterium One-celled, living things. When seen under a microscope they look like balls, rods, or spirals.

Black Death/Plague One of the oldest identifiable diseases known to man; a disease of wild rodents spread from one rodent to another by flea ectoparasites and to humans either by the bite of infected fleas or when handling infected hosts.

cholera An infection of the small intestine that causes a large amount of watery diarrhea, caused by the bacterium *Vibrio cholerae*.

communicable disease An infectious disease that can be passed from one person to another person.

epidemic Outbreaks of a disease in a community or region that is more than usual.

fungi An organism that can be found throughout nature in plants, soils, trees, vegetation, and in and on animals, including humans; can be beneficial or deadly to humans.

hepatitis An inflammation of the liver, most commonly caused by a viral infection. There are five main types: hepatitis A, B, C, D, and E. (*Source: Definition on Hepatitis from http://www.who.int/csr/disease/hepatitis/en/index.html, accessed September 20, 2013. Used by permission of the World Health Organization.*)

Human Immunodeficiency Virus (HIV) A virus that damages a person's body by destroying specific blood cells: CD4+ T cells. It can lead to acquired immune deficiency syndrome (AIDS).

influenza A contagious respiratory illness caused by viruses. It can cause mild to severe illness, and at times can lead to death.

influenza-like illness (ILI) The flu until proven otherwise.

novel virus A virus that has never previously infected humans, or has not infected humans for a long time.

outbreak When a communicable disease is recognized to be spreading at rates that are unusually high or is atypical in nature in a given location.

pandemic An outbreak of a disease in a community or region that is more than usual.

parasite An organism that lives in or on and off of a host.

polio A crippling and potentially fatal infectious disease with no cure, but there are safe and effective vaccines.

quarantine The act of isolating a person from the public to stop or limit the spread of disease.

Severe Acute Respiratory Syndrome (SARS) A syndrome that appeared in 2003 with symptoms including fever, malaise, chills, headache, myalgia, dizziness, rigors, cough, sore throat, and runny nose.

smallpox An acute contagious disease caused by variola virus. It was one of the world's most feared diseases until it was eradicated by a collaborative global vaccination program led by the World Health Organization. The last known natural case was in Somalia in 1977. (*Source: Definition of Smallpox from http://www.who.int/csr/disease/smallpox/en/index.html, accessed September 20, 2013.*

Used by permission of the World Health Organization.)

surge capacity The ability to manage a large volume of patients unexpectedly at any given time.

tularemia An infection common in wild rodents that is passed to humans through contact with infected animal tissues or by ticks, biting flies, and mosquitoes.

Universal Precautions OSHA's required method of control to protect employees from exposure to all human blood and other potentially infectious material (OPIM).

viral hemorrhagic fever A group of illnesses caused by several distinct families of viruses. The term is used to describe a severe multisystem syndrome in which, characteristically, the vascular system is damaged, the body's ability to regulate itself is impaired, and hemorrhage is present.

World Health Organization (WHO) A United Nations agency established to coordinate international health activities and to help governments improve health services.

CHAPTER 6

Vehicle Extrication

Jeffrey Lindsey

Jim Logan

Objectives

After reading this chapter, the student should be able to:

6.1 Differentiate between the processes of disentanglement and extrication and the decision-making processes associated with directing patient care activities and different methods of transport.

6.2 Explain how patient care priorities and extrication procedures must be managed and integrated through teamwork and communication with other extrication activities with fire, law enforcement, and EMS.

6.3 Ensure appropriate personal protective equipment is used during patient-care activities and extrication processes.

6.4 Facilitate patient protection during extrication.

6.5 Explain how to minimize the risk of injury from extrication hazards, such as airbags that have not deployed, fuel leaks, traffic, weather, and other hazards.

6.6 Describe the processes used to stabilize a vehicle prior to beginning extrication and how it may affect patient access and treatment.

6.7 Discuss the impact of damage to specific parts of the vehicle on extrication procedures.

6.8 Explain specific extrication safety considerations for hybrid vehicles.

6.9 Discuss the uses of particular types of hand and hydraulic extrication tools, such as striking, prying, cutting, and lifting tools.

6.10 Identify the safest, most effective ways of gaining access to patients in given MVC scenarios.

Key Terms

cribbing
cutting tools
disentanglement
extrication
extrication teams
extrication tools
hand tools
hydraulic tools
manual hydraulic tools
pneumatic lifting tools
power-driven hydraulic tools
prying tools
rigging
shims
shoring
striking tools
windshield survey

WHAT WOULD YOU DO?

"Hot" did not describe the temperature outside or the type of day Chris Simmons was having. Chris was in prehospital care for 10 years and had seen his career in EMS moving forward after his promotion to EMS officer last spring. Chris was one of five EMS supervisors in the midsize metropolitan area where he grew up. Chris had seven ambulances and three first response units he was responsible for on a daily basis and was a well respected leader in the prehospital and health care community.

As the sun set, the break in the hellish heat had started to become forgiving, but it produced thunderstorms as his shift welcomed the evening hours. The temperature outside was now 90 degrees Fahrenheit, and for the last few hours the shift had been strangely quiet. The tones sounded over the station speaker just after dinner was finished. Chris and the crew at the station were dispatched for a one-car motor vehicle collision (MVC) about 3 miles from their station on a busy stretch of interstate. After an extended response time due to the weather, road conditions, and rush-hour traffic exacerbated by the accident, they arrived at the scene.

Upon arrival and parking in a safe manner, the crew approached the scene and Chris gave a disposition of the scene to communications and advised the incident command that he had control of the medical branch of the operations. Fire suppression units had arrived a few minutes prior and had established command. Chris's crew radioed that one vehicle had left the road, hit a utility pole, and slid down a 10-foot embankment. The front and driver's side of the vehicle had significant damage. Chris made his way to his crew. With flashlights aimed at the vehicle, they could see at least one patient in the driver's compartment as extrication was begun by the rescue. Chris was the EMS officer charged with both prehospital care and extrication.

Questions

1. What would you consider to be related to this MVC and extrication of the patient?
2. What issues need your primary attention for effectively managing this scene and assisting with your crew's operational success and safety?
3. What additional resources would you consider?

INTRODUCTION

In 1966, the National Academy of Sciences National Research Committee on Trauma and Shock (1966) published a report entitled "Accidental Death and Disability: The Neglected Disease of Modern Society," which is more commonly called the "White Paper." It reported that in the previous year, 52 million accidental injuries occurred in the United States that killed 107,000 people, temporarily disabled 10 million, and permanently impaired 400,000 others.

> **Side Bar**
>
> Today, according to the National Highway Traffic Safety Administration (NHTSA) approximately 2.9 million people are injured each year in vehicle crashes in the United States. In 2008, 37,261 people were killed in these types of incidents, and roughly 40 percent of fatal crashes were alcohol related.

The White Paper is considered to have provided a critical impetus to the development of modern EMS. It also began the journey toward improving the survivability of trauma sustained on roads across the United States. In the decades since The White Paper was published, the number of vehicles on U.S. highways has increased by 3.69 million per year. A highway system has been developed that moves millions of people each day. Yet we have decreased morbidity and mortality by building safer vehicles, bringing health care to the scene of the emergency, and improving and formalizing the operational aspects of vehicle extrication, rescue, and prehospital care.

Procedures in vehicle extrication have evolved from when rescuers simply pulled the victim out of the car by his shirt collar after using a crowbar to shatter the window and pry open the door. Today's rapid extrication procedures—using advanced hand, hydraulic, and pneumatic tools—provide access to the patient sometimes in minutes. Combined with simultaneous patient stabilization and care, these procedures have dramatically decreased death and disability from highway crashes. However, the EMS manager must be reminded that some incidents are complicated and require precise techniques to properly stabilize the vehicle to extricate the patient without further harm. Sometimes this involves extended scene times and using every resource available to assist the crews in delivering quality patient care under the worst of conditions and circumstances (National Highway Transportation Safety Administration, 2009).

THE ROLE OF THE EMS MANAGER DURING VEHICLE EXTRICATION

The EMS manager's primary responsibility during vehicle extrication is the safety of the crew and welfare of the patient or patients. Personnel assigned to a dedicated rescue team will perform the majority of vehicle extrications. The EMS manager will use his critical thinking skills in order to create the plan for the **extrication** or **disentanglement** of patients.

Upon arrival, a **windshield survey** and on-scene briefing from the rescue unit leader will assist the EMS manager in making critical decisions on what medical equipment will be required by the crews, how the extrication will proceed, and what additional resources will be needed to perform a successful rescue that will end with a positive outcome and viable patient. The EMS manager may also be required to serve in the role of medical branch director in the incident command structure (ICS) if the incident is a mass casualty incident (MCI).

Side Bar

Additional Resources to Be Considered During Extrication

- Power company for control of power lines and poles
- Fire suppression units
- Hazmat for fuel leaks or spills
- Law enforcement for traffic safety
- Air evacuation for critical patients or prolonged extrications
- Additional ambulances
- Rotor Wing Air Evacuation – for prolonged extrications and/or critical patients
- Additional Ambulances – for multiple patients or Mass Casualty Incidents (MCI)
- School Bus or Van – for alternative means of patient transportation for multiple patients

Extrication teams focus on rolling the dash or cutting a post to flap the roof and may forget that a person with injuries is inside the vehicle. Ensuring and providing optimum care for the injured person requires constant communication between the EMS manager and the extrication officer. The EMS manager will direct how the extrication will proceed, or pause, as the patient's condition dictates, taking cues from personnel and circumstances related to the progress of the removal of the patient. During the rescue, the extrication technique that was initially agreed upon must be altered to mitigate the effects of force applied to the entrapped victim.

Along with being a patient's advocate during the rescue, and while ensuring operational safety with proper personal protective equipment (PPE), the crews must begin treatment of the patient according to local standing orders and protocol. This is often a challenge because of the patient's entanglement, limited space in which to work, and distractions such as noise. At times, personnel will be forced to climb through a broken back window and into the back seat of the vehicle to be in a position to both provide manual stabilization of the patient's head and spine and to effectively manage patient care. Airway, breathing, and circulation treatment modalities may have to be performed from a compromising or contorted position. Techniques learned in the classroom setting may have to be modified, but actions must be carried out in an aggressive fashion to ensure the best outcome for the patient. Treatment may be interrupted during the attempt to free the patient and restarted when the rescue team resets its equipment and technique during the extrication attempt. A well-prepared EMS manager must feel comfortable suggesting the use of all tools in his crews' toolbox in complicated extrications with a critical patient.

Once the patient is extricated from the vehicle, the focus should be on continued patient care and patient packaging. The mechanism of injury (MOI) will dictate how rapid assessments, treatment, and transport will be handled. The EMS officer is responsible for facilitating this all-hands approach to patient care and providing the crew with the necessary resources to accomplish the mission. The speed and choice of the transport location in relation to the most appropriate care facility are of the essence and are crucial to the outcome of the patient.

PERSONAL PROTECTIVE EQUIPMENT

The use of PPE must be paramount at every scene. Proper application of PPE is vital to every crew's safety. It is well-known that noncompliance in using body substance isolation (BSI) procedures, such as gloves, mask, gown, and other Universal Precautions, can lead to a transfer of disease. It is also true that compromising the use of PPE during vehicle extrication

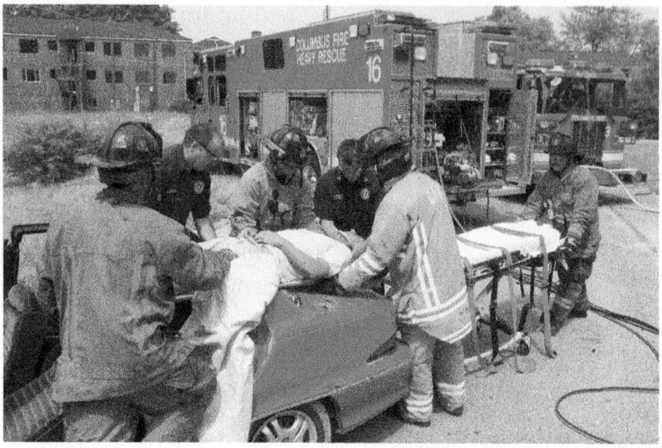

FIGURE 6.1 ■ Those who are not in compliance with PPE should not be permitted to operate at the site of extrication.

can lead to injury or even death of the rescuer. The use of both BSI and PPE specific to vehicle extrication must be utilized for protection of all involved at scenes requiring extrication. (See Figure 6.1.) The EMS manager must insist on safety and refocus personnel not wearing appropriate PPE. Those who are not in compliance with PPE should not be permitted to operate at the site of extrication.

HEAD AND FACE PROTECTION

At all vehicle extrications, proper head protection must be worn. Helmets protect crews from flying debris and provide protection from protruding sharp objects that have the potential to cause skull fractures and soft tissue injuries. All helmets used for extrication should meet all NFPA 1971 requirements. The face and eyes must be protected from vehicle fluids as well as the patient's fluids. Helmet shields, safety glasses, and goggles will also provide protection for an EMS provider during extrication. Using safety goggles with the helmet shield is strongly recommended, as debris can fly up from below and cause eye damage to the paramedic who is using only a helmet shield.

EAR AND HEARING PROTECTION

An extrication scene can be extremely loud. Amplified sound of the extrication symphony includes engine noise from multiple rescue vehicles, generators, hydrolytic and pneumatic extrication tools, and the combined voices of all those involved in the rescue. Ear protection should be in the form of headsets, earmuffs, or earplugs inserted directly into the ear canal.

HAND PROTECTION

Leather gloves provide the best protection against the twisted metal and broken glass that EMS providers will encounter during a vehicle rescue. Firefighting gloves are acceptable, but they may prove to be too bulky and restrict the dexterity needed to perform patient care. In most situations, EMS personnel should wear close-fitting leather gloves that provide the dexterity to provide unrestricted patient care but are sturdy enough to protect hands from soft tissue injuries. Again, BSI and PPE go hand in hand; therefore, medical exam gloves should be worn beneath the protective leather gloves to provide protection from blood and body fluids.

FOOT PROTECTION

Consider the hazards and potential injuries that may be present at all scenes when mandating or selecting footwear for an EMS service. Leather boots with steel toe and metatarsal protection are recommended, and a proper fit is necessary to reduce fatigue and blister formation.

BODY PROTECTION

Firefighting turnout coat and pants will provide EMS personnel protection against flying debris, sharp objects, and other hazards at the extrication scene. However, not all EMS personnel are fire based, or they find that this form of protection is too cumbersome and does not allow sufficient entry into the vehicle while performing patient care. Regardless, this type of gear is the best protection against the hazards present; however, it is true that it is restrictive, bulky, and hot.

An acceptable alternative for EMS personnel are extrication jumpsuits. The suits are manufactured by all of the structural firefighting turnout gear companies and are made from a cotton/Nomex blend for protection from flame. The jumpsuits are outfitted with reflective striping for high visibility. The greatest advantage of this type of protection is its lightweight construction and better fit, giving the EMS provider better mobility.

PATIENT SAFETY

After the EMS crew is safe and protected, the patient must be shielded from the same elements. The following are some items that will help to create a safe environment for the patient:

- Wool blankets for warmth and to protect from debris
- Helmet
- Hearing protection
- Goggles
- Dust mask, unless patient is having difficulty breathing and/or is on oxygen
- Shielding, such as a backboard used to form a barrier between the patient and sharp objects or equipment (Goodson, 2001)

TECHNOLOGIES, BENEFITS, AND HAZARDS

Modern vehicle technology has created features that are designed to improve the chances of drivers and passengers surviving a high-velocity impact. Some of these safety features also have potential hazards. The following segments describe some of these technologies and the associated hazards.

AIR BAGS

Along with the advent of the seat belt, supplemental restraint systems (SRS), or front-impact air bags, have provided increased collision protection. Many new vehicles are equipped with additional air bags throughout. Crews must consider the following while in the vehicle providing care:

- Side-impact protection systems (SIPS)
- Head protection systems (HPS)
- Knee bolsters

Air bags have saved many lives and have reduced the injuries once realized during high-velocity collisions. According to a report conducted by the NHTSA between 1987 and 2005, 19,659 lives have been saved with the use of airbags (National Highway Traffic Safety Administration, 2005).

Accidental activation of air bag systems can occur during vehicle extrication, injuring crews and patients. Deactivation of these devices is essential for a safe extrication. All air bags can be identified by words or the initials of the restraint system that are displayed at various points in the interior of the vehicle. Listed here are some basic suggestions regarding deactivation of supplemental restraint systems:

- Turn off the ignition.
- Turn off the SRS. Some autos have an air bag switch.
- Disconnect the battery, negative cable first.
- Tape the ends of battery cables.
- Wait for the reserve power to drain down during equipment staging and extrication preparation.

In electrical restraint systems, an electrical impulse of as little as .5 volt may cause a system to be accidentally activated. For vehicles with mechanical systems, it is important to know where sensors are located and to avoid excessive pressure or force in those areas. There have been many reports of air bags that were not deployed in frontal or near-frontal crashes. Treat all nondeployed air bags as if they are live, even following proper disconnection. Proper distancing is the best way to reduce personal injury of crews and patients from a nondeployed air bag. Many fire services employ a rule-of-thumb air bag distance directive called the "5-10-20-inch rule," a general estimation that improves awareness of the SRS and provides a cushion for safety:

- Stay 5 inches from a side-impact air bag.
- Double the figure (10 inches) for the driver's frontal air bag.
- Double the figure again (20 inches) for a passenger-side front air bag.

Nondeployed air bags pose a serious risk to crews and the patient during extrication. Front-impact air bags can expand at speeds in excess of 200 miles per hour. Side-impact air bags deploy at even higher rates.

Some common injuries after deployment of an airbag system are soft tissue injuries to the upper extremities, and blunt force injuries to the face and head. It is not unusual for a patient to experience fracture of the nose, especially if wearing eyeglasses or sunglasses.

FUEL CYLINDERS

Adding a flammable product to an MVC increases the potential for danger. Passenger vehicles run on a variety of fuels. Today, the most common fuels are gasoline and diesel. Fuel cylinders are most likely to be found in the trunk area of a passenger car or the bed of a pickup truck. These areas must be evaluated for the presence of fuel and managed by the appropriate extrication team. As a measure of safety related to fuel leaks during vehicle extrication, a fire engine company must be utilized for potential fire suppression activity. A charged (filled with water) hand-line (fire hose) should be on standby if needed.

ANIMALS AND EXTRICATION

Animals of all types may be traveling with their owners and may require special consideration during vehicle extrication. Here are some important factors to consider if an animal is involved during rescue procedures:

- Note the location of animals to avoid injuries to them or yourself.
- Avoid injury to animals.
- Use tools that produce the least noise and vibration to lessen the animals' irritation.
- Minimize actions that will create unnecessary vehicle movement that could upset animals.
- Use existing void spaces to assist animals to self-extricate.
- Be aware that animals may be affected by the odor of gasoline.
- Animals can react violently (bite, kick, scratch) due to fear. This reaction may result from them being constrained, possibly injured, or attempting to become free. Use all PPE to increase the crew's level of safety.
- Use personnel who are knowledgeable about animals, such as the local animal shelter personnel or the American Society for the Prevention of Cruelty to Animals (ASPCA), to assist during these incidents.

- Animals may require specialized care, including administration of sedatives by trained animal rescue personnel.
- Rescue personnel should assist and support animal rescue personnel if they are called to the scene. (Maryland Fire and Rescue Institute, 2010)

OTHER HAZARDS

Hazards at collisions can be caused by anything from road conditions to inclement weather. Here is a list of the most common hazards during vehicle extrication scenes:

- Ice
- Darkness
- Downed power lines (All lines should be considered charged with electricity—"live" or "hot"—and avoided.)
- Damaged poles or trees
- Traffic
- Loaded bumpers, particularly those with shock absorbers compressed after impact (Avoid these areas as they may spring with violent force at any time.)
- Hazardous materials released from their containers, fluid leaks
- Debris; jagged, sharp objects
- Glass

VEHICLE STABILIZATION

One of the most important tasks to be completed before a crew can extricate a patient will be the stabilization of the vehicle. Sudden movement caused by the use of tools and techniques or the shifting of weight can be dangerous and even fatal to the patient or your providers. Stabilization by the extrication team will provide an environment that will assist in keeping the crew safe while treating the patient and preventing unnecessary movement that may exacerbate the patient's injuries. It must be emphasized that the paramount purpose of vehicle stabilization is safety.

CRIBBING

Cribbing is the filling of void spaces to prevent the movement of the vehicle. (See Figure 6.2.) Prefabricated wood, plastic, or metal pieces are stacked in void spaces between the base (ground) and the underside of the vehicle and arranged in a fashion to create a tight fit between the auto and base. Achieving a

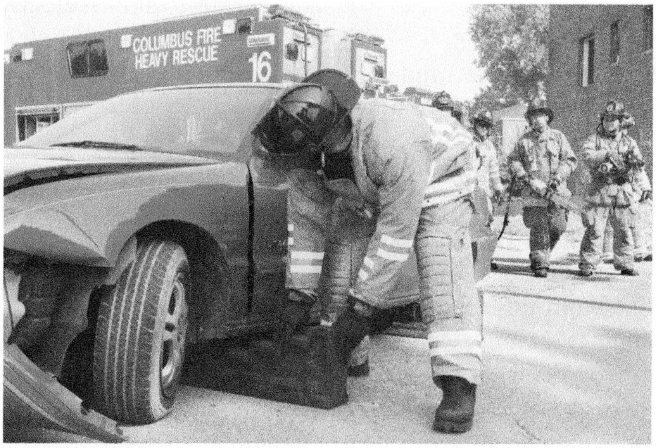

FIGURE 6.2 Cribbing is the filling of void spaces to prevent the movement of the vehicle.

tight fit can be assisted with **shims**, which are thinner cribbing pieces used to fill the gaps between the bigger pieces.

SHORING

Shoring is often utilized when cribbing cannot be accomplished in a practical way due to the opening or the span being too large. Large timbers or pneumatic devices are used to stabilize the vehicle during rescue and extrication operations. Shoring is often utilized with vehicles found in compromised positions, such as a vehicle found on its side.

RIGGING

Rigging is used to further stabilize the vehicle. Some of the more common materials used for rigging are ropes, chains, and webbing (Goodson, 2001).

VEHICLE ANATOMY

When dealing with vehicle extrication it is important to know what kind of vehicle is involved. There are two major vehicle anatomy structural types: nonhybrid vehicles and hybrid vehicles.

NONHYBRID VEHICLES

In the past, vehicles were manufactured on rigid substructures. Today, with the use of unibody construction, the substructures are integral parts of the vehicles. For example, if an extrication team begins with cuts to the roof of a nonstabilized vehicle that has structural damage, the chances are great that the vehicle will react in a way that will compromise safety and cause or worsen entrapment (Schmitz, n.d.).

Vehicle Top

Depending on how the vehicle came to rest, the top presenting part may or may not be the roof. The crew must be aware of any difficulties involved in gaining access into the patient compartment because of how the auto came to rest. If the vehicle is on its roof, the EMS crew and the extrication team must be aware of fluids that may be leaking into the patient compartment and contaminating the interior. The EMS provider must also be aware of the ever-present danger of power lines that may be on or around the vehicle.

Vehicle Bottom

In most situations, the bottom of the wreckage will be the floor or the underside of the vehicle, and all or most wheels will be on a firm surface, which will ease access into the patient compartment. However, crews must be wary of what may be beneath the vehicle. Leaking fuel, battery acid, or other substances could pose safety issues that must be addressed.

Driver and Passenger Sides

Impacts to the sides of the vehicle are of great concern related to mechanism of injury. The sides are some of the least protected areas and should prompt the EMS provider to consider the high index of suspicion of significant injuries. Advances have been made with the advent of side-impact air bags; however, any moderate-to-high-velocity impact to the side of the vehicle should alert the EMS provider to the possibility of severe injuries.

Vehicle Front

If the vehicle is moving forward, the front is the aspect that should arrive first and, therefore, is the most commonly damaged part. A number of engine-related hazards should be of concern to your EMS personnel and the extrication team. The most common concern is fire. Broken fuel lines and a compromised electrical system can lead to a fire in the engine compartment. Attention to disconnection of the battery and control of the fuel leak should be part of any extrication team's standard operating procedures. A precautionary hand-line from the first-arriving pumper should be employed as a safety precaution.

Vehicle Rear

In most front-engine vehicles, the fuel tank is located in the rear of the vehicle. Most collisions that suffer rear-end damage do not result in ruptured fuel tanks. However, design flaws do occur, and the extrication team must be alert to potential fuel leaks. A precautionary hand-line from the first-arriving pumper should be employed as a safety precaution.

Vehicle Interior

The interior is one of the most critical areas for removal of a patient from a vehicle. Interior components such as the dashboard, steering wheel, seats, and pedals must be removed from around the patient to accomplish extrication. The time it takes to remove these structures may also mean that the crews will have to spend extensive time with the patient inside the vehicle. It is expected that EMS providers will perform life-sustaining and lifesaving care even while the extrication is taking place. Ongoing assessment and monitoring of the patient during the extrication are of upmost importance. Continuing attention to airway management, fluid replacement, and spinal immobilization are also critical.

Vehicle Exterior

During the scene size-up upon arrival at an MVC, the exterior condition of the vehicle can provide the EMS officer and EMS crew with many clues. These clues include the probable severity of the injuries sustained by the patient, including the need for the appropriate equipment and additional resources. (See Figure 6.3 for components that are considered to be part of the vehicle exterior.)

HYBRID VEHICLES

More hybrid vehicles are being seen on the road every day. Attention to proper identification of hybrid vehicles and some basic safety procedures should be all that is needed to efficiently address the few differences between a hybrid and a nonhybrid vehicle.

Knowing the location and construction of the battery compartments and components that isolate the electrical system should help crews keep safe during extrication. Two of the most important aspects of disconnecting the electrical

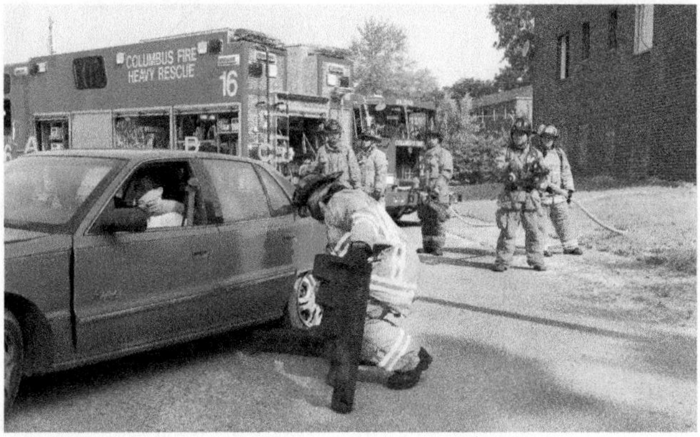

FIGURE 6.3 ■ Door posts, also known as pillars, are structural members that surround the door areas. These are usually referred to alphabetically from front to rear as the A, B, and C posts.

system of a hybrid vehicle, which contains high-voltage (HV) battery packs (see Figure 6.4), are no different from those for a nonhybrid. First, turn the ignition off and remove the key. Second, disconnect the 12-volt battery system. The high-voltage (HV) system has relays that automatically open and disconnect if the MVC is severe enough to deploy air bags. The HV system is also shut down as soon as the ignition is switched off or the 12-volt battery is disconnected.

Hybrid car manufacturers attempt to protect the HV systems from accidents by enclosing the HV batteries in metal cases and locating them near, under, or behind the rear seats. HV systems may remain powered for up to 10 minutes after the vehicle is shut off or the 12-volt system is disabled. To prevent serious injury or death, avoid touching, cutting, or breaching any HV power cable. These cables are bright orange in color.

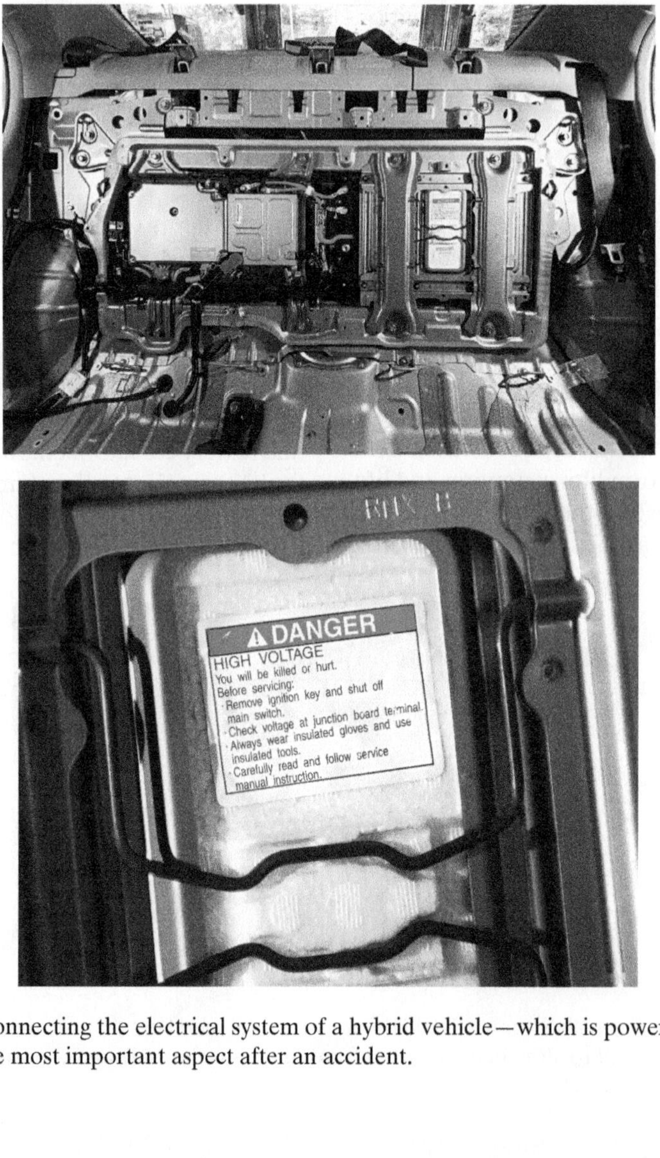

FIGURE 6.4 Disconnecting the electrical system of a hybrid vehicle—which is powered by high-voltage battery packs—is the most important aspect after an accident.

Side Bar

Guidelines for Working On or Near a Hybrid Vehicle

- Identify the vehicle as a hybrid.
- Stabilize the vehicle.
- Access the passenger compartment.
- Shift the gear selector to park.
- Turn the ignition off.
- Check the dash indicator for power.
- Disconnect the 12-volt battery.

As with all vehicle collisions, a precautionary charged hand-line from the first-arriving pumper should be deployed. If fire is present, copious amounts of water should be used to cool the metal case that houses the HV battery pack (Berman, 2006).

LIQUID PETROLEUM GAS VEHICLES

The availability of light-duty passenger vehicles fueled by liquid petroleum gas (LPG) is currently limited. A few light-duty vehicles—mostly larger trucks and vans—can be ordered from a dealer with a prep-ready engine package and converted to use propane. Existing conventional vehicles can also be converted for LPG use. Since propane is stored as a liquid in pressurized fuel tanks rated to 300 psi, LPG conversions consist of installing a separate fuel system if the vehicle will run on both conventional fuel and LPG or a replacement fuel system for LPG-only operation. Caution must be taken when a vehicle powered by LPG is involved in a vehicle crash. At incidents involving vehicles that use LPG for fuel, personnel or equipment should not be positioned in close proximity or to the rear of such vehicles. The gas cylinders/tanks are generally positioned in the rear compartment of the vehicle, which creates an explosion hazard.

EXTRICATION TOOLS

There are a variety of **extrication tools**. An EMS manager must educate his crew on the tools to perform extrication. Make sure crews "try before they pry," meaning try to see if they can gain access to a patient with simple procedures—such as through an unlocked door, window, or a void made by the accident—before utilizing any extrication tool. If tools are needed, it is essential to remember that extricating patients from vehicles may often be successful with basic hand tools and does not always require the use of complex power tools.

Best Practice

Heavy-Rescue Services

Pittsburgh EMS provides heavy rescue in the City of Pittsburgh. The personnel assigned to the Rescue Division are certified ALS providers with extensive training in rescue. Six paramedic crew chiefs and eighteen paramedics are assigned to the two heavy-rescue squads in the city. The City of Pittsburgh utilizes one of the few EMS heavy rescues found in large metropolitan areas in the United States. In comparison, most heavy-rescue units in the U.S. metropolitan areas are fire based and not operated by EMS personnel. The Pittsburgh EMS practice has demonstrated that EMS personnel can provide heavy-rescue services for an area and that it does not always have to be a fire-based service that provides such service.

HAND TOOLS

Common **hand tools** used during extrication are the same as those used in structural firefighting and other emergency or rescue work. Many EMS vehicles carry the basic hand tools on their units and can begin extrication prior to the arrival of a heavy rescue vehicle.

STRIKING TOOLS

The category of **striking tools** includes axes, hammers, mallets, battering rams, punches, and picks (see Figure 6.5.) These can be dangerous, and precautions must be taken when they are used near a patient. PPE must be worn at all times to prevent serious injury when striking tools are being used.

PRYING TOOLS

Prying tools are used to provide leverage and mechanical advantages by multiplying the force applied and are used to open hoods, trunks, and doors. Common prying tools are the Halligan tool, crowbar, and pry bar. When used correctly, prying tools are safer than striking tools.

CUTTING TOOLS

Cutting tools are used to cut through the different types of materials found at an extrication scene. Common types are saws, knives, cutters, axes, and snipping tools. Because these tools are constructed with a sharp cutting edge, appropriate PPE must be worn to avoid injury.

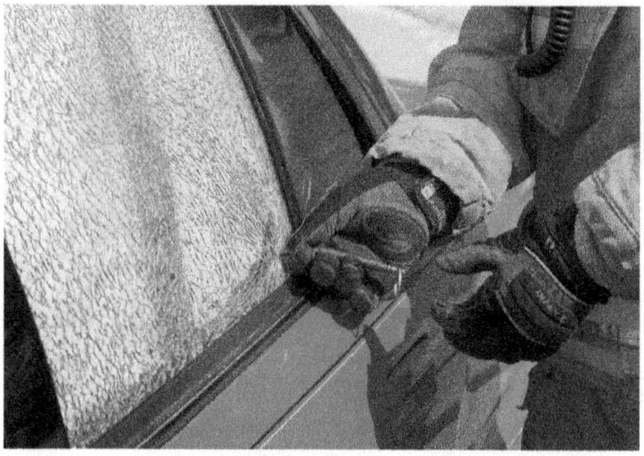

FIGURE 6.5 The category of striking tools includes axes, hammers, mallets, battering rams, punches, and picks.

HYDRAULIC TOOLS

Hydraulic tools employ the force that is exerted by a high-pressure liquid. They are many times referred to as the "Jaws of Life." In reality, Jaws of Life is a specific brand of hydraulic tools. Hydraulic tools come in various forms and have various uses. It is critical for you and your crews to understand the benefits and hazards associated with using hydraulic tools.

MANUAL HYDRAULIC TOOLS

Manual hydraulic tools are powered by someone operating a pump lever to activate the tool. These tools work well in areas where space is limited. However, it must be noted that manual hydraulic tools operate more slowly and within a more limited range than their power-driven counterparts. Some common manual extrication devices used today are the Porta-power and other hydraulic jacks. The Porta-power comes with many accessories for various applications that will assist with extrication in limited space. It operates with pressure from a hand pump compressor, which allows for operation in narrow space.

POWER-DRIVEN HYDRAULIC TOOLS

Power-driven hydraulic tools have a wide range of uses. Their power and speed are superior to manual hydraulic tools. Most are operated by electric motors or gas-powered engines that keep the tools' hydraulic fluid under pressure for operation. Some of the more common power-driven hydraulic tools are these (see Figure 6.6):

- Spreaders—used for pushing or pulling
- Shears—used for cutting roof supports or posts

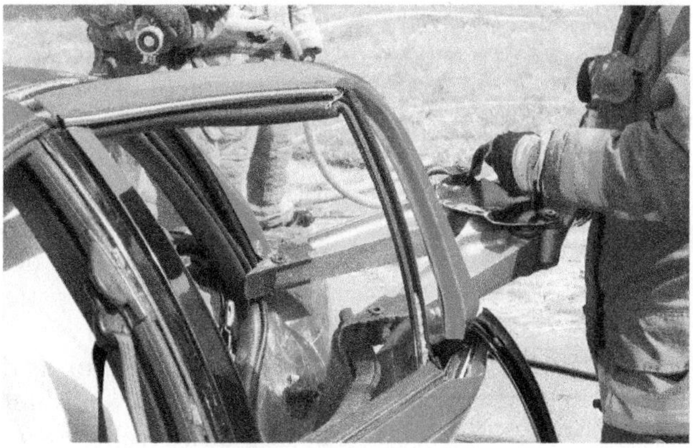

FIGURE 6.6 ■ These are some of the more common power-driven hydraulic tools.

- Pedal cutters—used for cutting pedal arms
- Extension rams—for pushing operations

PNEUMATIC LIFTING TOOLS

Pneumatic lifting tools are used to lift or displace objects that cannot be moved by conventional means (see Figure 6.7.) Pneumatic lifting bags are categorized as high, medium, or low pressure. The largest of the high-pressure bags can lift up to 75 tons and operate at 116 to 145 psi. Low- and medium-pressure bags are used to temporarily lift or stabilize large objects. Some low- and medium-pressure bags can lift objects up to 6 feet and operate on 7 to 15 psi. EMS personnel may find themselves working with the heavy-rescue team and these pneumatic lifting bags. Common uses of these bags are to lift vehicles off patients. The EMS manager may have to assist with balancing patient care and assisting in the rescue depending on the responsibilities of the agency at the scene of the incident. Patient care will be happening simultaneously as the air bags are inflated and deflated during the extrication process of the patient. These bags can also assist with stabilization so other tools can be used to free the patient.

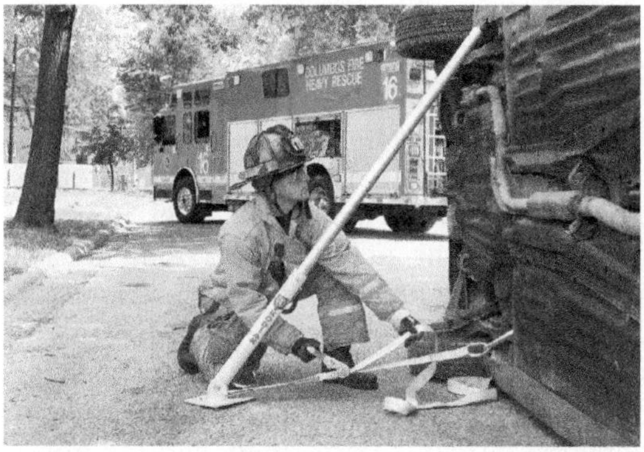

FIGURE 6.7 ■ Pneumatic lifting tools are used to lift or displace objects that cannot be lifted by conventional means.

OTHER EXTRICATION TOOLS

Many common construction tools are used in combination with the extrication tools mentioned in the preceding paragraphs. Some of the more common tools used during extrication operations are these:

- Power saws
  - Reciprocating
  - Rotary
  - Chain

- Thermal cutting tools
  - Plasma cutters
  - Cutting torches
- Lifting and pulling tools
  - Winches
  - Come-alongs
  - Block-and-tackle (Anderson, 2005; Goodson, 2001)

PATIENT CARE DURING EXTRICATION

EMS crews should begin performing patient care upon initial contact with the patient unless the scene is unsafe to do so. During extrication, patient care should continue uninterrupted to the best of the crew's ability. There will be instances during which extrication will supersede patient care. The patient should be treated to the level that is safe for EMS providers, the patient, and the extrication crew. Any time EMS providers are providing care for the patient still in the vehicle, they must be wearing the proper PPE. The patient also must be provided with protection from sharp objects and flying debris. The use of the following items may be considered to protect your patient during extrication:

- Tarp
- Blanket
- Eye protection
- Turnout coat
- Helmet with face shield (Bledsoe, Porter, and Cherry, 2003)

GAINING ACCESS

Removal of MVC victims is a critical function of fire services, rescue departments, and ambulance services. Vehicle extrication can be quite a simple or extremely complicated procedure. As a critical function that affects patient outcome, it requires individual proficiency in conjunction with teamwork. Gaining access to the patient after controlling hazards and proper stabilization of the vehicle is critical (Bledsoe, Porter, and Cherry, 2003).

In vehicle extrication, it is very common for the caregiver to gain access by whatever means necessary. It may be as simple as opening the opposite door and positioning himself next to the patient to perform primary and secondary assessment, treatment, and reassessment, or as difficult as crawling through a back windshield or window of an upside-down vehicle to perform the same care on an inverted patient. Whatever the circumstances, the patient's condition and the extent of entanglement must be relayed to those officers, and clear objectives must be set. All involved must be aware of the "big picture."

The patient's condition often will change quickly during the rescue. Anticipation of changing conditions in both the patient and the environment will allow for the needed equipment and treatment modalities to be available. In some situations, the best approach may be rapid stabilization and removal of the patient. The situation may call for this technique because of the need to get away from an immediate danger. In these cases, rapid removal to an area of safety before providing definitive patient care is justified. In these circumstances, deviations from or alterations of standing orders and protocols may occur due to special circumstances related to lengthy times, entrapment issues, or hazardous conditions. On-line medical direction may be required as time ticks away. Extended-care issues can be common in heavy vehicle extrication situations.

Given the patient's exposure to the stress of the accident, pain from the injuries sustained, treatments performed, and the noise and uncertainty of the extrication, this may be the time to provide some psychological support. Establishing a rapport early will help in alleviating fears. Make sure crews consider the following:

- Use the patient's name, and be sure the patient knows yours. All extrication team members, including EMS personnel, should know and use the patient's name. The benefits are twofold, as this practice fosters better communication and reminds the extrication team members that they are dealing with a human being.
- Make sure the patient knows that the crew will not abandon him.
- Explain treatments, extrication procedures, and any PPE that must be applied to the patient.
- Explain any delays.
- Never lie.

REMOVAL

Removal of the patient may be one of the most difficult tasks involved in extrication. Determining the best means of egress, including the best method of patient packaging, is critical. These will be determined by the patient's condition. Commercial devices for full spinal immobilization should be employed. As disentanglement occurs, additional care for soft tissue and musculoskeletal injuries that are being uncovered must be provided. Also, be prepared for issues related to hypovolemia, as blood and fluid loss may cause your patient to become hemodynamically challenged, resulting in shock.

CHAPTER REVIEW

Summary

Today, motor vehicles are more complicated and have more hazards than in past years. As technology evolves, the EMS manager must keep informed about the safe and effective means to extricate and care for patients at the scene of an MVC. The extrication process is typically performed by a designated rescue team; however, as an EMS professional and leader, it is important to understand the process and, in certain instances, direct the extrication of patients from motor vehicles.

WHAT WOULD YOU DO? Reflection

When arriving at an MVC, such as this incident, the EMS manager must consider any special equipment that is needed. In this situation, a rescue unit was on scene providing extrication. In addition, concern about scene safety would also include the utility pole. If the pole had an energized line, the power utility company must be notified to respond to the scene prior to making contact with the vehicle. Also, since the patient is over the embankment, provisions must be made to get the patient up the embankment to the ambulance. Plus, consideration must be taken to get personnel to the patient. Lighting on the scene is also a consideration.

Since the incident occurred during a weather event, proper safety measures must be implemented and monitored. Personnel working during an electrical storm is always a concern. Additional resources would include the rescue team (both for the vehicle and the embankment issue), law enforcement, the utility company, at least one transport unit, and fire as needed for any fuel leaks and hazards.

Review Questions

1. Differentiate between the processes of disentanglement and extrication.
2. Explain how patient care priorities and extrication procedures must be managed and integrated through teamwork and communication with fire, law enforcement, and EMS.
3. Explain how to minimize risk of injury from extrication hazards, such as air bags that have not deployed, fuel leaks, traffic, weather, and other hazards.
4. Describe the processes used to stabilize a vehicle prior to beginning extrication.
5. Explain specific extrication safety considerations for hybrid vehicles.
6. Identify the safest, most effective ways of gaining access to patients in given MVC scenarios.

References

Anderson, B. G. (2005). *Vehicle Extrication: A Practical Guide*. Tulsa, OK: Penn Well Corporation.

Berman, B. (2006, April 4). "Hybrids and Emergency First Responders." Hybridcars.com. See HybridCars website.

Bledsoe, B. E., R. S. Porter, and R. A. Cherry. (2003). *Essentials of Paramedic Care.* Upper Saddle River, NJ: Pearson Prentice Hall.

Goodson, C. (2001). *Principles of Vehicle Extrication,* 2nd ed. Oklahoma City: Fire Protection Publications, Oklahoma State University.

Maryland Fire and Rescue Institute. (2010, June 2). "Vehicular Rescue Involving Animals." See Firehouse website.

National Academy of Sciences, Division of Medical Sciences, Committee on Trauma and Committee on Shock. (1966, September). "Accidental Death and Disability: The Neglected Disease of Modern Society." Washington, DC: National Academy of Sciences–National Research Council.

National Highway Traffic Safety Administration. (2005). "Traffic Safety Facts 2005 Data." (Washington, DC: NHTSA's National Center for Statistics and Analysis.)

National Highway Traffic Safety Administration, Center for Statistics and Analysis. (2009, June). "2008 Traffic Safety Annual Assessment–Highlights." (Washington, DC: NHTSA's National Center for Statistics and Analysis.)

Schmitz, R. (n.d.). "New Vehicle Technology." See Firefighting in Canada website.

Key Terms

cribbing The filling of void spaces to prevent the movement a vehicle.

cutting tools A type of tool used to cut through the different types of materials found at an extrication scene.

disentanglement The removal of debris and vehicle parts that trap a person in a vehicle.

extrication The process of removing a patient from a vehicle.

extrication teams A group of individuals who are trained and equipped to remove and disentangle patients from a vehicle.

extrication tools A type of equipment used to remove and disentangle a patient from a vehicle.

hand tools A type of tool used during extrication; these tools are the same as those used in structural firefighting and other emergency or rescue work.

hydraulic tools A type of tool in which force is exerted by a high-pressure liquid.

manual hydraulic tools A type of tool powered by someone operating a pump lever to activate the tool.

pneumatic lifting tools A type of tool used to lift or displace objects that cannot be lifted by conventional means.

power-driven hydraulic tools A type of tool that has a wide range of uses and power and speed superior to manual hydraulic tools.

prying tools A type of tool used to provide leverage and mechanical advantages by multiplying the force applied; used to open hoods, trunks, and doors.

rigging A technique used to further stabilize the vehicle.

shims Thinner cribbing pieces used to fill the gaps between the bigger pieces.

shoring A technique often utilized when cribbing cannot be accomplished in a practical way due to the opening or span being too large.

striking tools A type of tool that includes axes, hammers, mallets, battering rams, punches, and picks.

windshield survey The assessment of the scene that personnel do as they arrive on the scene of an incident.

CHAPTER 7

Structural Collapse

DAVID HARRINGTON

Objectives

After reading this chapter, the student should be able to:

7.1 Identify the need for structural collapse search and rescue operation.
7.2 Identify the steps required to initiate the response to a structural collapse event.
7.3 Describe the necessary steps for proper size-up of a structural collapse event.
7.4 Identify and describe the steps necessary for initiating site control and scene management.
7.5 Identify the general hazard associated with a structural collapse incident.
7.6 Identify the indicators for the potential for secondary collapse.
7.7 Identify the five different types of construction, and the categories and expected behaviors of components and materials in a structural collapse.
7.8 Identify the resources required to conduct a structural collapse search and rescue operation.
7.9 Identify and describe the five types of void space collapse patterns and four types of nonvoid space collapse patterns.
7.10 Describe the methods for conducting visual and verbal searches at structural collapse incidents.
7.11 Identify and describe the FEMA Task Force Search Rescue Marking System, Building Marking System, and Victim Location Marking System.
7.12 Conduct a proper scene size-up at a structural collapse event.
7.13 Remove readily accessible victims from a structural collapse incident.

Key Terms

approach hazards
Authority Having Jurisdiction (AHJ)
awareness level
canine search team
collapse patterns
concentrated load
control zones
dead load
design load
distributed load
extrication
Federal Emergency Management Agency (FEMA)
FEMA Resource Typing System
force
hazardous materials
impact load
incident action plan (IAP)
incident command system (ICS)
incident commander
live load
loads
National Fire Protection Agency (NFPA)
operational capacity
operations level
physical search team
resources
secondary collapse
standard operating procedure (SOP)
structural collapse
technician level

WHAT WOULD YOU DO?

Your supervisor's truck has been dispatched along with an ambulance to a report of an explosion and possible fire at an apartment complex that is known for its drug activity. Your unit is the first to arrive on scene, where you discover that while SWAT was serving a warrant at the location, an explosion occurred on the first floor of a three-story apartment. There has been a pancake collapse of the two upper floors, possibly trapping multiple victims. You safely park your vehicle away from the debris that is strewn around the scene. You observe heavy grey smoke emerging out of what used to be a Type 3 Ordinary Construction building. Police officers covered in blood come running up to tell you that you will need more help and in a hurry.

Questions

1. What are the first steps you should take to effectively begin managing the scene?
2. During your initial size-up, what should you be looking for during a structural collapse incident?
3. What types of resources should be requested to assist in hazard mitigation and the operation?

INTRODUCTION

Every EMS manager will be faced with challenging situations he has never experienced outside of a classroom or on the drill field. Even though structural collapses are not a routine response, the potential for one is a lot more common than many think. There is not any community that is immune from the causes of a structural collapse. Providers trained to the awareness level in structural collapse rescue should be familiar with their communities and the potential of a structural collapse event within those communities. When responding to a structural collapse it is important to conduct a size-up, gain control to make the scene as safe as possible for all responders, gather the appropriate **resources**, provide as much rescue and patient care as safely possible, and integrate the operation into the much larger picture with other resources as they arrive.

By having a basic understanding of the common causes that can result in a collapse in the different types of construction, an EMS manager can be better prepared. It is also important to understand the process of safely responding to such a event which includes, the departmental or local response guidelines and the process for requesting the required resources to effectively mitigate this events. As an awareness-level provider, it is necessary to know not only the limitations based on training received but also the limitations of a specific department. Too many unintended consequences occur when personnel or departments that lack proper training or equipment resist calling for help early. This can lead to a long delay in rescue and care to victims who otherwise could have been saved. This has resulted in needless injuries to department rescuers who are not properly prepared to function safely or efficiently on the scene of a structural collapse.

CAUSE OF STRUCTURAL COLLAPSES

There are a variety of reasons, both manmade and natural, for a **structural collapse** to occur. Manmade factors that can lead to a collapse of a structure include engineering miscalculation in design leading to a load being placed on the structure that is beyond its capacity, poor construction, and poor quality of material and craftsmanship. Other factors can include impact loads being imposed upon the structure that are caused by events such as a vehicle or aircraft crashing into the building. An explosion from a natural gas leak, industrial accident, or even a terrorist event can also lead to collapse of a structure.

Natural causes leading to a structural collapse can include weather events that result in heavily weighted snowfall, and severe storms with heavy wind and tornados that bring additional flooding. Excessive rainfall in some areas can lead to landslides and mudslides. Earthquakes and their aftershocks inflict heavy damage upon structures, especially those that have not been properly designed to withstand those forces. Fire can lead to extensive damage to a structure, resulting in a partial or complete collapse. Although fire is considered a natural phenomenon, it can result from both natural and manmade acts.

STANDARDS AND REGULATIONS FOR A STRUCTURAL COLLAPSE RESCUE TEAM

For a structural collapse rescue team to function efficiently and safely, it must meet an established set of requirements dictating its level of **operational capacity**. These requirements encompass the minimal and continual training, documentation of activities, standard operating procedures, and response.

In 1994, the Technical Committee on Technical Rescue along with the **National Fire Protection Administration (NFPA)** Standards Council issued the original NFPA 1670 document that contains the standards on Operations and Training for Technical Search and Rescue Incidents. This document was created for the fire service, and also other emergency response agencies such as EMS, and law enforcement. The standards within the NFPA 1670 identify and establish levels of functional capability for organizations that currently are or are considering conducting operations at technical search and rescue incidents. As stated from this document, "the requirements of the standard shall apply to organizations that provide response to technical search and rescue incidents". (*Source: Reprinted with permission from the NFPA's website. www.nfpa.org. Copyright © 2013, National Fire Protection Association, Quincy, MA. All rights reserved.*) NFPA 1670 encompasses six additional disciplines besides structural collapse rescue: confined space rescue, trench and evacuation rescue, vehicle and machinery rescue, wilderness search and rescue, rope rescue, and water rescue. (*Source: Reproduced with permission from NFPA 1670-2004, Standard on Operations and Training for Technical Search and Rescue Incidents. Copyright © 2004, National Fire Protection Association. This reprinted material is not the complete and official position of the NFPA on the referenced subject, which is represented only by the standard in its entirety.*)

> **Side Bar**
>
> **NFPA 1670**
>
> The purpose of NFPA 1670 is to assist the Authority Having Jurisdiction in the following areas:
>
> - Assessing the structural collapse rescue hazard (the potential for occurring) within an agency's response area
> - Identifying the level of operational capability of personnel and agencies
> - Establishing operational criteria

NFPA 1670 is a tool that guides an organization through the process of assessing its own capabilities in both preparation and operational readiness for a structural collapse response. A department, organization, work group, committee, or person who makes the decisions and enforces the policies for the structural collapse rescue team, department, or agency is known as the **Authority Having Jurisdiction (AHJ)** (National Fire Protection Administration, 2009). The AHJ is responsible for ensuring that the personnel who make up the team conducting technical rescue operations meet the standards within this document. This will assist the AHJ in establishing its desired level of operational capability at a structural collapse incident. The AHJ teams' level of training translates into its level of capability, which strongly dictates the team's ability to effectively identify and manage hazards associated with a specific incident. Aside from these qualities, another portion that has to be factored in is the team's accessibility to available resources, both internal and external.

NFPA 1670 separates the provider levels of capability for structural collapse into three classifications: Awareness, Operations, and Technician. An AHJ, based on its functional capabilities, will make the determination about which level of operations it has the ability to operate. Once the decision is made, the AHJ should establish a written **standard operating procedure (SOP)** that encompasses its level of functional capability to provide structural collapse rescue (NFPA, 2009).

AWARENESS LEVEL

The **awareness level** "represents the minimum capabilities of organizations that provide technical search and rescue incidents". (*Source: Reproduced with permission from NFPA 1670-2004, Standards on Operations and Training for Technical Search and Rescue Incidents. Copyright © 2004, National Fire Protection Association. This reprinted material is not the complete and official position of the NFPA on the referenced subject, which is represented only by the standard in its entirety.*). This level of training prepares the personnel within the department or team to conduct a proper size-up of the scene, hazard recognition, scene management, and a safe basic search and rescue of victims that are readily accessible. The minimum training for an organization shall be at the awareness level (NFPA, 2009). A provider trained in awareness level and responding to a structural collapse incident may be faced with being the first-arriving resource to a structural collapse incident. (See the sidebar for a list of objectives as specified within the NFPA 1670 for the awareness level trained provider.)

Side Bar

Objectives for an Awareness Level Provider (NFPA 1670)

5.2 Awareness Level:

5.2.1 Organizations operating at the awareness level for structural collapse incidents shall meet the requirements specified in Sections 5.2 and 7.2 (awareness level for confined space search and rescue).

5.2.2 Organizations operating at the awareness level for structural collapse incidents shall implement procedures for the following:

(1) Recognizing the need for structural collapse search and rescue
(2) Identifying the resources necessary to conduct structural collapse search and rescue operations
(3) Initiating the emergency response system for structural collapse incidents
(4) Initiating site control and scene management
(5) Recognizing the general hazards associated with structural collapse incidents, including the recognition of applicable construction types and categories and the expected behaviors of components and materials in a structural collapse
(6) Identifying the five types of collapse patterns and potential victim locations
(7) Recognizing the potential for secondary collapse
(8) Conducting visual and verbal searches at structural collapse incidents, while using approved methods for the specific type of collapse
(9) Recognizing and implementing the FEMA Task Force Search and Rescue Marking System, Building Marking System (structure/hazard evaluation), Victim Location Marking System, and Structure Marking System (structure identification within a geographic area)
(10) Removing readily accessible victims from structural collapse incidents

OPERATIONAL LEVEL

The **operations level** "represents the capability of organizations to respond to technical search and rescue incidents and identify hazards, use equipment and apply limited techniques specific in this standard to support and participate in technical search and rescue incidents". (*Source: Reproduced with permission from NFPA 1670-2004, Standards on Operations and Training for Technical Search and Rescue Incidents. Copyright © 2004 by the National Fire Protection Association.*) This level of training prepares the responders within with the department or organization to do what is listed above as well as shoring and rescues from light frame, ordinary, reinforced, and unreinforced masonry construction.

TECHNICIAN LEVEL

The **technician level** "represents the capability of organizations to respond to technical search and rescue incidents, to identify hazards, use equipment, and apply advanced techniques specified in this standard necessary to coordinate, perform, and supervise technical search and rescue incidents". (*Source: Reproduced with permission from NFPA 1670-2004, Standards on Operations and Training for Technical Search and Rescue Incidents. Copyright © 2004 by the National Fire Protection Association.*) This advanced level of training gives the responder the ability to conduct shoring and rescue operations from concrete tilt-up, reinforced concrete, and heavy steel construction.

Best Practice

Mutual Aid Box Alarm System

It is not practical to have a response team for every single event that might occur. However, various agencies have capabilities that may be needed during certain events. One of the most creative and useful processes came out of the Chicago area. A group of innovative fire captains and chiefs seeking to automate mutual aid in their region created the Mutual Aid Box Alarm System (MABAS) in Illinois in 1970. From its inception in the Chicago suburbs, MABAS has grown to a statewide, nondiscriminatory mutual aid response system for fire, EMS, and specialized incident operational teams. Other states are adopting MABAS procedures and structure because, quite simply, they work well—every day, for all hazards, and in disasters near and far. The system is well tested, standardized, and refined by experience.

MABAS officials will assist those who want to learn more about this system and adopt something similar in another state. This willingness to share information and serve as advisors is a hallmark of MABAS in Illinois. Sharing the MABAS effort in Illinois are representatives from the Office of the State Fire Marshal, Department of Public Health–EMS Division, and the Illinois Fire Chiefs Association. The system defines a resource response plan to any location within the state when the governor issues a Declaration of Disaster. MABAS signed a Memorandum of Understanding with the Illinois Emergency Management Agency on January 16, 2001, which was a first in Illinois history.

You can also obtain a book specific on the story of MABAS and an overview of the system—what it is, why it works, and what it can do for your fire department and state from the International Fire Chief's Association. For more in-depth study, MABAS has volumes of information on its website, including contact information and details and documents on the association's structure, deployment and operations, special teams, and assets.

As a structural collapse rescue provider progresses to the technician level, additional NFPA standards must be followed. NFPA 1006 "Standard for Rescue Technician Professional Qualifications" outlines the job performance requirements that must be met prior to a structural collapse rescue provider's certification as a technician-level provider. These requirements cover extensive knowledge in scene size-up, capabilities and limitations of search instruments and resources, types of building construction, occupancy classifications, collapse patterns, victim behavior, and potential areas of survivability. Additional requirements are placed on personnel who go on to specialize in the different functions within the team, such as those who fill positions within the command structure such as the task force leader. Other specialty tracks include logistics leader, plans leader, search specialist, and rescue leader.

BUILDING CONSTRUCTION

Search and rescue operations may occur within a variety of structures built with different materials. It is important to understand that every type of material and construction type has its own unique characteristics. These factors must be considered when preparing to conduct any search and rescue operation. Depending on the age, size, and demographics of the community, construction types can be extremely varied, all bringing their own unique challenges to the emergency services that support that community. Having this knowledge ahead of time will provide information to predict collapse patterns and determine where likely void spaces may be. In situations where a building may have suffered only a partial collapse, then the possibility of further movement of the structure can be predicted. It is highly recommended that further study on this subject should be conducted continually as the dynamics of engineering constantly change.

LOADS

An engineer designs a building to transfer **loads** displayed by the building down to the earth. In structural design, a **design load** in most cases will be greater than the load that the structure is expected to support. This is because structural engineers will incorporate a safety margin into their design of the structure to ensure that the structure will be able to support weights beyond the expected load. The two different loads factored into the design are dead load and live load. The intended use of the building helps determines the **live load**. The live load includes the weight of all the furnishings and people in the building. This may include production equipment, furniture, stock, supplies, and the people who will either work, visit, or live inside. Invariably, there will be situations in which the use of the building changes dramatically from the original intended use, redefining the entire dynamic of the structure. In some cases, the live load may increase beyond the design parameters. This situation results in undesigned loads being imposed upon the structure. **Dead load**, also referred to as a **concentrated load**, has forces applied to a structural component at one point rather than being distributed uniformly across a span. An example of a concentrated load is a beam that crosses over a girder or a large HVAC unit located on a roof. Another factor that the engineer must consider is a **distributed load**. Examples of distributed loads are weight from rain water or snow spread out over a roof section. Engineers must also take into account **impact load**. An impact load is a dynamic load, as opposed to a static load. This can result from the motion of forces caused by heavy wind gust, seismic activity, machinery, elevators, vehicle movement, and large numbers of people who may occupy a structure. All of these examples defining the different types of loads that bear upon the components of a structure are examples of **force**.

COMPONENTS OF A STRUCTURE

A structure is built with different components that are designed to take the total design weight of the structure, and then transfer and distribute its mass. These components are designed to be subjected to the different loads and stresses placed upon them as they interconnect to one another, forming the skeleton of the structure, allowing the transfer, and distributing the load to the foundation that then becomes part of the earth. Other components, such as floors and ceilings, are later incorporated into the structure, providing additional strength. These components are made up of columns or pillars, beams, and walls.

A column or pillar is a structural component that transmits, through compression, the weight of the structure above downward and parallel through its center to other structural components below. In communities located around seismic zones, columns and pillars are designed to resist lateral (side to side) forces that may be imposed during an earthquake. Columns and pillars are typically used to support beams or arches on which the upper parts of walls or ceilings rest. Some columns or pillars are only designed as a decorative feature and not needed for structural purposes.

In many cases, walls may be incorporated and built into a column or pillar. Walls will typically connect columns together. These may be designed as load-bearing or nonload-bearing walls. Walls should, for all practical purposes, be considered a slender narrow column or pillar, but if they are of load-bearing design, they most likely will be supporting the load of the beams, walls, floors, roofs, and other components above them. This is a very important detail for a collapse rescue team to note when deciding where to place shores to support the load from a certain section of a structure. Nonload-bearing walls are very weak and only designed to support their own weight.

A beam is designed to transfer loads perpendicular to its long axis. Beams are supported by columns, pillars, and walls. Additional walls and columns may be placed onto the top of a beam, further creating compression force and tension force to the bottom of the beam. Beams are designed to accomplish many different purposes in construction and can be built or formed from a variety of materials, such as steel, concrete, and wood. (See the sidebar for some of the most common types of beams.)

Side Bar

Common Types of Beams

- A *cantilever beam* is supported at only one end. The beam carries the load directly over the top of the support where the unsupported ends overhang. This design places the top of the beam in tension and the bottom of the beam in compression.
- A *continuous beam* is a horizontal beam placed on top of several supports or columns.
- A *girder* is a beam constructed of steel, wood, or reinforced concrete and used as a main horizontal support in a building or bridge that supports other beams.
- A *joist* is a beam constructed from wood, steel, or concrete that is set parallel, connecting two or more walls or across a butting girder designed to support a floor or ceiling.
- A *lintel* is a horizontal beam constructed of wood, metal, or stone that spans an opening, as between the uprights of a door or window or between two columns or pillars.
- A *purlin* is a horizontal beam placed along the length of a roof that rests on the main rafters and supports the common rafters or roof decking.
- A *long beam* is constructed from wood or metal and designed to span an opening or room, usually to support the roof or floor above.
- A *truss* is a framework composed of beams, girders, or rods commonly constructed of wood or steel. A truss usually takes the form of a series of triangles, ensuring greater rigidity where there are large spans and heavy loads are expected, especially in bridges and roofs.

Building components are assembled with connectors. Rigid connectors are created by welding components, such as columns or walls to beams. Connectors also may fall into the pinning category, such as screws, bolts, nails, and rivets. Some components are held in place with nothing more than gravity, such as parking garages.

BUILDING MATERIALS

Building components and connectors come together in five common construction types: wood, steel, concrete, reinforced masonry, and unreinforced masonry.

WOOD

The most common material used in the construction of residential and commercial buildings is wood. Wood is a tough, yet inexpensive, option that can be manipulated into nearly any shape to support style of construction. Wood can be attached to components using pinning devices such as nails, bolts, and screws. If done correctly, this makes the structure very resistant to the forces that can be created by earthquakes and high winds. However, in cases of exposure to intense heat from fire, wood will begin to lose its integrity and fail over time. Trusses, particularly I-beams constructed from wood and plywood, will fail in as little as 20 minutes if exposed to high heat.

STEEL

Steel is commonly used in the construction of commercial buildings because of its versatile nature. Steel is known for being very strong and tough against different forces, yet lightweight and modifiable. Steel is also very ductile, allowing it to be stressed beyond its elastic limits and to bend excessively while still maintaining its resistance to fail. Many modern residential structures are now being constructed with lightweight steel columns, beams, and trusses. By themselves, these components can be very flimsy, but once connected together they create a very solid and strong framework that forms the building. Steel components are connected by either pinning, such as rivets and bolts, or by rigid methods such as welding. Steel is most commonly built and formed into girders because of its tensile, compression, and shear strength. If not laterally braced, a steel beam can buckle or twist along its long axis. Steel-framed structures must be designed properly, proportioning to avoid overloading of the vertical columns. When exposed to heat, steel has a tendency to lose its strength. Further exposure to extreme temperatures will cause elongation of the steel, causing the structural components to deform and buckle and leading to the eventual collapse of the building.

CONCRETE

Concrete is used to construct many different structures due to its strength. Concrete is essentially created by using a precise mixture of cement, sand, gravel, and water. Depending on the proportions of these ingredients, the final strength of the concrete will vary. Although concrete maintains very high compression strength, it lacks tensile and shear strength unless sufficient steel can be added to give it adequate strength and ductile properties, making it more similar to steel. Steel bars are cast into sections of concrete to provide for greater tensile strength along the long axis of the slab. These bars, referred to as rebar, are enclosed with steel ties and stirrups that also increase the shear resistance. Concrete is then poured over the rebar, surrounding it and making it part of the slab as it cures. Cables may also be placed throughout the slab prior to curing only to be tensioned later after the curing process. Adding tension to the cables compresses the concrete, giving it added strength. Concrete may be precast, meaning that it is formed and poured at the factory and then delivered to the construction site.

Although concrete is tremendously strong, it too is susceptible to different stressors. Extreme heat exposure from flame impingement can cause spalling, a condition that occurs when natural moisture imbedded inside of the concrete expands due to the heat, causing the concrete to crack. When this occurs, large pockets of concrete will crack into very small particles, leaving large masses of concrete missing. This can be even more catastrophic when the rebar heats up, transferring extreme heat deep inside the concrete slab and causing complete failure of the structure. Under normal conditions over time, concrete will shrink and crack, but that is not the same as spalling.

MASONRY

Masonry can be separated into two categories: reinforced and unreinforced. Reinforced masonry include masonry units such as clay bricks or hollow concrete blocks, in conjunction with steel rebar or cables, grout, and/or mortar combined to strengthen the masonry structure. These walls are built for their load-bearing compression strength. Reinforced masonry walls, when adequately built, possess excellent ductility and are commonly used in communities prone to seismic activity.

Unreinforced masonry does not have steel rebar reinforcements imbedded into the masonry, making it very susceptible to forces. Veneer brick walls are an example of unreinforced masonry and are not designed to be load bearing.

THE FIVE CATEGORIES OF BUILDING CONSTRUCTION

The fire service recognizes five categories of building construction.

TYPE I: FIRE-RESISTIVE CONSTRUCTION

Type I construction is built with noncombustible or limited combustible materials with a fire-resistant rating. This rating gives the material the ability to withstand the effects of fire and prevent its spread. Material used in Type I construction consists of reinforced concrete and monolithic-poured concrete slabs. Buildings constructed from precast or post-tensioned concrete slab can be from one to thirteen stories high. Examples of this type of construction are large multistory structures such as office buildings, apartments, and parking garages.

TYPE II: NONCOMBUSTIBLE CONSTRUCTION

Type II buildings are constructed with steel. Three methods of Type II construction are steel moment framing, braced framing, and light metal construction.

Steel moment frame construction consists of beams and columns joined by a combination of welding and bolting the components together. This method results in resistance to lateral loads caused by wind and mild to moderate earthquakes since the frame is designed to bend and remain elastic, allowing it to return to its original position after the load has been removed. In the case of a major earthquake exhibiting strong ground motion, permanent deformity is likely to occur due to the ductile properties of the steel members. Steel moment frame buildings can be from one to more than a hundred stories with glass and other veneer material attached to the exterior.

Diagonally braced steel framed structures add cross-members to give the structure additional strength. These buildings are typically built from one to twenty stories in height. For the same reasons as in steel moment frame construction, these diagonal braces are susceptible to conditions ranging from distortion and—in extreme cases—buckling, causing catastrophic failure of the columns. Complete collapse is rare; more often, shedding of the exterior veneer, glass, and precast concrete walls can occur due to the distortion.

Light metal buildings are typically preengineered, one- or two-story structures. Examples of light metal structures include garages, storage warehouses, modern office buildings, and, more recently, residential homes. Metal siding and roofing make up the sheathing that covers the exterior. When built well, these structures, can endure small to moderate earthquakes due to the flexibility of the components. However, this is not the case when exposed to heavy windstorms. These forces of nature can cause damage, such as the loss of a wall and roof sheathing, along with the buckling of the purlins and girts that were protected by the sheathing. A pulin is a longitudinal component of the roof frame that typically supports the rafters that connect to the ridge of the roof. The girts acts as a bracing that connects the corner posts of a structure. Progressive collapse can result from further damage, such as tie-rod bracing being stretched and broken as well as the lower cord bracing at the end walls buckling. All of these occurrences can ultimately lead to total collapse of the structure.

TYPE III: ORDINARY CONSTRUCTION

Ordinary construction exhibits exterior load bearing walls made of noncombustible material. However, the roof, floors, and interior framing are constructed primarily or partly of wood along with wood sheathing, such as paneling. Most often, the exterior walls are reinforced masonry, such as brick or concrete block. Examples of older Type III construction include the buildings that line main streets through the older sections of a town or village. These structures were built to accommodate a business, such as a restaurant or small retail store, on the bottom floor and a residential townhouse or apartments on the upper floors. Modern examples of ordinary construction include some strip malls, churches, and other structures built with reinforced block walls and wood truss roofs.

TYPE IV: HEAVY TIMBER CONSTRUCTION

Heavy timber construction is characterized by the utilization of wood structural members of specified minimum size, as well as wood floors and roofs of specified minimum thickness and composition. The load-bearing walls are constructed of reinforced masonry and the non-bearing exterior walls are typically constructed of noncombustible material. Special fasteners and adhesives are used to attach the exposed floor and roof beams, eliminating any concealed spaces. Although this type of construction is considered quite stout, collapse is common in situations where the timbers have been exposed to intense heat from a fire. Prior to the floor or roof collapse, the timber will begin to sag, pulling free from the wall. Without the compression weight from the floor and roof sections, freestanding walls can become unstable and are likely to collapse soon afterward. Examples of Type IV construction include churches and older warehouses and manufacturing facilities.

TYPE V: WOOD FRAME CONSTRUCTION

Wood frame construction is the most common of the five different types of construction. This type of construction is built with wooden studs that rise vertically from the foundation to the top of the structure. The roof and floors are then attached to the vertical studs. The term *lightweight construction* describes the newer type of wood frame structures that are built with lightweight wood trusses for roofs and floors. These trusses are put together with a gusset plate, a type of connector. Gusset plates are square, rectangular, or triangular metal plates with one side displaying hundreds of small spikes that are driven into the joints where the trusses connect together. The trusses rely on the grid system of the truss for its strength. Other types of trusses are constructed using high-strength glue. Although these trusses are strong under normal conditions, exposure to intense heat from a fire can cause both the gusset plates to fail and glue to melt away, causing early failure resulting in collapse. Light frame structures can also collapse when the lower wood frame walls do not possess sufficient strength to resist lateral forces. Examples of Type V construction include single and double occupancy homes, commercial retail buildings, apartments, and some hotels.

TYPES OF COLLAPSES

The type of collapse depends largely on the event, the types of forces imposed, and the type of construction. Each construction type discussed in the preceding sections will tend to exhibit somewhat different collapse patterns depending on several factors. There are four common **collapse patterns**.

LEAN-TO FLOOR COLLAPSE

A lean-to collapse occurs when a roof or floor support fails on one side of the structure, leaving the opposite side of the floor still connected to the adjoining wall. It results in a void space that is close to the wall opposite where the failure occurred, just below the floor or roof of the supported side. (See Figure 7.1.) Due to the increased lateral load being pressed against it, there is an amplified risk of the still-standing wall failing where the floor or roof is still attached.

V-SHAPED FLOOR COLLAPSE

A V-shaped collapse occurs when lower walls or floor joists fail, due to heavy loads located in the

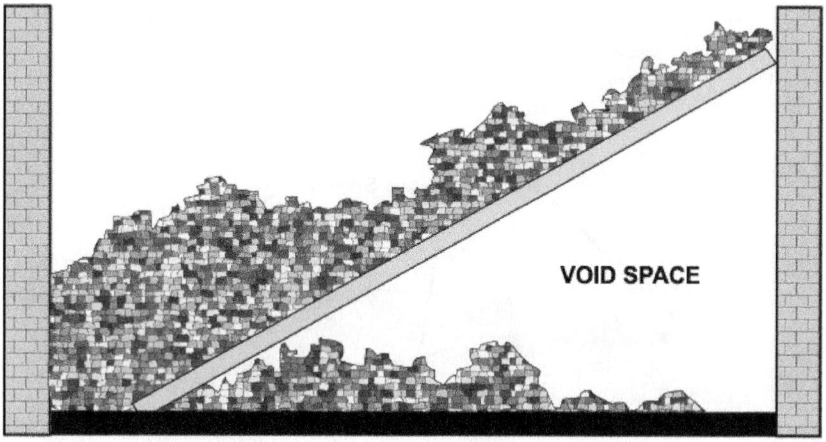

FIGURE 7.1 ■ A lean-to floor collapse. *Source: Reproduced with permission from David C. Harrington, City of Oak Ridge, Tennessee, Fire Department.*

center of the floor overstressing them. This can result in two void spaces being formed on the two walls outside where the collapse occurred. (See Figure 7.2.) This type of collapse is often found in buildings that have experienced chronic decay of the building material along with overload of the area where the collapse occurred.

PANCAKE FLOOR COLLAPSE

A pancake collapse occurs when a complete compromise of the load-bearing walls occurs, causing the floor supports to fail, in turn dropping the floors and the roof on top of each other. (See Figure 7.3.) Limited void space can be created between the floors due to the debris being relocated and allowing space to be created between the floors and roof sections.

CANTILEVER FLOOR COLLAPSE

A cantilever collapse occurs when one or more walls have failed, leaving the other end of the floor(s) attached to the other bearing

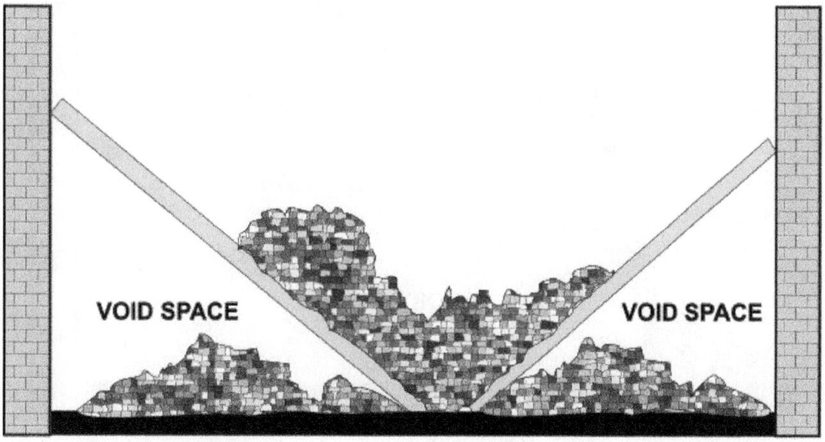

FIGURE 7.2 ■ A V-shaped floor collapse. *Source: Reproduced with permission from David C. Harrington, City of Oak Ridge, Tennessee, Fire Department.*

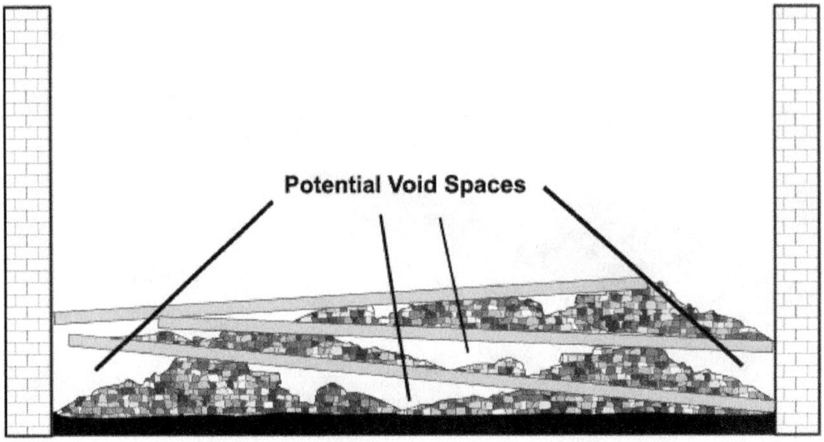

FIGURE 7.3 A pancake floor collapse. *Source: Reproduced with permission from David C. Harrington, City of Oak Ridge, Tennessee, Fire Department.*

wall. (See Figure 7.4.) Voids will be sporadic throughout the debris. Because of the nature of this type of collapse, shoring operations must be completed prior to search and rescue operations.

A-FRAME FLOOR COLLAPSE

An A-Frame collapse, also referred to as a tent-style collapse, occurs when the floor or roof separates from the exterior bearing walls but is still supported by one or more interior walls or partitions. (See Figure 7.5.) Voids are typically created near the center of the structure with the debris above sliding to the exterior walls.

OTHER TYPES OF COLLAPSE

Other types of collapse that can occur do not typically create natural void spaces. With this type of collapse, extreme caution must be

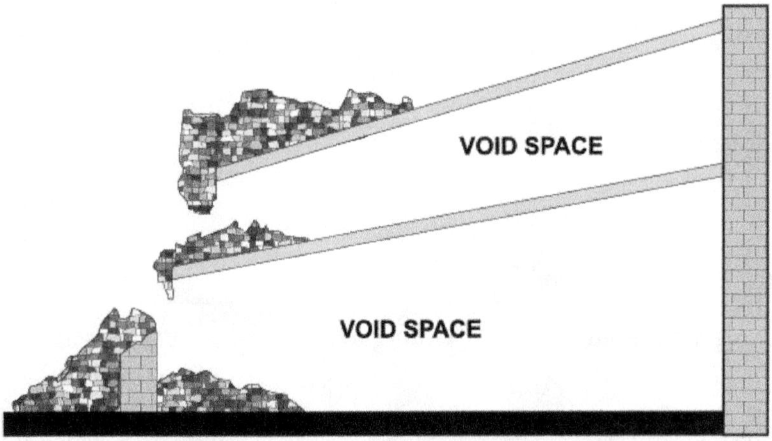

FIGURE 7.4 A cantilever floor collapse. *Source: Reproduced with permission from David C. Harrington, City of Oak Ridge, Tennessee, Fire Department.*

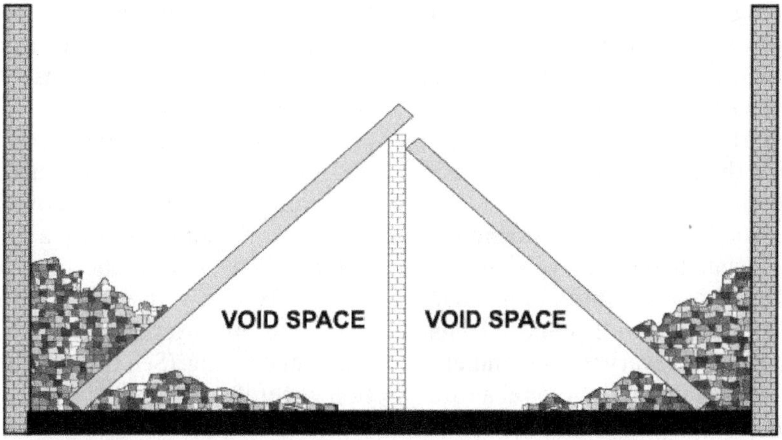

FIGURE 7.5 An A-Frame floor collapse. *Source: Reproduced with permission from David C. Harrington, City of Oak Ridge, Tennessee, Fire Department.*

given to keep resources well outside of the collapse zone as a precautionary measure. A good rule of thumb is to maintain an exclusion area of 1.5 times the height of the building as a potential collapse zone. Many emergency responders have been injured, and even killed, and equipment lost due to unanticipated collapses of exterior walls or structural elements of buildings.

90-Degree Collapse

A 90-degree, or total-wall, collapse occurs when the entire full height of the exterior wall falls outward and over as one unit. This is very common in masonry walls but can also occur in Type V structures with attached veneer walls.

Inward-Outward Wall Collapse

An inward-outward wall collapse occurs when the exterior wall separates horizontally into two sections, with the bottom section of the wall falling outward away from the structure, and the upper section of the wall falling inward. This type of collapse can occur without warning in braced framed buildings and more commonly in wood-frame buildings.

Curtain-Fall Wall Collapse

A curtain-fall wall collapse occurs when a masonry wall collapses literally straight down, resulting in a large rubble pile close to the original structure. This is often associated with brick veneer walls.

Lean-Over Wall Collapse

A lean-over collapse occurs when the building's center of gravity shifts at an upper floor area, resulting in the structure leaning to one side or the other, onto adjacent buildings, or totally collapsing sideways. This type of collapse is more common with Type V construction.

SAFETY

During structural collapse, rescue conditions can change continually, making the operation extremely unpredictable for the responders who are working the scene. However, the risk can be reduced significantly by being aware of all the hazards that can be associated with a structural collapse incident. Safety begins with having a good understanding of all the different facets of a structural collapse incident. A responder must be familiar with the different types of building construction. This knowledge allows for the responder to predict collapse patterns and determine the likelihood of where potential victims may be located.

A major part of any structural collapse rescue mission is the nonnegotiable utilization of operational discipline and teamwork. This is built around a solid **incident command system** within the rescue team itself, working as a component of a much larger incident management team. Following a well-prepared **incident action plan (IAP)**, every team member is responsible for maintaining situational awareness and being committed to looking for unsafe acts and conditions that can affect the safety of all responders on the scene.

Hazards can fall into either of two categories: existing and potential. Existing hazards can be detected with either human senses or by specialized monitoring equipment. This equipment is designed to identify dangers that may not be detectable by our senses, such as an oxygen-deficient or oxygen-enriched, explosive, and toxic atmosphere. Potential hazards are hidden dangers that could present themselves under certain conditions and are very situational depending on the type of incident.

As the operation commences, the **incident commander** may appoint a primary safety officer. The safety officer is responsible for making sure the overall operation is conducted in a safe manner. Depending on the size and complexity of the incident, multiple safety officers may be assigned as lookouts at designated sectors around the site. Depending on the type and location of the involved structure, a site-specific safety officer may also be assigned to assist with identifying and mitigating hazards that are specific to a particular site. These safety officers should be considered subject matter experts on the process or contents within a particular site. Despite the fact that the incident commander or his operations officer may have control of the rescue operations, the safety officer has the authority to cease rescue operations if he identifies a safety concern that requires attention. Once the safety concern is addressed, the rescue operation may continue.

The details addressing the existing and potential hazards of a particular incident are outlined in the incident command system (ICS) forms completed by a contingency of personnel located at the base of operations (BoO). Typically, the safety officer will conduct a safety briefing as part of the overall incident briefing. (See the sidebar for information generally included in a safety briefing.)

Side Bar

The Safety Briefing: Identification of Important Information

- Assigned safety officer(s)
- Safe zones
- Existing and potential hazards
- Mitigation measures
- Escape routes
- Signals used to communicate immediate evaluation, cease rescue operations, and resume rescue operations

The safety plan should constantly be reevaluated and adapted to changing conditions. Any change that may affect the overall safety of an operation must immediately be communicated to the safety officer and the incident commander. These changes must also be communicated during the next safety briefing for the upcoming work period.

RESPONSE

While en route to a structural collapse event there are many **approach hazards** that must be considered. These can include traffic issues especially around congested downtown districts, high winds, high water, washed-out roadways, and downed trees and power lines. It also is important to be aware of other agencies that may be responding to the structural collapse.

The initial response to a reported structural collapse incident can be extremely daunting even for a seasoned veteran. There are many unknowns to consider, both during the response phase and throughout the rescue operation itself. It is recommended that job aids, such as resource guides that contain simple step-by-step procedures and guidelines to help a responder or team manage a complex situation. Typically, these job aids come in the form of a field operations guide (FOG) or manual and are published by different groups depending on the discipline. Structural collapse rescue teams most often refer to the "National Urban Search & Rescue (US&R) Response System: Rescue Field Operations Guide" (FEMA, 2006).

Once on scene, the first step should be to perform a rapid, but thorough, size-up of the scene to recognize and begin mitigating existing hazards, including gas, electrical, water, and **hazardous material**. Scene control should start immediately by establishing a perimeter around the scene. The initial distance away from the collapse for parking an emergency vehicle should be no less than 100 feet. Then **control zones**, referred to as the hot zone, warm zone, and cold zone, can be established. (See Figure 7.6.) (See the sidebar for a description of each of the zones.)

Control zones should be cordoned off with border tape and protected by law enforcement, if possible. Emergency responders can be the target of violence and their equipment stolen, especially during a large catastrophic event. **Federal Emergency Management Agency (FEMA)** urban search and rescue (US&R) teams, if deployed, are now required to have a security force attached to their team for protection. Many state-level US&R teams have followed this trend, creating a security

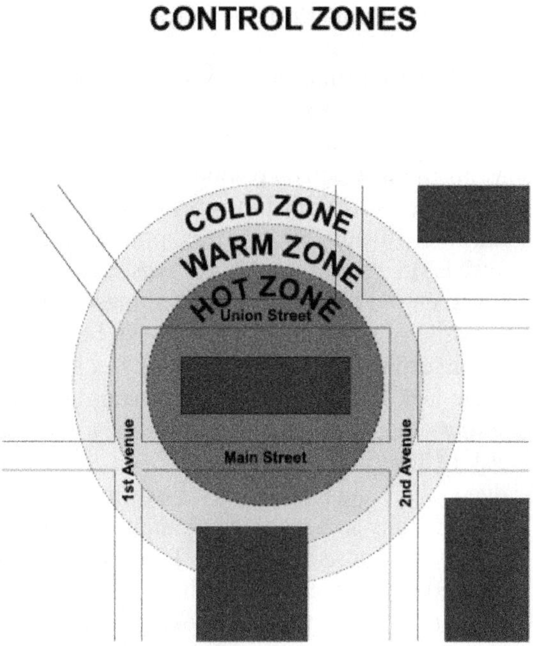

FIGURE 7.6 ■ Control zones are created around an incident to designate safety boundaries.
Source: Reproduced with permission from David C. Harrington, City of Oak Ridge, Tennessee, Fire Department.

Side Bar

Control Zones

Hot Zone—This area includes the collapse zone and area around the structure where existing and potential hazards exist. This area is also where the majority of the search and rescue operation occurs.

Warm Zone—This area surrounds the hot zone and is where some of the support operations occur. Depending on the operation, certain equipment may be staged in this area so that it is available for immediate use.

Cold Zone—This area is where personnel, apparatus, and equipment are staged until needed.

attachment made up of their local and state law enforcement resources.

The first phase of any disaster involves the arrival of the spontaneous rescuers. These rescuers are members of the community. Many of these citizen responders are unskilled in rescue operations but want to help. Others may be off-duty firefighters, police officers, and EMS providers. Many lives have been saved due to the quick actions of these heroes. However, extreme caution must be taken when utilizing these resources. Because of their lack of formalized rescue training and safety equipment in most instances, a greater risk of additional injuries and death can occur due to their failure to recognize existing hazards.

In many communities, Community Emergency Response Teams (CERTs) have been formed. These teams are trained and have the ability to conduct surface search and rescue, meaning that they can call out or hail for victims and, if found, rescue the those victims not trapped in structures. It is not recommended that untrained personnel conduct void space rescues within a structure. However, this does occur without the knowledge of the emergency services having command of the scene, especially on large-scale incidents without enough oversight.

SIZE-UP OF A STRUCTURAL COLLAPSE INCIDENT

Once the command structure is in place and the scene is secure, size-up of the structure can begin. Size-up begins with proper training. Initial training begins with the awareness level, continues to the basic operations level, and progresses through the technician level. Knowing how to predict how structures and materials will react to different external factors, and how to make an unstable situation safe, will help in calculating the potential and existing hazards and what resources will be required to tackle the situation.

PREPLANNING FOR A RESPONSE

Many teams have created preplan books or databases similar to fire preplans that contain detailed drawings and other important information on the specific structures within their jurisdiction. These preplans should provide information for individual structures on the type of building along with the type of material primarily used, floor plans, all types of utilities used, and where their shutoffs are located.

Depending on response guidelines for a specific department or jurisdiction, an initial response to a structural collapse should include fire, rescue, EMS, and law enforcement resources. Public utilities for electric, water, and gas should also be requested immediately in the likelihood that the utilities have been compromised or perhaps caused the incident. If a large number of injured victims is suspected, the local or regional medical control center should be notified as soon as possible so that it can begin making preparations with local hospitals for the possibility of incoming casualties.

Once a disaster is declared, the appropriate plan is implemented and carried out by the participating authorities. Some incidents, however, may be much smaller in magnitude, such as an event affecting only a single residential structure, requiring only a minimal response. It must be remembered, though, that when in doubt one should call early for resources. It is much easier to cancel than to delay calling and have to wait longer for the arrival of assistance.

APPROACHING THE SCENE

On the approach toward the scene, the size-up involves looking for potential and existing hazards that could include downed power lines, smoke plumes, water main breaks that may undermine the roadway, and other indicators that could endanger emergency responders. Environmental factors should also be considered in the size-up. These factors include ice, high water, mud, and other debris that may hamper access to the incident site.

The goal should be to gain control of the scene early and establish secondary staging areas for nonessential apparatus and personnel. This will accomplish several objectives. First, it will allow EMS providers to get the right resources to the right places at the right times. Second, it will allow for the quicker implementation of the accountability system. Third, by restricting direct access to the area around the collapse zone, the potential for a **secondary collapse** of the unstable structure caused by the transfer of vibrations from movement of heavy vehicles is reduced.

THE SIX-SIDED APPROACH

When approaching the collapsed structure, EMS providers should observe the involved structure using a six-sided approach. This 360-degree approach includes all four sides of the building as well as an assessment of the top and bottom of the structure. Seeing the bottom of the structure refers to assessing the ground in and around the structure. Assessing the condition of the structure is the process known as structural triage. Observing and making notes about the following details will assist in determining the action plan:

- Building and Construction Type—Begin by determining what type of construction the building is, along with the type of materials used in the construction process. This information is very important in determining what type of collapse patterns to expect and the potential hazards that will more than likely be found.
- Type of Occupancy—What is the building used for? This information will offer additional insight as to what types of processes are performed within a facility as well as what hazardous material may be stored inside.
- Time of Day the Event Occurred—This assessment gives additional insight as to how many potential victims there may be.
- Age of Structure—The age of a structure, along with its condition, will add to the risk profile of the operation. Older structures that are in a state of disrepair may already be exhibiting compromised structural integrity, even prior to the event that has occurred. Special caution must be taken when working around older structures to keep resources outside of potential collapse zones.
- Structural Integrity of the Building—Are the corners of the building straight? Are there any visible openings such as doors or windows and, if so, are they straight or twisted? Is there the potential for a secondary collapse? Signs of secondary collapse include formed cracks in masonry or block walls, out-of-plumb walls, unconnected beams, and other dangling debris.
- Extent of the Collapse—Is the collapse partial or complete? Partial collapses will have a greater likelihood of victims being trapped in void spaces within the collapsed area. Victims may also be inside unaffected areas but with their egress from the structure compromised. Special care must be taken not to compromise exiting structural components, which in turn could lead to additional collapses.
- Mechanism of Collapse—Is there a determination based on the collected information as to what led to the collapse? The mechanism of collapse, such as a single load-bearing wall collapsing leading to a lean-to collapse, will define what type of void spaces and potential victim locations to expect.
- Other Buildings or Structures That Are Involved—Is this event going to be on a larger scale than originally thought? If so, more resources will be required.
- Additional Hazards—Are any additional hazards noted that were not seen during the approach to the scene? Situational awareness is a must on any emergency scene due to the fluid nature of the situation. Every effort has to be made to not only recognize the existing hazards but also to think ahead about potential hazards that have yet to surface.

THE "GO–NO GO" RISK/BENEFIT ASSESSMENT

As a rescue team conducts an assessment of a collapse, team members will take into account the factors in the preceding list and will conduct a "go–no go" risk/benefit assessment. This assessment guides EMS providers in determining if the risk profile of a specific collapsed structure is truly worth the benefit that can be gained from placing rescuers in harm's way. The "go–no go" risk/benefit factors include many of the same things considered during any other rescue incident.

- Type of Event, When It Occurs, and Occupancy Type—This will determine the potential for victims being trapped inside the structure.
- Type of Collapse—This can define the type and condition of potential void space that may exist. A small probability of void spaces translates into a small probability of survivable victims.
- Time Required to Access Victims—This is determined by estimating the time it will take to gain access to the first victim. To calculate this time, first consider the time it will take to cut through the floors, walls, roof sections, and debris, then shore and brace the passageways as you proceed.
- Likelihood of Secondary Collapses—Indicators of a secondary collapse include cracked or missing mortar on masonry or block walls, walls that are displaced and not attached to the main building framework, creaks or noises coming from the structure, and any pieces of building material peeling off or dangling from the structure. This potential may be amplified by aftershocks from an earthquake or structural integrity compromise from other related factors.
- Intelligence Reports—Are there credible witness reports of trapped victims? Additional indicators may be found by search specialists using listening devices or cameras and by search dogs hitting on any sounds or scent indicators.
- "No Go" Conditions—Are there any "no go" conditions? These conditions, which would automatically stop or delay a rescue operation, can include anything that could compromise the safety of the rescuers. This would include unmitigated hazardous material, fire, aftershocks, high water, unsecured utilities, and security issues. Once the recognized issue has been mitigated, operations may continue.

SEARCHING FOR VICTIMS

The search for victims begins during the building triage phase of the size-up process. Victims who escaped the structure should be gathered in an area well outside of the collapse zone and interviewed. This allows for collecting information about who may still be inside the structure. This can be a critical step in how the operation may proceed once rescue teams arrive. If it is possible that victims are still trapped within a partially or fully collapsed structure, rescue teams will weigh the risk and benefit of conducting a more aggressive search and rescue operation. If it can be established early that all occupants of the structure were able to escape, then rescue teams will not have to be needlessly put at risk by searching the unstable structure.

Many companies, through their emergency procedures, have an accountability plan in place. This plan will normally address an escape plan, an employee staging area or assembly point, and a person or series of people who are appointed to maintain a list of the employees for whom they are responsible at that assembly point. If someone is missing, the responsible person must report it immediately to his supervisor, the head of security, or the company's safety director. Preventing employees from leaving the premises makes it easier to account for those who may still be missing.

Victims who are injured should immediately be triaged, treated, and transported in accordance with local protocols. Uninjured victims can be moved to a safe area, such as a bus or another building, outside of the collapse zone.

Part of the size-up process includes interviewing victims who have been evacuated from the collapse. It may be possible for them to provide valuable information about unaccounted-for persons and what may have happened just prior to the collapse. They should be asked the following questions:

- Was there a smell of natural gas or any other odor prior to the event?
- Was there an explosion or fire?
- Are there any hazardous materials stored inside the structure? If so, what, where, and how much?
- Did the business or an occupant receive a bomb threat prior to the event?

A 360-degree search should be conducted for injured victims who are accessible from outside the structure or lightly trapped by debris that may be lying around the site. In stable structures that are deemed safe to enter, physical searches may occur. Working in teams of two, rescue personnel should simultaneously conduct a right-side and left-side search of each room. Search teams should look for victims trapped under any debris and listen for any sounds that could indicate a trapped victim. These sounds may include cries for help, moans, and even knocking noises created by the victims. If it can be safely done, victims who are lightly trapped should be accessed, triaged, immobilized, and removed to a medical treatment area that has been established by EMS. From there, EMS should further assess, stabilize, and transport in accordance with their mass casualty incident (MCI) protocols.

When dealing with a collapse situation, there may be a confined space situation as well. A confined space is enclosed and has limited access and egress, is not designed for continual human habitation, may present with engulfment hazards, and is likely to have the potential for a hazardous atmosphere. A hazardous atmosphere can potentially contain contaminants as well as low oxygen levels. Many would-be rescuers—professionals and citizens alike—are killed each year in confined spaces while attempting to rescue a victim who may already be dead. It must be understood that rescue services can be held accountable to the Occupational Safety and Health Administration (OSHA) when a rescuer is injured or killed in a confined space, especially if state and federal regulations were not followed. Technical-level structural collapse rescue teams are trained and equipped to function safely inside confined spaces.

The incident commander or task force leader will assign a recon team, also referred to as a triage team, to assess the damaged structures within a geographical area. During this process, the recon team will determine what structures will be searched and in what order. Greater priority will be given to those structures that have suffered only a partial collapse due to a greater likelihood of survivors and the greater speed at which these structures can be searched and cleared. A series of building triage forms are completed by the recon team that grades each structure, along with attached notes and diagrams of the building in question. The forms describe in detail the probable locations of void spaces, shoring requirements, and so on. These teams will make recommendations based on their findings, and they may determine that the structure may be too hazardous for search and rescue operations to be conducted. This information is forwarded to the physical search teams that will be sent in to conduct a physical search of the structure. The **physical search team** is tasked with conducting interior searches without the use of specialized equipment. They may assist victims out of the building if found and not trapped.

GEOGRAPHIC LOCATIONS: TERMINOLOGY

Based on the layout of the structure, the recon team will use a rather simple but standard method for describing the geographic locations of the building. The terms are used consistently by all emergency services to identify the different sides and levels of a building.

EXTERNAL VIEWS

Each of the four sides of the building is just that: a *side*. The front of the building is referred to as "Side A." From there, the other sides are labeled in a clockwise motion around the building. As you move to the left around the building, you will be on "Side B." The rear of the building is "Side C," and "Side D" is the right-hand side. (See Figure 7.7.)

INTERNAL VIEWS

The building itself is further broken into five internal quadrants. To do this, the building is divided into four equal imaginary squares, with a fifth small square quadrant placed in the center of the building. The internal quadrant that represents the left half of Side A and the right half of Side B is referred to as Quadrant A. The left half of Side B and the right half of Side C are referred to as Quadrant B. Quadrants C and D are referred to in the same manner. The center fifth quadrant that makes up the core of the building is referred to as Quadrant E. (See Figure 7.8.)

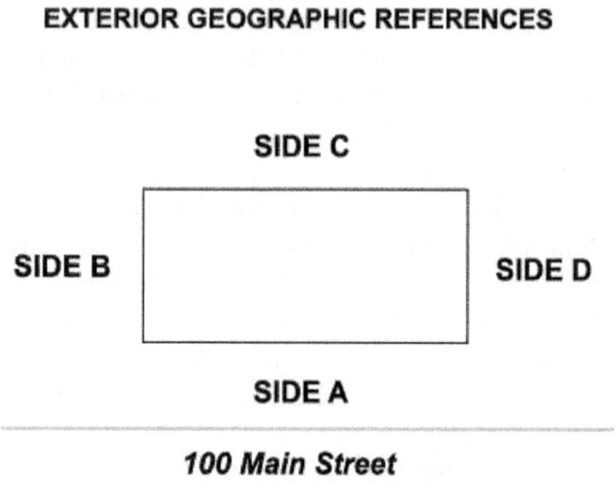

FIGURE 7.7 Common references are used to designate the different sides of a structure. *Source: Reproduced with permission from David C. Harrington, City of Oak Ridge, Tennessee, Fire Department.*

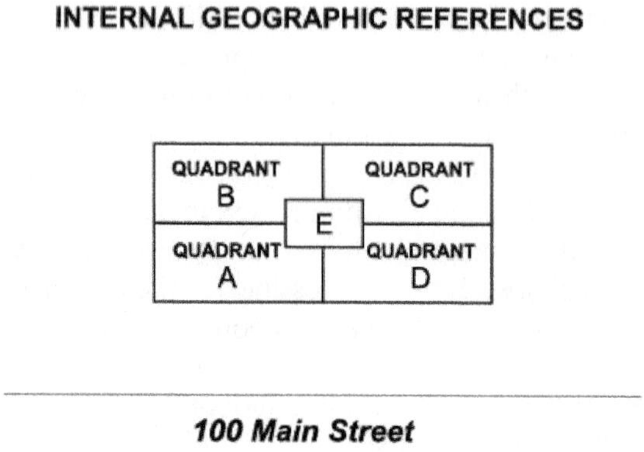

FIGURE 7.8 Common references are used to designate the interior areas of a structure. *Source: Reproduced with permission from David C. Harrington, City of Oak Ridge, Tennessee, Fire Department.*

DIFFERENT LEVELS WITHIN A STRUCTURE

Stories are referred to as *divisions*. The first floor is Division 1. The second story is Division 2, and so on. Basement divisions are designated by their levels below ground. The first lower level just below ground is referred to as Division B1. The second floor below ground is referred to as Division B2, and so on. (See Figure 7.9.)

STRUCTURAL COLLAPSE MARKING SYSTEMS

Structural collapse rescue teams utilize standardized FEMA Structural Collapse Marking Systems as part of a procedure for identifying

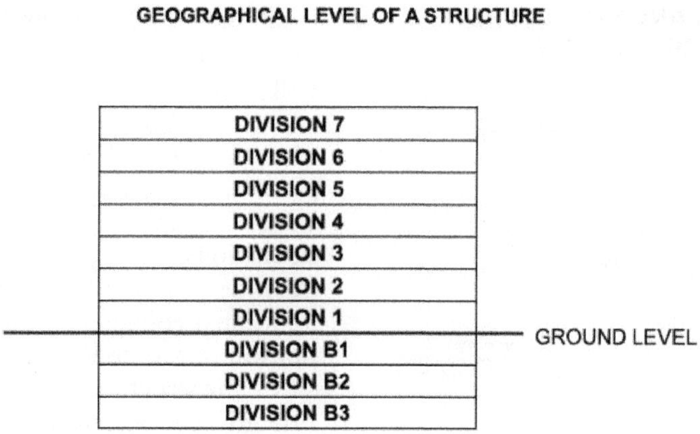

FIGURE 7.9 Elevation references designate the different levels both above and below ground. *Source: Reproduced with permission from David C. Harrington, City of Oak Ridge, Tennessee, Fire Department.*

and communicating hazards and search results of buildings involved in widespread disasters:

- Building and Structure Marking System
- Search Assessment Marking System
- Victim Location Marking System

THE BUILDING AND STRUCTURE MARKING SYSTEM

The Building and Structure Marking System is used to identify the buildings within a geographic area that have been affected by widespread devastation where many of the normal indicators that we use, such as street signs or house numbers, may be gone. The marking system allows teams to re-create the layout of a geographic area and then deliver this information back to the command post where it is documented, evaluated, and prioritized for decision making. Other markings may be added to the area to indicate street names and addresses. The building and structure markings also identify what was found during the assessment of the building. This would include any hazards such as stability issues, hazardous materials, rodents, and so on. This information determines if the building is safe for rescuers to enter and search.

The US&R teams rely on these markings as communication mediums that assist them in determining what buildings have been assessed and are safe to search, which buildings have been searched, and any problems that were encountered. This also reduces the likelihood of buildings being searched twice due to miscommunication.

The building and structure markings begin as a 2-feet-square box that is placed on an exterior wall adjacent to the primary entry point or, if the building is mostly collapsed, on a rubble pile. This square is only placed on the wall or debris pile after a hazard assessment is conducted and documented on the hazardous assessment form.

A square is typically spray-painted on the wall or a visible debris pile near the entrance of the structure in an international orange color. A painted single box or square with nothing painted inside the marking indicates that the structure is relatively safe for search and rescue operations to be conducted with little danger of further collapse. A square with

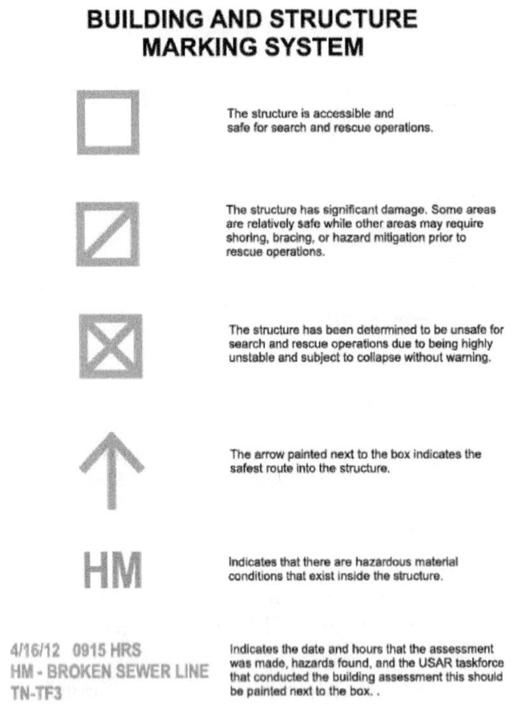

FIGURE 7.10 A building and structure marking system indicates which buildings have or have not been assessed, which are safe or unsafe, and what problems have already been encountered. *Source: Reproduced with permission from David C. Harrington, City of Oak Ridge, Tennessee, Fire Department.*

a diagonal line painted from the top right corner down to the bottom left corner indicates that the structure has been significantly damaged. Although some areas within the structure may be safe, other areas will require some sort of shoring, bracing, and possibly removal of hazards prior to additional search and rescue operations. A single square with an "X" painted in it indicates that the structure has been deemed unsafe for search and rescue operations, meaning that the structure has been determined to be highly unstable and additional collapses are likely to occur without warning. (See Figure 7.10.)

If the structure has been determined to be safe for operations, a single arrow will be painted adjacent to the square on the left or right side of the square that indicates to rescue personnel the location of the safest travel entry into the structure. Additional information may be added, such as the letters "HM," which indicate that a hazmat condition may exist either inside or on the outside adjacent to the structure. (See Figure 7.11.)

THE SEARCH MARKING SYSTEM

The Search Marking System used by the physical search team is designed to let other rescue teams know that a search is actively being conducted or has been completed. It also communicates who conducted the search, when it was completed, what if any hazards were identified, and the results of the search. Again, this system is used to reduce any redundancy.

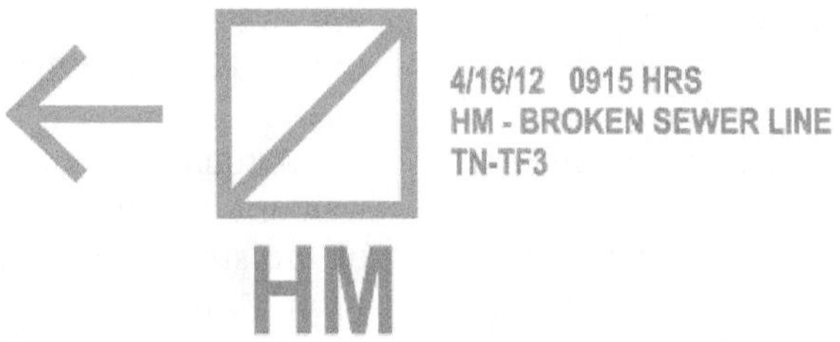

FIGURE 7.11 This marking indicates the level of damage, potential hazards, point of entry, by who and when the assessment was conducted. *Source: Reproduced with permission from David C. Harrington, City of Oak Ridge, Tennessee, Fire Department.*

When search and rescue personnel prepare to enter a structure, they will first paint a single diagonal line creating a half of an "X" from the top right down to the bottom left, indicating to other rescue teams that may come up on the structure that an active operation is being conducted inside. Once the interior operation is concluded, the search and rescue team upon exit will paint another diagonal line, completing the "X." (See Figure 7.12.)

Additional information will be painted inside each of the four sections of the "X." The top section lists the date and time the search and rescue team exited the structures. The left section names the US&R team that conducted the search and rescue operation. The bottom section provides a count of the number of live and deceased victims. The right section indicates the personal hazards found inside. The completion of this mark indicates to other search and rescue teams the completion and results of the operation. (See Figure 7.13.)

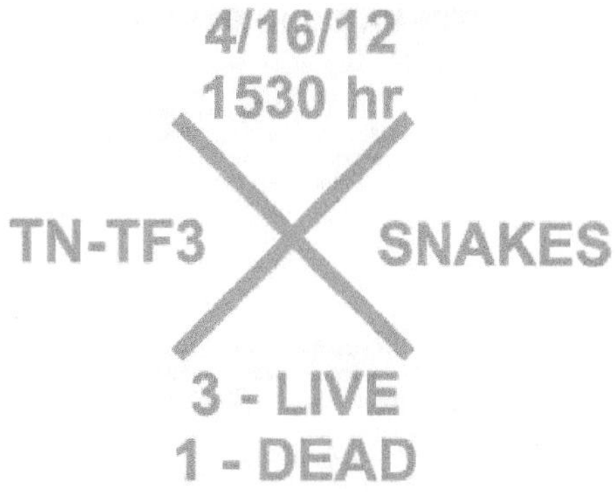

FIGURE 7.13 This marking indicates that a search team has conducted and completed an interior search of a structure, leaving the results of their findings. *Source: Reproduced with permission from David C. Harrington, City of Oak Ridge, Tennessee, Fire Department.*

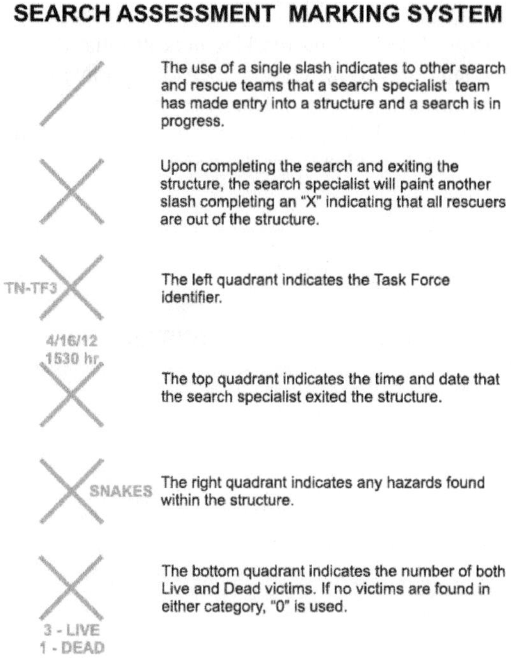

FIGURE 7.12 A search assessment marking system is used by search teams as they conduct an interior structural search. *Source: Reproduced with permission from David C. Harrington, City of Oak Ridge, Tennessee, Fire Department.*

VICTIM LOCATION MARKING SYSTEM

The victim location marking system is used to identify where victims are located within the structure. This marking indicator may be placed either on the exterior or interior of the structure in close proximity of where the victim is believed to be located, as well as whether it is believed that the victim is alive or dead. The painted "V" should be approximately 2 feet in height. A single arrow should also be painted to indicate the exact location of the victim. Above the "V," the task force identifier is painted—for example, "TN-1" (Tennessee Task Force 1). (See Figure 7.14.)

Once the victim location is confirmed, a circle will be painted around the "V." An example of this is if a search team hears a noise suspected of coming from a victim, a "V" may be painted in the area where the victim

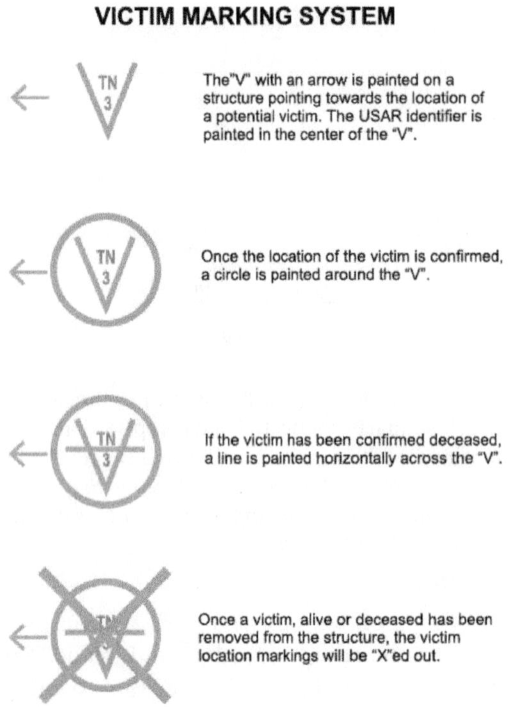
VICTIM MARKING SYSTEM
TN 3
The "V" with an arrow is painted on a structure pointing towards the location of a potential victim. The USAR identifier is painted in the center of the "V".
Once the location of the victim is confirmed, a circle is painted around the "V".
If the victim has been confirmed deceased, a line is painted horizontally across the "V".
Once a victim, alive or deceased has been removed from the structure, the victim location markings will be "X"ed out.

FIGURE 7.14 ■ A victim marking system is used by search teams to indicate where a victim has been located within a structure. *Source: Reproduced with permission from David C. Harrington, City of Oak Ridge, Tennessee, Fire Department.*

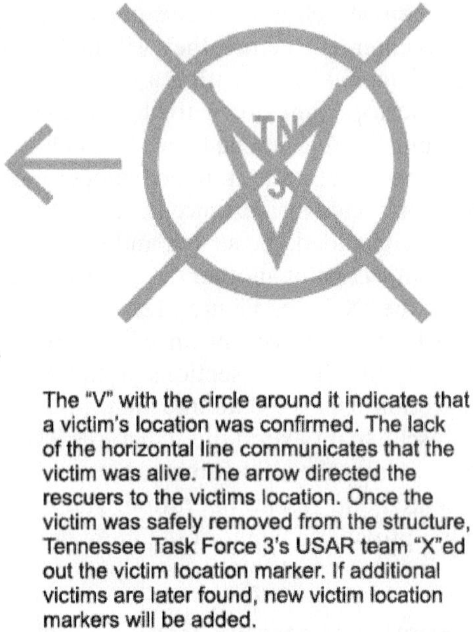
TN 3
The "V" with the circle around it indicates that a victim's location was confirmed. The lack of the horizontal line communicates that the victim was alive. The arrow directed the rescuers to the victims location. Once the victim was safely removed from the structure, Tennessee Task Force 3's USAR team "X"ed out the victim location marker. If additional victims are later found, new victim location markers will be added.

FIGURE 7.15 ■ This marking indicates that the rescue team has confirmed the location of a live victim and has removed them from the structure. *Source: Reproduced with permission from David C. Harrington, City of Oak Ridge, Tennessee, Fire Department.*

may be located. The team then can confirm that location when search cameras are used to see the victim. If the victim if found, the search crews will paint the circle around the "V" to confirm his location. (See Figure 7.15.)

If a victim is located and confirmed to be deceased, a horizontal line will be painted across the "V." Once rescue teams have removed the victim, a large "X" will be painted completely through the circle. This will signal to additional rescue teams that no additional rescue efforts are required at that location. (See Figure 7.16.)

Depending upon how many structures are damaged, this process will continue until every structure assigned to a specific team has

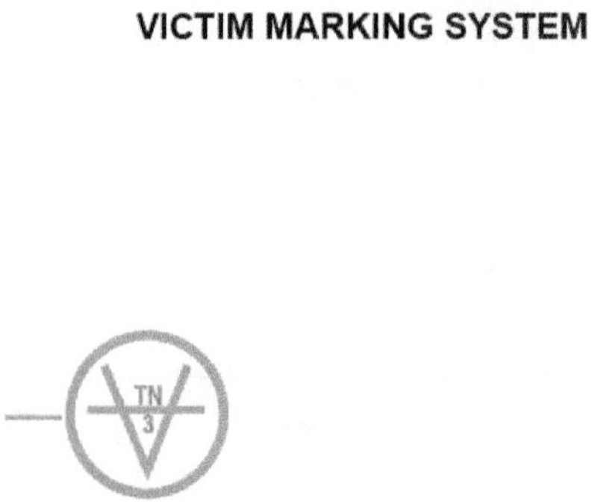

FIGURE 7.16 ■ This marking indicates that the search team has confirmed the location of a deceased victim within the structure. *Source: Reproduced with permission from David C. Harrington, City of Oak Ridge, Tennessee, Fire Department.*

VICTIM MARKING SYSTEM

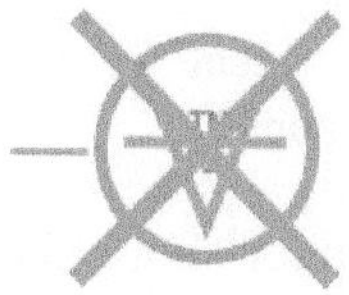

FIGURE 7.17 ■ This marking indicates that the rescue team has removed the deceased victim from the structure. *Source: Reproduced with permission from David C. Harrington, City of Oak Ridge, Tennessee, Fire Department.*

been triaged, prioritized, and searched, and all victims are removed. (See Figure 7.17.)

TREATMENT OF PERSONS INVOLVED IN A STRUCTURAL COLLAPSE

It is common during large structural collapse events for there to be multiple persons needing treatment. Many of them may be walking wounded suffering from a variety of injuries such as these:

- Musculoskeletal injuries: broken bones
- Soft tissue injuries: abrasions, lacerations, bruises, punctures, and impaled objects
- Internal injuries: internal bleeding
- Head injuries: skull fractures, concussions
- Burns: thermal, chemical, and radiological
- Respiratory distress

These persons should be removed quickly to safe areas outside of the collapse zone and triaged by EMS. Further steps should be taken to prevent shock by controlling bleeding and maintaining body heat.

SPECIAL MEDICAL CONSIDERATIONS

Crush syndrome is a re-perfusion injury resulting from a heavy object being released on top of a victim's limb or torso. As the weight of debris or an object sits on a patient's limb or lower torso, it restricts the blood blow to the portion of the body that is on the opposite side of the object. The lack of perfusion to the limb or limbs prevents oxygenated blood from getting to the cells and also prevents the carbon dioxide that is carried away from the cells from getting back to the lungs, where it would be exchanged with oxygenated air as part of the respiratory process. As a result, the stagnated blood begins to build up lactic acid, myoglobin, potassium, and phosphorus, which are all products of the process of rhabdomyolysis. Rhabdomyolysis is the breakdown of skeletal muscle damaged by this ischemic condition. When released into the system, these by-products can cause sudden cardiac arrest and renal failure in its victims.

In some cases, patients who are still trapped can present with normal vital signs because the body is compensating. Victims may present with or complain of the following:

- Numbness in the limb or limbs distal of the weight
- Anxiety, restlessness, or a feeling of impending doom
- Difficulty breathing with increased respiratory rate
- Normal to increased heart rate
- Pale, cool, clammy skin (diaphoresis)

Part of the treatment will include preparing to secure the airway and support the victim's respirations. The patient may be administered certain medications by intravenous (IV) or intraosseous (IO) infusion, which can reverse buildup of the by-product, in turn reducing some of the effects on the heart and renal system.

Compartment syndrome is a condition somewhat similar to crush syndrome and characterized by compression of the nerves, blood vessels, and muscles. This can include the limbs as well as the whole torso. Increased swelling in the compartment due to internal bleeding of the tissue or swelling of the muscle distal of the object trapping the limb compresses against the blood vessels, in turn decreasing perfusion to the tissues. Signs and symptoms of compartment syndrome include these:

- Pain early in the process
- Paresthesia (the feeling of pins and needles)
- Numbness in the extremity distal of the compression
- Swelling and discoloration of the affected limb
- Increased capillary refill time in the affected limbs, primarily the fingers

Treatments should be geared toward securing the patient's airway, assisting breathing with supplemental oxygen administration, bleeding control, fracture stabilization, and spinal immobilization. To immobilize and transport the patient through narrow openings and the tunnels of shoring, most rescue teams use a device called the Sked. The Sked is a single piece of pliable heavy-duty plastic that wraps around the victim, keeping him aligned. The victim is typically placed in a rappelling harness if he has to be raised vertically during the extraction and then secured into the device. While inside the Sked, the patient is hauled out of the space using a series of haul systems made up of rope and other rappelling hardware. Once outside of the collapse zone, the patient may be transferred to a ground or air ambulance for transportation to a trauma center.

RESOURCE MANAGEMENT

As the initial responder to a structural collapse incident, the questions that should be asked first are these:

- If a department does not have an in-house structural collapse rescue team, where is the nearest available team that has the qualifications to meet the challenges of the mission?
- Is there a mutual aid agreement in place with a team? If not, what procedures must be followed to request a team?
- How long will it take for the rescue team to prepare for departure and respond?

An awareness-level responder should be somewhat familiar with the potential target hazards within a community. A target hazard is defined as a structure or occupancy that poses a risk to the occupants as well as response personnel. These target hazards include hospitals, nursing homes, schools, large office buildings, apartment complexes, and manufacturing facilities, especially those with hazardous materials used and stored on site. Steps should be taken before an event occurs to have a written procedure that deals with a structural collapse incident.

Many communities have established mutual aid agreements through their county and state emergency management agency (EMA) to bring together a list of resources that are available to agencies across their region. These lists give very detailed summaries based on the **FEMA Resource Typing System** as to what resources each agency possesses and has to offer. Much like an insurance policy, these programs essentially become an agreement between all the agencies and the state that if called upon for assistance, based on that agency's ability to respond within a predetermined time frame, it can send specific resources.

Another consideration when requesting resources is the cost of bringing in the resources. When requesting resources, it is easy to take for granted the expenses incurred to cover operation expenses of heavy equipment, other services, and salaries to cover the overtime and backfill of other agencies. Although an unwritten agreement between neighboring communities may be in place that allows for assistance to be sent across lines without charging each other, most agencies do not have the budget to cover their personnel responding to another region, especially for extended periods of time. Many agencies have been faced with having to pay significant amounts of money from their own budgets to cover the operating cost of specialized teams and equipment brought in to conduct an operation. Although we should never consider price as a factor in making the decision to save a life, an incident commander should consider all options before making the request.

A responder should be knowledgeable about the local, state, and national laws that dictate how to acquire these resources. In some areas, a simple mutual aid agreement will address these issues. During large catastrophic events where local resources are completely overwhelmed, the county EMA should be asked to assist, calling in the state EMA as a resource. Providing that the event meets the criteria, much of the cost may be paid for by state funds.

RESPONSE PERSONNEL

The single most important resource is the response personnel who are coming to assist with the operation. A structural collapse incident is not only one of the largest types of incidents that a rescuer may face, but it is also one of the most time intensive. History demonstrates that an operation involving a single building can last anywhere from hours to days. This can depend on the size of the structure involved, the structure type, the size of the collapsed area, the number of missing victims that must be accounted for, and several other factors related to the hazards that must first be mitigated. Larger operations involving multiple damaged or collapsed structures can draw an operation out for weeks and perhaps months.

In the first couple of hours of a large event, it may be difficult to acquire technician level structural collapse providers. Depending on the qualifications of the local responding jurisdictions, many of the personnel seen early on in the incident may be responders who are not qualified in structural collapse rescue operations. Most likely, especially in a huge event that crosses large geographic areas, many of the first responders will be self-dispatched, creating a potential safety issue with increased incidents of freelancing.

It is important to establish an ICS as soon as possible and assign reliable and trained personnel to fill some key positions that can oversee your incoming resources. A staging area established well off site in a large parking lot is extremely useful for keeping arriving personnel and their equipment together until further assignments are given. If possible, law enforcement should be utilized to assist with traffic control and direct incoming units to the apparatus and personnel staging area.

Personal and operational self-control and discipline are required to prevent freelancers, including civilians as well as those trained in public safety who have come to the scene because they have the need do something. One of the most difficult things to do is to prevent responders from doing just anything, especially when the possibility of saving a life is in the balance. However, not gaining control early over such a situation increases the likelihood of more injuries and more lives lost.

During any event, rescuers will want to push themselves to the breaking point. This can create additional safety issues for the rescue team by increasing the likelihood of injuries occurring, heat and cold emergencies, and mistakes. A balance of assignments, rotation, and rest must be maintained throughout all work periods.

Most US&R teams are designed to be self-sufficient for up to 2 weeks. This includes bringing in their own provisions required to supply their personnel for that deployment. These provisions can include shelter, food, water, fuel, and any medical supplies needed to take care of the team. Other resources may be acquired as needed once the US&R team arrives at its BoO. This can be quite risky, however, especially if the local infrastructure has been compromised, leaving many of the local businesses shut down. In these situations, US&R teams will be forced to rely on the talents and resourcefulness of their logistical specialists to acquire needed supplies. (See the sidebar for resources that may be requested.)

Side Bar

Resources to Acquire in Advance of a Collapse

- Fuel to run apparatus and equipment
- Food for responders (Meals Ready to Eat (MRE) work fine, but a mobile canteen provided by the Red Cross or other agency is preferable for the base of operations.)
- Fresh drinking water
- Bathroom facilities (e.g., portable toilets)
- Wash and hygiene areas for responders
- Shelters for foul weather or team rest cycles
- Lighting equipment and generators
- Replacement parts for tools (cutting blades, drill bits, etc.)
- Certain over-the-counter medication for responders (acetaminophen, aspirin, antacids, etc.)

LOGISTICS RESOURCES

A qualified US&R team will have a logistics specialist and staff assigned to research these "what ifs" and make necessary arrangements to locate and acquire the needed resources to keep the team functioning during the entire deployment. In smaller operations, the operation may rely solely on one person assigned to accomplish these details.

To assist with this process, a resource manual should be created that can be routinely updated with the businesses and vendors that can supply specific items during an event. This guide should be structured to provide detailed information on not only the items but also what quantities can be provided and how long delivery to the scene would take. Round-the-clock contact phone numbers should also be included in case the event occurs during the overnight hours.

Prior agreements should be made before an event occurs between an agency and private vendors for acquisition at any hour, as well as payment arrangements for equipment and supplies. By properly preplanning for events such as a structural collapse, valuable time and effort will be saved during an actual emergency operation. Several states have created incident management teams (IMTs) within the different regions of their states. These IMTs specialize in assisting AHJ with the management of large-scale incidents like those caused by natural or manmade disasters. An IMT can only be activated through the state EMA upon request from a county EMA. In communities where resources are very limited, IMTs have the ability to bring in resources not only from around the region but also from around the state. This can be a very important resource that should not be overlooked if it is found that the magnitude of the event outweighs the AHJ's ability to manage it effectively.

TEAM RESOURCES

A structural collapse rescue team such as an organized US&R team will always deploy with their mobile toolboxes. This specialized equipment is normally organized and packaged with painstaking detail. A container numbering system specifies what is carried in every container and where each is located on the apparatus or trailer.

Whatever system a structural collapse rescue team uses to move the equipment to its destination, they must be sure that they have the proper tools to complete the job at hand. To maintain consistency among the federal US&R teams, FEMA plays a large role in determining what type, how much, and in some cases what brands of rescue equipment these teams will use. Many of the state and local structural collapse rescue teams also utilize the same system as the federal teams.

TOOLS AND EQUIPMENT

Many of the tools used to conduct shoring and rescue operations in light-frame construction, like what is found in most residential structures, are pretty much the same standard tools bought at any local hardware store, with a few exceptions. Much of the work conducted during light-frame rescue operation consists of stabilizing lightweight frame members, allowing rescuers to safely search for and extricate potentially live victims. The techniques used to accomplish these tasks utilize skills in shoring a structure with high-quality pressure-treated lumber.

The skills used to conduct basic shoring operations are taught in both theory and hands-on, approved, operations level structural collapse courses, taught by experienced instructors. Technician level structural collapse rescue personnel are trained to perform the same tasks on Type I and II structures. Their breaching and breaking tools consist of heavy-duty hydraulic, electric, and pneumatic jack hammers; hammer drills; and specialized chainsaws capable of cutting into reinforced concrete. (See Figure 7.18.) To gain entry into portions of the collapse that involve heavy steel-frame members, rescue teams will utilize a variety of cutting tools, such as gasoline or hydraulic rotary saws, electric reciprocating saws, acetylene torches, and plasma cutters. These breaching, breaking, and cutting tools are common in almost every team's inventory.

Technician level teams are not only trained to breach and shore up large sections of concrete and steel but also to secure and lift out large sections of both using basic makeshift and custom haul devices or cranes. These techniques are necessary to gain access to void spaces where potential victims may be located. It is routine for technician level teams to work and train closely with qualified crane

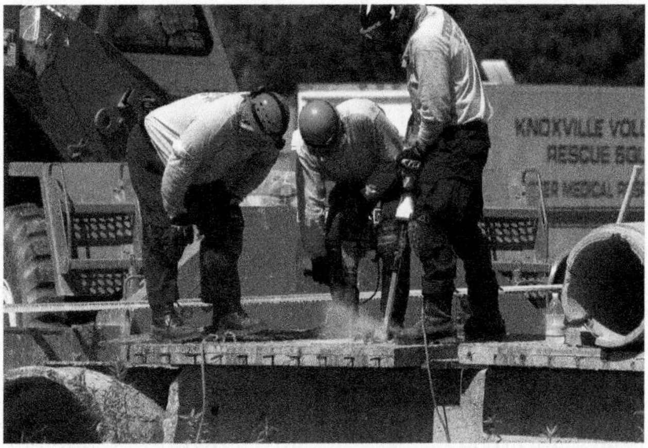

FIGURE 7.18 Hydraulic breakers are used to gain access through reinforced concrete. *Source: David C. Harrington.*

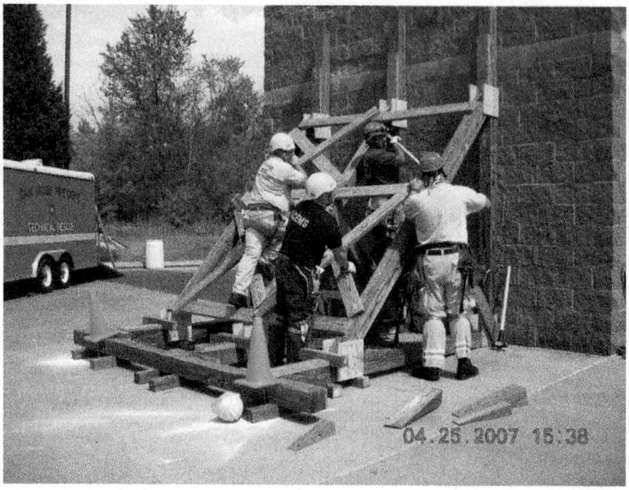

FIGURE 7.19 A shoring team builds a raker shore system to support a vertical wall. *Source: David C. Harrington.*

companies and their operators, giving them further capabilities when dealing with complex situations where they may have to lift out and move large sections of the structure.

As rescue teams enter into a partial or fully collapsed structure, they must shore it up as they proceed. Every breach or opening is shored to secure the access and egress for the rescuers and the victims. (See Figure 7.19.) As a team enters into void spaces, it may be necessary to build complex shoring systems that are capable of supporting weights up to 80,000 pounds, depending largely on the size of the lumber.

The shoring systems used by every structural collapse rescue team have been designed by structural engineers and tested under real-world conditions. To maintain consistency, rescue teams rarely deviate from the standard system design. To assist with this, team members refer to "The Urban Search & Rescue Field Operations Guide" published by the U.S. Army Corps of Engineers (2009).

Even at the technician level, structural collapse teams may be faced with complexities that are beyond their level of training. For this reason, many structural collapse rescue teams include a structural engineer. The engineer's knowledge is utilized to assess the stability of a structure and assist with designing and building advanced shoring systems. It is important to understand that conducting any rescue operation in or directly around a confirmed or potentially unstable structure cannot actively move forward without these safeguards in place.

SEARCH EQUIPMENT

The process of breaching, shoring, and searching a structure is a very methodical process that can take extended time to accomplish. Rescue teams possess a wide assortment of high-tech equipment that can decrease the time and effort required to conduct a search of every square foot of a building. Specialized search cameras, thermal imagery, highly sensitive listening devices, and search dogs trained to recognize victims by smell are the tools of choice when searching for victims inside of a collapsed structure. US&R teams employ within their ranks technical-search specialists who have attended specialized FEMA training in the utilization of this equipment.

Canine search teams use highly trained animals with a superior sense of smell, making them an invaluable resource at a collapse incident. Canines must go through a rigorous accreditation process that many do not successfully pass. (See Figure 7.20.) Those that have become accredited within the FEMA system may participate with multiple US&R task forces and are often part of international response teams. A canine will rely on both sight and smell to locate possible victims within a collapse zone. Once the canine hits upon the location of a potential victim, a second canine will be brought in to search the same area. If the second canine also hits on

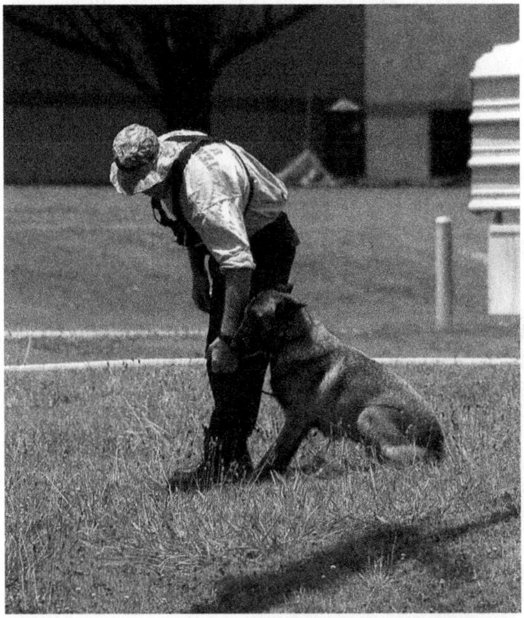

FIGURE 7.20 A US&R canine search specialist will rely on both sight and smell to locate possible victims within a collapse zone. *Source: David C. Harrington.*

the same location, this is considered a confirmed find. At this point, rescue teams will actively use additional detection equipment to locate the victim.

One of the first steps in attempting to locate victims should be to hail or call out to them in an attempt to get them to respond, which works well for conscious victims. For unconscious victims and those located farther inside a collapsed structure, acoustic and seismic technology can be used. These devices are initially deployed in an array around the collapse zone to listen for sounds created by victims from within the collapse. Detected sounds can be isolated and pinpointed by examining the individual probes and determining which identify the strongest sources. (See Figure 7.21.) From there, the individual probes are redistributed to allow for the rescue team to move toward the strongest signal and identify the location of a potential victim. However, acoustic and seismic devices cannot detect unconscious victims. In addition, these devices have limited range and signals can easily be interfered with by noises around the collapse zone.

Another tool that rescue teams use to work their way into the collapse area is a specialized search camera or fiber optics. Each brand and type has its own unique advantages, depending on the situation that may be encountered. The SearchCAM utilizes a 1.75-inch camera mounted on the end of a pole that can extend into a void space, allowing the operator to view what the camera sees on a 7-inch monitor screen. (See Figure 7.22.) The camera has its own light source that can illuminate the dark space. Rescuers using core drillers will create a 2-inch-diameter hole into concrete if no natural opening is available. The end of the pole where the camera is attached can also be articulated 90 degrees to the left or right, allowing the operator to see around corners and to all sides of the void space.

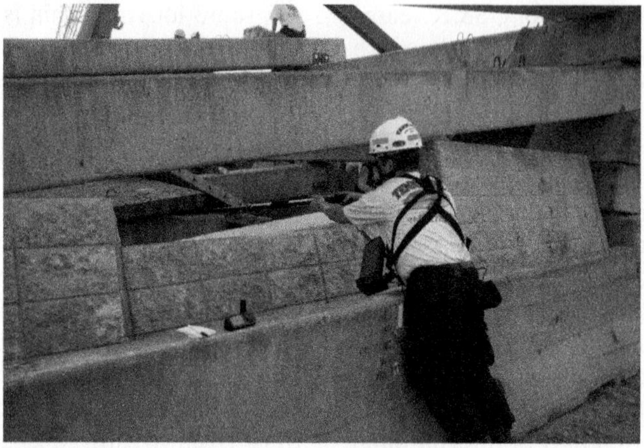

FIGURE 7.21 ■ US&R search specialists use a search camera to look into void spaces for victims.
Source: David C. Harrington.

Another type of camera is the SnakeEye. This 1.25-inch camera is also mounted on the end of a pole, allowing for insertion into the void space. The operator can view the space through a color LED monitor mounted at the controls. This camera also has the ability to articulate at the end. An additional feature of the SnakeEye is that the camera can be removed from the pole and mounted directly to the end of the cable. This allows the camera to be lowered vertically downward into a void space up to 100 feet. The camera is waterproof, making it usable in muddy and wet environments.

A more recent addition to the structural collapse cache of search cameras is fiber-optic viewing equipment. This technology is much

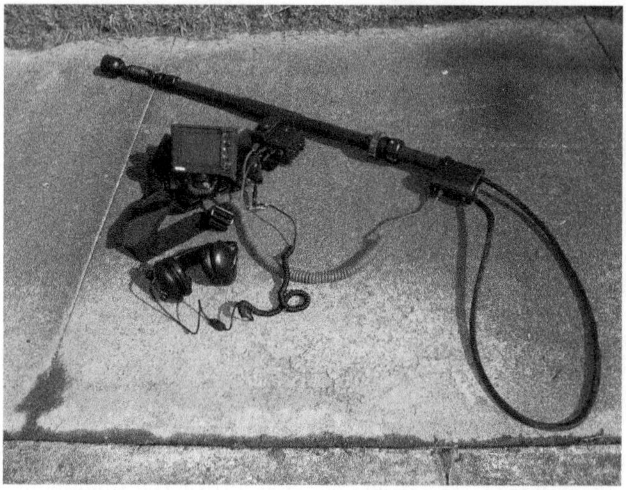

FIGURE 7.22 ■ This search cameras features an extendable boom and articulating camera head.
Source: David C. Harrington.

like the devices used by physicians to view the interior regions of the heart as well as other parts of the body. In its application for structural collapse rescue, the device allows the operator to view extremely tight and restrictive void spaces to pinpoint the location of victims. The resolution of the camera can be limited, however, depending on the quality and number of fibers within the fiberscope's cable bundle. The end of the fiberscope can articulate in all four directions, allowing the operator to direct the rescue workers more specifically as to where they may drill their next hole in attempting to locate a victim. Fiber-optic devices can be extremely expensive.

Another type of device that can be used as an alternative is the rigid borescope. This device has been in use by the manufacturing industry for many years to assist in seeing inside of machinery, such as engines or other castings. The rigid borescope uses long tubes that have integrated lenses and mirrors similar to a prism. Along with an adequate light source, this device can allow the operator to see inside the void space with great detail and resolution.

MEDICAL RESOURCES

Once victims have been located, they must be assessed for a variety of conditions that can affect their health. Some medical conditions are beyond the injuries usually associated with trauma that are specific to structural collapse incidents and must be considered prior to **extrication**. If victims are conscious and responding appropriately, it can be assumed that their airway is patent, they are breathing, and their circulation is presently intact. If not, there are limited actions that can be taken, especially if the victim is severely trapped in the debris.

Many structural collapse teams have personnel who are trained to the level of medical specialist. These individuals are usually paramedics but can also be doctors and nurses. The intense training involved to certify to this level involves learning the theories and treatments for conditions, such as crush syndrome and compartment syndrome.

HAZARDOUS MATERIALS RESOURCES

As part of the process for sizing up the scene, special attention should be paid to not only the type of structure involved but also who and what occupied the structure. For example, many industrial manufacturers, laboratories, and chemical supply companies maintain large quantities of chemicals as part of their operation. These chemicals can be flammable, corrosive, explosive, radioactive, and toxic. Great suspicion should be aroused regarding the possibility that the containers these chemicals are stored in could be compromised due to the collapse. Up-to-date preplans giving detailed lists of specific chemicals and quantities can usually be obtained from the local fire department. Individuals who work at the facility who may be familiar with what's stored on site may also be able to give you this information. Unless your team is equipped and qualified to mitigate these hazards, a hazardous materials team should immediately be requested to be on site.

Other potential hazardous materials that should be considered present at every collapse incident are those associated with disrupted infrastructure. Gas lines, sewer lines, steam lines, fuel lines, and other chemical distribution lines can create a hazardous situation for rescuers as they attempt to locate and rescue victims.

Rescuers should never enter a structure without prior testing for dangerous atmospheres. If it has been determined that a suspected release has occurred, a hazardous materials

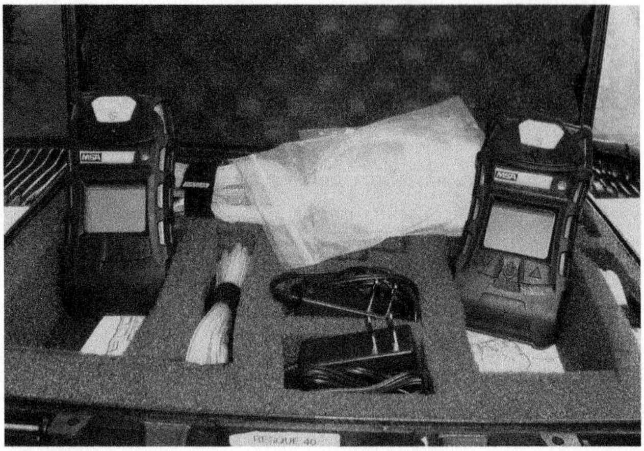

FIGURE 7.23 Multigas monitor capable of detecting oxygen level, hydrogen sulfide, methane, and LEL. *Source: David C. Harrington.*

survey team will conduct an assessment of the scene using atmospheric monitors to identify any hazardous product. (See Figure 7.23.) If any hazardous material is detected, control zones will be established based on the type of product, concentration in the atmosphere, and prevailing weather conditions. Further research will be conducted to determine the type of respiratory protection and personal protective equipment needed. When the presence of a hazardous material is suspected, be sure to approach the scene from the uphill and upwind side. Always place staging areas and the command post away from the established hot and warm zones, uphill and upwind of the scene. Deny entry to all personnel until it has been determined to be safe by the hazardous materials team.

After 9-11, the world changed in many ways. The likelihood of a terrorist event becomes greater and greater as time goes by. The use of improvised explosive devices (IEDs) and other weapons—including chemical, biological, radiological, nuclear, and enhanced conventional (CBRNE) weapons of mass destruction—should always be considered in the foreground of any event, unless proven otherwise. As for hazardous materials, teams are specifically trained to mitigate CBRNE events. It is very likely that first responders will be targets of opportunity during a structural collapse incident caused by a terrorist event.

LAW ENFORCEMENT RESOURCES

As a structural collapse incident unfolds, the scene can quickly become very chaotic and difficult to manage under the best of conditions. Controlling the scene should become the first priority in creating a safe working environment. Law enforcement can play a vital role in accomplishing this task. If it is suspected that the incident was the result of a criminal act, law enforcement will play the lead in collecting evidence and conducting the investigation.

CHAPTER REVIEW

Summary

No other type of incident is as challenging as a structural collapse. The decisions made by an awareness-level provider within the first few moments can make the difference between a successful or failed operation. Not only must the scene be controlled and a command presence established, but a responder must have the ability to acknowledge the gravity of the situation and request the additional resources needed to tackle the complex rescue needs. It is necessary to recognize and mitigate a variety of hazards within the scope of an individual's training and take the steps necessary to avoid or deny access to those known hazards that can ultimately injure or take the lives of fellow responders and civilians. Even with the limitations of awareness level training, many lives can be spared by effectively sizing up the situation and searching for victims who are accessible or lightly trapped by debris.

EMS special operations teams who work at the scene of structure collapse typically perform the rescue and then transfer care to EMS providers. EMS can further assess, treat, and transport victims to appropriate health care facilities.

The knowledge gained from the material within an awareness level structural collapse course is only the beginning. It is the foundation for additional more advanced training within the discipline of structural collapse rescue.

WHAT WOULD YOU DO? Reflection

The first steps that should be taken to effectively manage the scene are to initiate the incident command system and begin the size-up process by assessing for any existing and potential hazards. Next, you should establish control zones around the collapse site to protect resources from secondary collapse. Once you have been able to access the scene, immediately request any additional resources that may be required to mitigate the situation. It is also important to assign someone to establish an accountability system in order to keep track of resources. As you begin searching for victims, assess for any ambulatory patients and those who are lightly trapped. Be sure to assign the next-arriving EMS unit to begin triage of all accessible patients. If applicable, transfer command to the highest-ranking fire official upon their arrival.

During the initial size-up, observe for existing and potential hazards such as downed electric lines, natural gas leaks, smoke plumes from fires or hazardous materials, undermined roadways from broken water lines, unstable buildings and debris, and the possibility for secondary collapse. Also observe for the type of construction, number of buildings involved, type of collapse, and victims.

Based on the information provided for this scenario, the requested resources should include the fire department if not already on scene, a hazardous materials team, additional EMS transport units, an operational-level structural collapse team at a minimal, a technician-level structural collapse team (preferred), additional law enforcement, and utilities.

Review Questions

1. What are the five types of void space collapse patterns?
2. What are the indicators of a secondary collapse?
3. Which NFPA document contains the standards pertaining to the operational and training requirements for technical search and rescue incidents?
4. What provider level possesses the minimal training that allows for them to conduct the size-up of the scene, assess for and identify hazards, manage the scene, conduct basic search, and perform the rescue of victims who are readily accessible?
5. Identify the five types of construction.
6. Identify the "no go" conditions that would automatically stop or delay a rescue operation.
7. A person experiencing crush syndrome exhibits what signs and symptoms?
8. What are the advantages and disadvantages of attempting to locate victims by hailing or calling out to them?
9. What is the basic information that should be gathered by the 9-1-1 dispatcher when receiving a call for a structural collapse incident?
10. Identify the different types of hazards found around the collapse area.

References

Brannigan, F. (1992). *Building Construction for the Fire Service,* 3rd ed. Quincy, MA: National Fire Protection Association.

Daley, M. (2010, July 29). "Building Collapse Operations, Part 2. "*Firehouse Magazine*. See the organization website.

Eady, M. (2006, September). "The Rescue Technician and NFPA Standards." *Fire Engineering*.

FEMA. (n.d.). "Structural Collapse Technician Course: Student Manual." See the organization website.

FEMA. (2006). "National Urban Search & Rescue (US&R) Response System: Rescue Field Operations Guide." See the organization website.

National Fire Protection Association. (2003). "NFPA 1006: Standard for Rescue Technician Professional, Qualifications for Structural Collapse Rescue." (Quincy, MA: National Fire Protection Association.)

National Fire Protection Association. (2009). "NFPA 1670: Standard on Operations and Training for Technical Search and Rescue Incidents." (Quincy, MA: National Fire Protection Association.)

U.S. Army Corps of Engineers, Urban Search and Rescue Program. (2009, February). "Urban Search & Rescue Shoring Operations Guide." See the Disaster Engineer website.

Key Terms

approach hazard A hazard that may be encountered EMS personnel while responding to the scene of an incident.

Authority Having Jurisdiction (AHJ) The organization, office, or individual—such as a fire chief; fire marshal, chief of a fire prevention bureau, labor department, or health department; building official; or electrical inspector—who is responsible for approving equipment, an installation, or a procedure.

awareness level The minimum capability of a responder who could be called upon to respond to, or could be the first on the scene of, a technical rescue incident. This level can involve search, rescue, and recovery operations.

canine search teams Search dog teams trained for search and rescue operations for living and deceased victims in a variety of environments and conditions.

collapse patterns The expected characteristics that are demonstrated by a structure during a specific type of collapse.

concentrated load A load that is applied to a structural component at one single point rather than being distributed uniformly across a span.

control zones An area created on an incident scene outside of an established perimeter that surrounds an area determined to be extremely hazardous.

dead load The total weight of the building materials, equipment, and fixtures that are permanently attached to the building itself.

design load The maximum load that a structure and its components are designed to handle.

distributed load An external force or load that is spread over a region of length, surface, or area as opposed to a single point.

extrication The process of removing or disentangling a victim from an entrapment.

Federal Emergency Management Agency (FEMA) An independent agency of the United States government that is responsible for federal emergency preparedness and mitigation and response activities.

FEMA Resource Typing System The categorization and description of resources commonly utilized in large incidents to assist emergency management personnel to identify, locate, request, order, and track outside resources to the jurisdiction that needs them.

force The strength or energy of the different types of loads that bear upon the components of a structure.

hazardous materials A dangerous product in the form of a solid, liquid, or gas that can harm people, other living organisms, property, or the environment.

impact load A dynamic load that results from the forces created by the movement of operating machinery, elevators, cranes, vehicles, heavy winds, seismic activity, and similar moving forces.

incident action plan (IAP) A formalized document that includes the incident goals, operational period objectives, and response strategy defined by incident command during the response planning phase.

incident command system (ICS) Allows for organizations to work together effectively by establishing common terminology and advocates a management-by-objectives philosophy.

incident commander The person responsible for overseeing every aspect of an emergency response, including development of incident objectives, managing all incident operations, and management of resources.

live load The forces created by the weight from the items that furnish a structure.

loads A weight or a mass that is supported.

National Fire Protection Administration (NFPA) An international nonprofit organization whose mission is to reduce fire and other hazards by providing and advocating codes and standards, research, training, and education.

operational capacity An agency's ability to perform at a specific operational level based upon its ability to meet specific requirements and standards.

operations level The capability of hazard recognition, equipment use, and techniques necessary to safely and effectively support and participate in a technical rescue incident. This level can involve search, rescue, and recovery operations, but usually operations are carried out under the supervision of technician-level personnel.

physical search team A team that specializes in conducting a physical search for victims in a collapse environment without the use of specialized search equipment.

resources A variety of assets, such as personnel equipment, teams, and supplies, utilized to meet the needs of an incident.

secondary collapse An additional partial or complete collapse initiated from the damage inflicted by a primary event.

standard operating procedure (SOP) An established departmental procedure or process that should be carried out in response to a specific operation or in a given situation.

structural collapse The loss of the load-carrying capacity of a component or member within a structure due to the material being stressed beyond its strength limit, resulting in a fracture or excessive deformations and subsequent structural failure.

technician level The capability of hazard recognition, equipment use, and techniques necessary to safely and effectively coordinate, perform, and supervise a technical rescue incident. This level can involve search, rescue, and recovery operations.

Confined-Space Rescue

8 CHAPTER

David Harrington

Objectives

After reading this chapter, the student should be able to:

8.1 Identify the criteria for an enclosure to be classified as a confined space.
8.2 Identify the criteria for an enclosure to be classified as a permit-controlled confined space.
8.3 Identify the different types of confined spaces.
8.4 Identify the need for a confined-space rescue operation.
8.5 Identify the hazards that are associated with a confined-space incident.
8.6 Identify the different levels of response personnel for confined-space incidents.
8.7 Describe the need and methods required for management of the confined-space incident scene.
8.8 Identify the resources required to conduct a confined-space rescue operation.
8.9 Describe the methods and equipment for controlling existing and potential hazards during a confined-space operation.
8.10 Identify the non-entry methods for conducting a confined-space rescue.

Key Terms

access and egress equipment
air management officer
attendant
concentration
engulfment
entrant
entrapment
flash fire
gate-valve lockouts
immediately dangerous to life and health (IDLH)
lockout hasps
lower explosive limit (LEL)

National Incident Management System (NIMS)
packaging
parts per million (ppm)
personnel accountability report (PAR)
pipe blanks
upper explosive limit (UEL)
ventilation

WHAT WOULD YOU DO?

You are dispatched to a farm located in the rural part of your county for an unknown medical problem. On arrival, you are met by a frantic woman who is trying to explain that her husband has experienced a possible heart attack while working on a pump down inside their well. Their son, who was helping, came to tell her to call for an ambulance. He then climbed down inside of the well to assist his father. Neither man came out or responded to her repeated calls. She tells you that her husband was using a gasoline water pump to siphon out the water. When the pump shut down, he climbed down to see if he could find the problem. Several neighbors are now beginning to gather in the yard after hearing her cries. Based on your training, you suspect that both men have become victims of a confined-space accident. As you begin your size-up, you assess the situation.

Questions

1. What should you look for during your size-up of a confined-space incident?
2. What hazards should you consider that may be associated with this scene?
3. What steps should you take to properly manage the scene? What resources would be required to manage the incident?

INTRODUCTION

Every day, processes must be conducted inside and around enclosures that bring workers in close proximity to a variety of hazards. Locations such as industrial and chemical facilities, farms, utilities or public works locations, communications facilities, energy-producing facilities, and even residential properties harbor enclosures that require performance of routine tasks in order for ordinary processes to function normally. More often, workers must go into confined areas within the structure for that work to be conducted. In most cases, the worker can make the entry, conduct the necessary work, and exit the space without incident.

While not every enclosure is by definition a confined space, an enclosure that possesses specific characteristics or associated hazards is classified as a confined space. Confined spaces are considered to be silent killers that lure their unsuspecting victims into a false sense of security. This is because the inherit danger that lurks within a confined space is invisible and can have a negative effects before victims can detect them.

This is easy to understand when we consider that a simple entry into what appears to be an otherwise harmless environment can possess the ingredients with the potential to create a deadly combination. Most victims of confined-space incidents likely never had any idea they were in trouble because in many cases there were no obvious visible hazards. The one thing that all these groups had in common was their lack of knowledge about the dangers involved in attempting a rescue of a victim inside of a confined space.

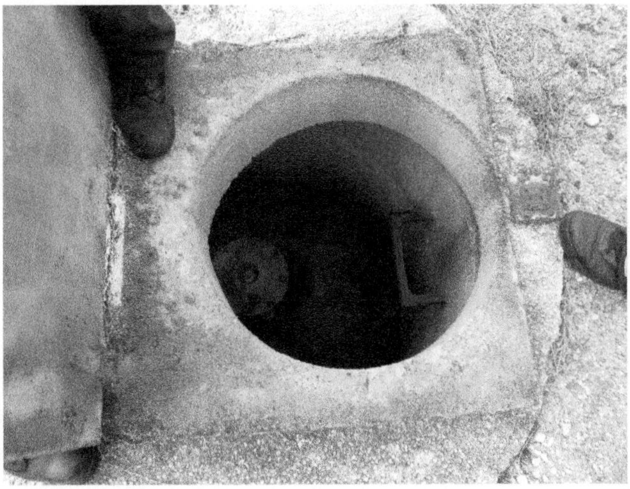

FIGURE 8.1 ■ A confined space has limited or restricted means of egress. *Source: Photo courtesy of David C. Harrington.*

CONFINED-SPACE IDENTIFICATION

An emergency responder should be familiar with what a confined space is, the associated hazards, and the OSHA regulations that apply. A confined space by definition must have three characteristics:

- A space that has limited or restricted means of egress
- A space that is large enough for a person to enter to perform assigned tasks
- A space that is not designed for continuous occupancy (See Figure 8.1.)

Confined spaces are also found within the areas of operation involving urban search and rescue responses. Heavily damaged and collapsed structures will inherently possess many of the same conditions and hazards of a permit-required confined space.

A permit-required confined space must meet additional criteria as defined by the Occupational Safety and Health Administration

Side Bar

Examples of Confined Spaces

- Grain hoppers
- Silos (See Figure 8.2.)
- Manure pits
- Wells
- Septic tanks
- Chemical storage tanks (See Figure 8.3.)
- Railroad tank cars
- Manholes and storm drains
- Sewer system
- Electrical vaults
- Industrial smokestacks, furnaces, and boilers
- Open trenches and excavations deeper than 4 feet
- Sanitary sewer pump lift stations
- Industrial transformers
- Automobile repair pits
- Large storage lift bins
- Chimneys
- Cargo ship holds
- Hoppers

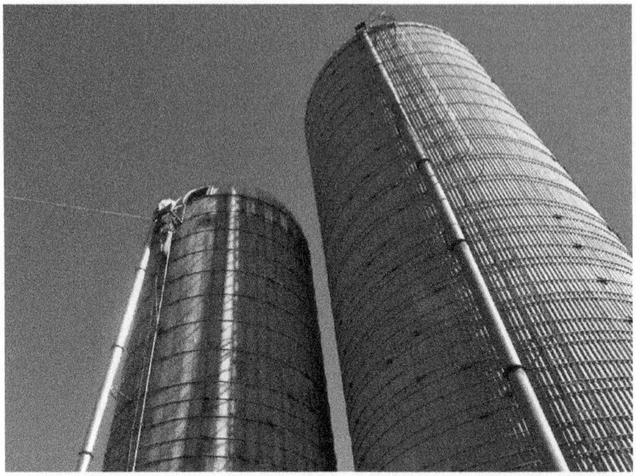

FIGURE 8.2 Silos can contain a material, such as grain, that can create an engulfment hazard for workers. *Source: Photo courtesy of David C. Harrington.*

(OSHA). To be a permit-required confined space, the space must also possess at least one of following characteristics:

- The potential to contain a hazardous atmosphere
- Contains a material that has the potential for **engulfment** of the entrant
- Has an internal configuration that might cause an entrant to be trapped or asphyxiated by inwardly converging walls or by a floor that slopes downward and tapers to a smaller cross section
- Contains any other recognized serious safety or health hazards (OSHA, 2011a)

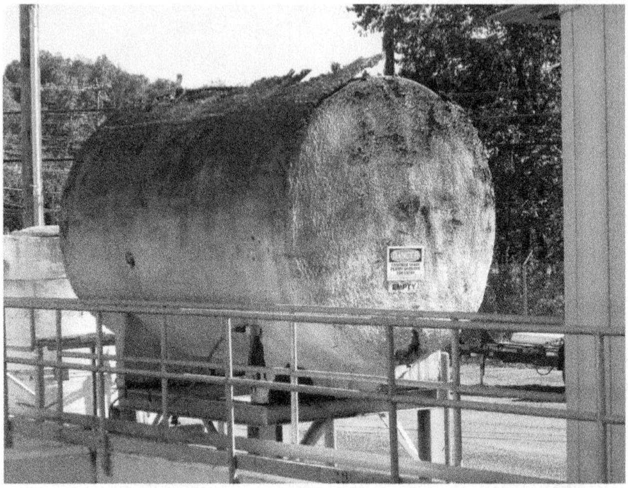

FIGURE 8.3 Chemical storage tanks may contain hazardous substances. Even when empty, they may contain explosive or toxic vapors. *Source: Photo courtesy of David C. Harrington.*

For an awareness-level provider, every confined space should be considered to possess these characteristics unless proven otherwise.

OSHA REGULATIONS

Regulations that apply to confined spaces were created in 1971 by OSHA under authority granted by sections within the Occupational Safety and Health Act of 1970. This act established federal standards applicable originally to ship repairing, building, and breaking operations. Over the next several years, OSHA began to address the growing trends of accidents resulting in injuries and deaths within the industry. Much of this research was based on accident data filed by the National Institute for Occupational Safety and Health (NIOSH) outlining the numbers and types of accidents that occurred in confined spaces.

Along with these findings, NIOSH instituted standards that included provisions for required permits to authorize an entry by workers, the testing and monitoring of the space prior to and during the entry, additional precautions to be initiated to include continual ventilation, purging of the space, lockout/tagout procedures, and pre-entry medical surveillance of the entry personnel. Further recommendations included training on the labeling and posting of confined spaces as well as entry procedures to include the stationing of standby persons, communications, and rescue. The recommendations for personal protective equipment and rescue equipment along with standardization of recordkeeping were also submitted.

In 1993, OSHA submitted its final rule and OSHA Standard 29 CFR 1910 was adopted. This standard specified the safety requirements for entry into confined spaces, and it designated permit-required confined spaces, which pose special dangers for entrants because their configurations hamper efforts to protect entrants from serious hazards, such as toxic, explosive, or asphyxiating atmospheres. This new standard continues to provide a comprehensive regulatory framework within which employers can effectively protect employees who work in permit spaces. Although the rules and regulations within this standard were originally written for industries within the public and private sector, they also apply to public safety agencies. Any public safety agency assuming the responsibility to perform confined-space rescue operations must also comply with the federal OSHA Standard 29 CFR 1910.146, Permit-Required Confined Spaces (OSHA, 2011a).

The National Fire Protection Association (NFPA) developed codes and standards, similar to the OSHA regulations, through the consensus of volunteer committee members who offer their professional expertise in the fire and rescue industry. These codes and standards are designed to minimize the risk to response personnel while in the performance of their duties. NFPA standards 1670 and 1006 both apply to confined-space rescue operations. NFPA 1670 (Standard on Operations and Training for Technical Search and Rescue Incidents) defines the requirements that rescue agencies use to operate at technical rescue incidents. This standard identifies the requirements for written procedures for response and safety, personal protective equipment, risk and hazards assessment, and establishment of operational response levels, and resource considerations. NFPA 1006 (Standard for Technical Rescuer Professional Qualifications) establishes the job performance requirements for emergency response personnel to perform technical rescue activities. These activities include knowledge and cognitive objectives, such as preplanning confined spaces within an agency's jurisdiction, site assessment, hazard recognition and control, atmospheric monitoring, entry team preparation, victim assessment, packaging and transfer techniques, and incident termination procedures (NFPA, 2013, p. 21). It must be noted that these standards have some overlap with certain OSHA guidelines; however, the Authority Having Jurisdiction (AHJ) can choose to adopt or ignore them, unlike the OSHA regulations.

LEVELS OF TRAINING

There are specific levels of training that qualify rescue personnel for participating in confined-space rescue operations.

AWARENESS-LEVEL RESPONDER

Awareness-level responders in confined space are required to be trained and familiar with the following:

1. The need for confined-space search and rescue
2. Initiating contact and establishing communications with victims where possible
3. Hazards associated with non-entry confined-space incidents
4. The different types of confined spaces
5. Performing a non-entry retrieval of a victim where possible
6. Implementing the emergency response system for confined-space emergencies
7. Implementing site control and scene management

It is important for awareness-level responders to be fully mindful of limitations in both their knowledge and ability. Awareness-level response personnel should not perform rescues even from outside of a confined space without proper training and specialized equipment.

OPERATIONS-LEVEL RESPONDER

Operations-level responder training further adds to the awareness-level knowledge base. In this level of responder, as with an awareness-level provider, making entry within a confined space is not specified. Further training, knowledge, and skill sets are required for this level of response. In addition to what an awareness-level responder needs to know, operations-level responders must be trained to be able to do the following:

1. Conduct atmospheric monitoring of the confined space
2. Conduct preparation for entry into the confined space
3. Possess the ability to make entry into the confined space
4. Package and prepare the victim for removal from the confined space
5. Remove all entrants from the confined space

TECHNICIAN-LEVEL RESPONDER

The technician-level responder is trained in not only the areas listed above but also in much more advanced knowledge and skills. This can include advanced hazard mitigation, command and control at the scene of a confined-space incident, planning the actual rescue, and making entry into more complex spaces.

CONFINED-SPACE HAZARDS

Each confined space is unique in its own way. Each space possesses its own hidden dangers that can be ultimately fatal to the unsuspecting **entrant**. Although the vast majority of deaths associated with confined-space incidents are related directly to a factor within the space itself, it must not be overlooked that victims can also suffer from medical-related events resulting from cardiac or other serious conditions. Hazards can classified into generalized categories: atmospheric hazards, hazardous materials, engulfment hazards, thermal hazards, falling objects, slip and trip hazards, electrical energy hazards, and mechanical energy hazards.

ATMOSPHERIC HAZARDS

Atmospheres that are contaminated with a toxic vapor or lack adequate oxygen are one of the most common causes of fatalities in confined spaces. Normal air contains between 20.8 percent and 21 percent oxygen. An oxygen-deficient atmosphere is a situation in which the oxygen concentration drops below 19.5 percent.

> **Side Bar**
>
> **Effects of Decreasing Oxygen Content**
>
> - 20.9 percent: Normal percentage of oxygen found in normal air. No effect.
> - 19.5 percent: Minimum permissible oxygen level. No effect.
> - 15 to 19 percent: Decreased ability to work strenuously. May impair coordination and may induce early symptoms with nonprotected workers.
> - 12 to 15 percent: Respiration and pulse increase; impaired coordination, perception, and judgment occur.
> - 10 to 12 percent: Respiration rate and effort increase. The unprotected worker will begin to exhibit poor judgment and further changes in level of consciousness. Worker will begin to present with cyanosis around the lips.
> - 8 to 10 percent: Symptoms can include altered level of consciousness, syncope, unconsciousness, cyanosis to the face and lips, possible nausea, and vomiting.
> - 6 to 8 percent: Fatal if not corrected within 6 minutes.
> - 4 to 8 percent: Worker will be comatose, experience convulsions, eventual respiratory failure, then cardiac arrest.

An oxygen-deficient atmosphere can be caused when an inert gas is introduced into the space, in turn displacing the oxygen. Inert gases can include nitrogen, carbon dioxide, or argon. Processes such as the cleaning of a space and automatic fire suppression systems typically use inert gasses. Oxygen can also be consumed by natural processes such as simple combustion, bacterial activities, ripening fruit, and rusting metal. Other processes that consume oxygen include drying paint or coatings.

When the oxygen **concentration** is increased above 23.5 percent, the atmosphere is considered to be oxygen enriched. This can occur due to certain chemical reactions, leaking oxygen hoses, or torches. An oxygen-enriched atmosphere will increase the risk of fire and explosive potential. Both of these conditions can only be found during the air monitoring process that should always be conducted both before an entry is made and continuously throughout the entry.

Flammable or combustible gases or vapors also fall into this category of atmospheric hazards. Flammable or combustible contaminants are measured on a scale that is based on its **lower explosive limit (LEL)**. The LEL of a specific gas or vapor is the lowest concentration of the gas or vapor that will ignite if an ignition source is present. Air monitoring instruments designed to detect combustible gases or vapors will sound an alarm when 10 percent LEL of a gas or vapor is detected. As the concentration increases towards 100 percent LEL, the risk of explosion also increases.

Toxic gases and vapors such as hydrogen sulfide and carbon monoxide can also be found inside confined spaces. The concentrations of these types of gases are measured in **parts per million (ppm)**. This can be described as the concentration of a specific contaminant within a million parts of air. In addition, it should be recognized that if an LEL of a contaminant is detected, it is very likely that the oxygen in the air has been displaced, resulting in an oxygen-deficient atmosphere. Each chemical or contaminant has its own specific level of concentration that makes it highly dangerous. Some chemicals may be dangerous, if not lethal, at less than 1 ppm, whereas other chemicals may not be dangerous until they reach a concentration of up to several thousand ppm. (We discuss air monitoring in greater detail later in this chapter.)

An initial reading gives an ambient baseline of the air quality prior to initiating **ventilation** of the confined space. Even if the air is within normal ranges for oxygen and without contaminants, ventilation should be initiated as soon as possible and continued throughout the entire operation. If a flammable gas or vapor is detected and found to be beyond its **upper explosive limit (UEL)**, ventilation should not occur until the source of the explosive vapor is contained. Once ventilation has been initiated, close monitoring of the LEL should continue. By ventilating the confined space, the concentration of the flammable or combustible gas or vapor will drop into its flammable or explosive range between the LEL and UEL. If this occurs, ventilation should continue until the concentration is brought below the contaminant's LEL. All ignition sources should be eliminated before this process is initiated to reduce any risk of explosion. Ventilation should only be conducted with an intrinsically safe electric fan.

HAZARDOUS MATERIALS

Confined spaces could contain a variety of chemicals used for different processes depending on the use of the facility. If the space is part of a water treatment facility, raw sewage is not only a hazardous material risk but should be considered an engulfment hazard. Prior to testing the oxygen concentration, responders should test for corrosives that could permanently damage detection equipment. Combustible or flammable liquids or gases should be tested next. Other classifications for hazardous materials include toxins and irritants. Hazardous material technician-level responders should only be utilized to mitigate these hazards.

ENGULFMENT HAZARDS

In facilities that have containers—including storage bins, silos, vats, tanks, bunkers, and hoppers—the risk for engulfment hazards increases. An engulfment occurs when a worker falls into a containerized product—such as sand, gravel, grain, flour, sawdust, seed, soil, or a liquid—and is engulfed.

The force of the product falling on the worker creates an **entrapment** that results in a traumatic injury caused by severe constriction of the torso, followed by traumatic asphyxiation. A patient's respiratory system can also be affected by the crushing effects. Further respiratory insult can result from the patient being suffocated by product entering the patient's mouth and filling the lungs. First responders should be cautious about approaching these containers until railings and foot boards have been installed around them. All responders working around an open trench or container should wear fall-protection harnesses along with retrieval lines.

THERMAL HAZARDS

Many facilities within the manufacturing and public sectors possess confined spaces directly associated with complex processes. A power production facility is a good example of a site that can have several enclosures requiring entry to be made for routine maintenance where the thermal temperatures can reach well beyond 100°F. (See Figure 8.4.) These temperatures obviously can present thermal insult to workers as well as to rescuers who have to make an entry. Even if a facility can be temporarily shut down, it may take days if not

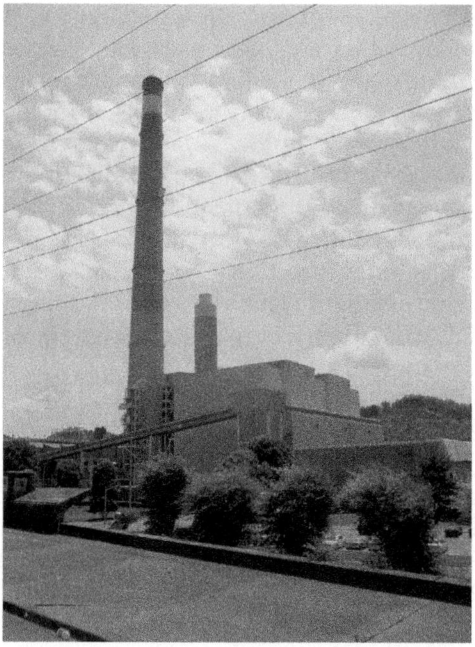

FIGURE 8.4 Facilities such as energy power plants present extreme thermal hazards in multiple confined spaces where maintenance is routinely conducted by entrants. *Source: Photo courtesy of David C. Harrington.*

weeks for the temperatures to drop to comfortable levels. The potential for further thermal injuries is enhanced with the personal protective equipment that the rescuer must wear within a space. Great care must be taken to properly assess entry personnel before, during, and after an entry.

FALLING OBJECTS

While working inside of a confined space, one should always be careful not to place tools or other objects above the heads of yourself or other rescuers. For example, a vibration or a person can knock an object off a ledge, causing it to fall and injure someone. To reduce the risk of injury, rescuers should always wear an approved rescue helmet.

SLIP AND TRIP HAZARDS

Depending on the type and use of the enclosure, slippery surfaces may be found both inside and outside of a confined space. Whether it is a ladder leading from the entrance to the base of the enclosure or the floor surfaces, moisture, oil residue, mud, and other film can coat surfaces upon which a worker may be walking, crawling, or climbing. Fall protection is a must when working around an elevated position, even when outside the space. Tools left on walkways, low pipe, and wire chases create a tripping hazard, especially in low-visibility spaces. Adequate lighting and cautious movement should be taken around the outside of such spaces.

ELECTRICAL ENERGY HAZARDS

Electrical components within a space can present an increased risk of electrical shock to workers and rescuers alike. Electrocution can result from the worker coming in contact with energized electrical wiring, defective cable conduits, or situations in which the space may be flooded with submerged electrical components. Prior to rescue teams entering into a confined space, all nonessential electrical power should be shut off. The exception to this rule would be when shutting off a particular piece of safety equipment or process requiring electrical power could create additional safety hazards.

Maintenance staff or other personnel who are familiar with the equipment and processes are good resources to guide rescue teams through the particulars of a certain site. All electrical power sources should only be deenergized by qualified personnel. Once power has been deenergized, it is important for the rescue team to employ lockout/tagout procedures to prevent the power from being reenergized.

MECHANICAL ENERGY HAZARDS

Many types of equipment processes within a confined space can either create or store physical energy. Physical energy is categorized as potential energy or kinetic energy. Potential energy, or stored energy, can be released in either a controlled manner or spontaneously. Pressurized pistons, compressed springs, and cables under tension are examples of stored energy. Kinetic energy is created by movement. This can result from applied force, the movement of the machinery itself, or the release of energy that was once stored, such as a pressurized piston releasing. Like electrical energy, potential and kinetic energy must be either secured or blocked to prevent further movement prior to an entry. Once this is accomplished, steps must be employed so the object or machinery remains secured and proper notification is communicated to other workers or rescuers until the operation is complete. This process is referred to as lockout/tagout.

Lockout/Tagout Standard

Lockout/Tagout is the title for OSHA Title 29 CFR, Part 1910.147, Control of Hazardous Energy. Title 29 CFR, Part 1910.147, describes the procedures and practices required for controlling the hazards associated with electrical, hydraulic, mechanical, pneumatic, chemical, and thermal energies (Occupational Safety & Health Administration, 2011b). Workers who enter into confined spaces to conduct routine or unscheduled work are at high risk of being injured or killed by the hazards described throughout this section. The OSHA Lockout/Tagout standard dictates that it is the responsibility of employers to protect their employees from the energy sources created by machinery and equipment while it is being serviced and maintained. (See Figure 8.5.) Employers are required to create a working energy control plan that is specific to the needs of their facility or site as well as the types of machines and equipment that are subject to be serviced.

The goal of lockout/tagout is to isolate, deenergize, or otherwise prevent movement by the use of an appropriate safety device. These devices are made up of **gate valve lockouts**, **pipe blanks**, wall switch covers, circuit breaker lockouts, and other specially designed

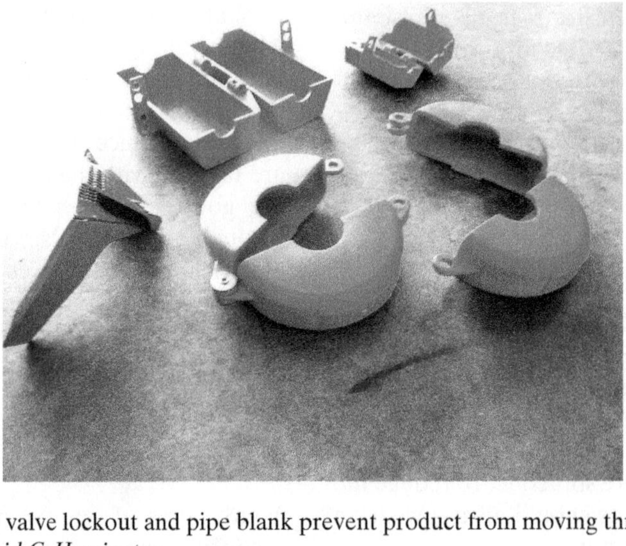

FIGURE 8.5 ■ A gate valve lockout and pipe blank prevent product from moving through pipes. *Source: Photo courtesy of David C. Harrington.*

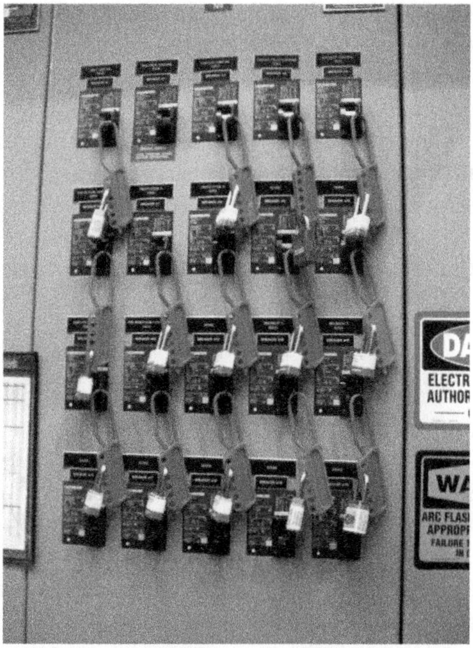

FIGURE 8.6 Circuit breaker lockouts prevent a worker from energizing a circuit. *Source: Photo courtesy of David C. Harrington.*

items that prevent the opening, closing, or activating of a piece of machinery or equipment. (See Figure 8.6.) Once the piece of machinery or equipment is shut down and secured, a **lockout hasp** is placed, allowing for each member of the entry team and backup teams to attach an issued padlock to the hasp that prevents it from being taken off. (See Figure 8.7.) Each entry team member keeps his key to the team's padlock on his person to prevent the lock and hasp from being removed until all entry team members have exited the space.

THE BASICS OF AIR MONITORING AND INSTRUMENTATION

Atmospheric hazards are one of the greatest threats to workers and rescue teams entering into confined spaces. Before an employee or rescuer enters into a confined space, the internal air must be tested using a direct-reading instrument. The purpose of monitoring the

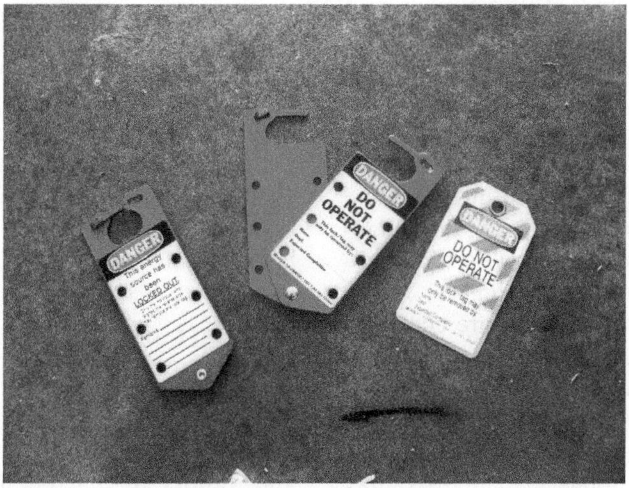

FIGURE 8.7 A lockout/tagout hasp is attached to a lockout device. Each worker attaches his own lock. *Source: Photo courtesy of David C. Harrington.*

atmosphere is to identify any contaminants that may occupy air in and around a confined space. Early identification is important as it drives operational decision making in several areas, including what types of protective equipment will be worn by response personnel, the areas where protection is required, predicting the potential health effects of an exposure, and the determination for further medical monitoring.

Air monitoring for confined-space rescue operations is typically conducted with direct-reading instrumentation. Direct-reading instruments are the first line of defense for preventing a response team from walking into an unsafe atmosphere. As gas enters into the sensor inside the instrument, it undergoes an electrochemical reaction that results in a change in the electrical output of the sensor. The concentration of the gas is based on the difference in electrical output. These highly sensitive instruments have the ability to identify not only high concentrations of contaminants in the air, but also concentrations down to 1 ppm. However, these devices can only detect specific classes or family groups of chemicals, as opposed to the specific individual chemical compounds. This can also be a disadvantage as it can result in false positives due to the detection of substances that may interfere with what the instrument is designed to detect. These instruments, despite their abilities, are only as good as the person operating them and their ability to interpret the readings. All devices require initial and ongoing training for the user; otherwise the likelihood of user error is extremely high.

Air monitoring instruments are classified as high-maintenance items because of the extreme sensitivity of the sensors within the instrument. Routine calibration has to be done in accordance with the manufacturer's recommendations. Some instruments may require calibration prior to each use, whereas other instruments require calibration on a regular monthly schedule. Some devices require that the instruments be sent to the manufacturer annually for routine maintenance and calibration. This ultimately relates to an expensive prospect for agencies that rely on these devices. For this reason, lesser equipped confined-space rescue teams rely on a hazardous materials team that possesses these instruments and can respond in support of the rescue operation.

COMBUSTIBLE GAS INDICATOR

Combustible gas indicators (CGIs) detect combustible gases and vapors. A filament inside of the instrument, usually made of platinum, is heated by burning the combustible gas or vapor. The amount of heat created within the chamber is then measured, allowing for the concentration of the combustible gas or vapor to be measured. The limitations of the device include accuracy, depending on the actual chemical being detected versus the calibration gas. Remember that readings taken in an oxygen-deficient atmosphere will be inaccurate.

FLAME IONIZATION DETECTORS

Flame ionization detectors (FIDs) are designed to detect the concentration of specific organic gases and vapors. This type of instrument pulls gases and vapors into the chamber, ionizing them in a flame. This, in turn, creates an electrical current that translates into how much concentration is present.

PORTABLE INFRARED SPECTROPHOTOMETER

Portable infrared spectrophotometers determine the identity and concentration of gases and vapors by the chemical being passed through different frequencies of infrared (IR). The specific frequency absorbed determines the specific chemical. This instrument is not recommended for use in potentially flammable atmospheres due to it not being intrinsically safe.

ULTRAVIOLET PHOTOIONIZATION DETECTOR

Ultraviolet (UV) photoionization detectors (PIDs) detect the total concentrations of many organic and some specific inorganic gases and vapors. PIDs accomplish this by ionizing the molecules of a gas or vapor using ultraviolet radiation.

DIRECT-READING COLORIMETIC INDICATOR TUBES

Colorimetric tubes measure concentrations of specific gases and vapors by creating a chemical reaction with a chemical indicator inside of a small glass tube. A stain is produced whose length throughout the tube or extent of color change observed is proportional to the compound's concentration. (See Figure 8.8.) There are different tubes for each specific gas or vapor requiring the user to know ahead of time what the expected type of vapor or gas is prior to using a specific tube set.

OXYGEN METER

Oxygen meters use an electrochemical sensor to measure the partial pressure of oxygen in the ambient air, in turn giving an oxygen concentration in percentage. It is important to remember that these devices must be calibrated in clean air prior to each use. Remember, oxygen sensors are susceptible to false readings if exposed to certain contaminants, such as ozone or carbon dioxide.

TECHNIQUES OF AIR MONITORING

OSHA requires that an atmosphere within a confined space be tested remotely prior to rescue crews making entry into the confined space. This allows for the team to mitigate any known hazards prior to placing crews into a deadly atmosphere. The priorities of air

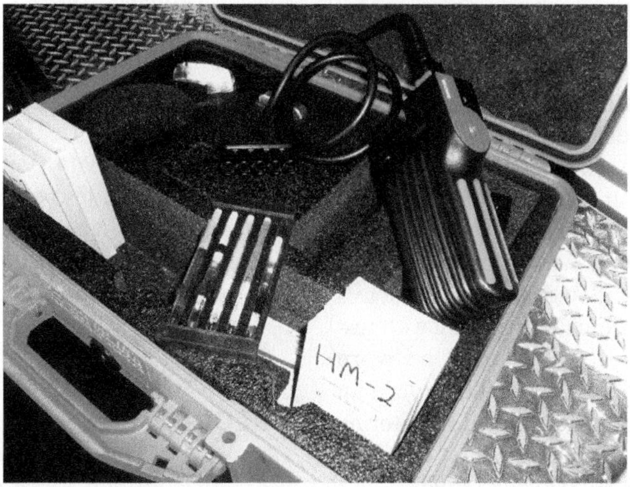

FIGURE 8.8 Direct-reading colorimetric indicator tubes can detect specific contaminants. *Source: Photo courtesy of David C. Harrington.*

monitoring should be based on the existing hazards and other information that is gathered during the size-up phase of the rescue operation. This information will dictate the types of detection equipment that will be used for the remainder of the operation and will guide the rescue team's decision as to what minimal level of personal protective equipment (PPE) will be employed during the air monitoring process. Because an inadequate concentration of oxygen may affect air monitoring instruments, oxygen should be tested for first. Then monitoring for what is **immediately dangerous to life and health (IDLH)** is conducted, followed by general on-site monitoring, perimeter monitoring, and periodic or continual monitoring.

When testing the atmosphere within the confined space, an initial reading should be taken first at the top of the space, second in the middle, and last at the bottom. Some concentrated gases may be lighter than air, causing them to accumulate at the top of the space, whereas gases that are heavier than air will tend to accumulate at the bottom of the space. Other gases that are more evenly mixed with air may hover toward the middle of the space. Remember, gases can exit through the entrance of the confined space, placing unprotected rescuers who may be gathered around the opening in danger of inhaling those toxins.

As the site assessment continues, great care must be taken to identify any possible sources that could generate these airborne contaminants. If the incident site is outdoors, initial measurements should be taken upwind, working around the site to the downwind portion of the incident site. This will allow for safety perimeters to be established. Adequate PPE along with respiratory protection always should be worn whenever collecting this information. Once an outer perimeter is determined, fixed monitoring instruments should be employed to establish where the use of PPE is no longer required.

Once the initial testing has been completed, the continuous air monitoring of the confined space can be conducted by the confined-space **attendant**. The attendant is stationed outside of a permit-required confined space while an entrant is conducting work inside of the space. It is recommended that personal air monitoring instruments capable of continuous monitoring should also be worn by rescue entry personnel while they are inside the confined space.

Side Bar

Responsibilities of a Confined-Space Attendant

- Performing no other duties that interfere with the attendant's primary duties
- Remaining outside the permit space during entry operations unless relieved by another authorized attendant
- Knowing the existing and potential hazards, including information on the mode of exposure, signs, or symptoms
- Maintaining communication with and keeping an accurate account of workers entering the permit space
- Ordering evacuation of the permit space when one of the following occurs:
    - A prohibited condition exists.
    - A worker shows signs of physiological effects of hazard exposure.
    - An emergency outside the confined space exists.
    - The attendant cannot effectively and/or safely perform required duties.
- Summoning rescue and other services during an emergency
- Ensuring that unauthorized people stay away from permit space (OSHA, 2011a)

PERSONAL PROTECTIVE EQUIPMENT

PPE for confined-space rescue operations is based on the existing and potential hazards found within a confined space. It should be concluded that bulky clothing such as structural firefighting gear should not be utilized in confined spaces due to the increased risk of getting hung on obstacles inside small enclosed spaces. If a potential flash hazard is possible, flame-resistant clothing such as brush gear is an excellent alternative. This not only gives the wearer an added level of protection from a **flash fire**, but it also gives the wearer some protection from sharp objects. (See Figure 8.9.) If a flammable or explosive atmosphere exists, an entry should not be made until the hazard is mitigated.

The entrant should also wear a low-profile rescue helmet similar to what is worn during vertical rescue operations. Steel-toed boots will protect the entrant's feet from being crushed by heavy objects. Durable rescue gloves designed for vertical work will give the wearer better dexterity for handing the vertical rope and hardware required to extract the victim. Safety glasses should always be worn to protect the rescuer's eyes. If loud sounds are an existing or potential issue, ear plugs or headphones are recommended to protect the entrant from hearing damage. An additional piece of important equipment that every rescuer should carry is at least one and preferably two good intrinsically safe flashlights. One of these lights should be mounted directly to the rescue helmet and the other carried in or attached to the rescuer's gear.

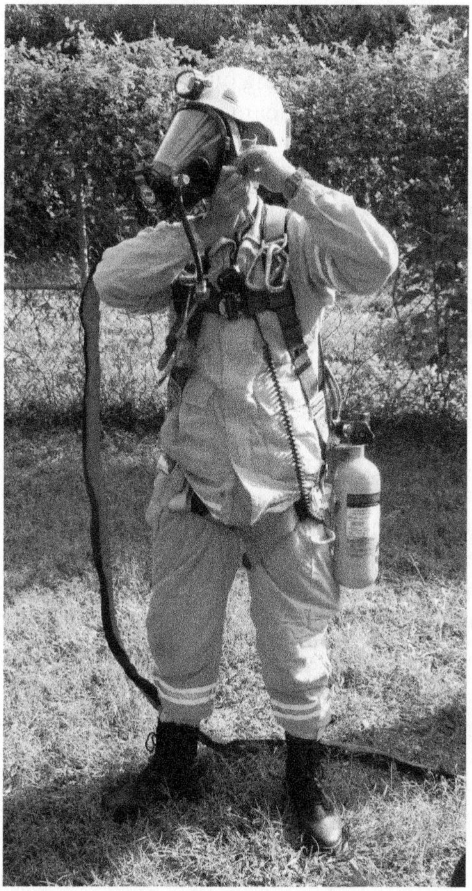

FIGURE 8.9 ■ Flame-resistant clothing—such as brush gear, rescue helmet, gloves, and eye and respiratory protection—gives responders standard protective equipment when entering into a confined space. *Source: Photo courtesy of David C. Harrington.*

RESPIRATORY PROTECTION

Respiratory protection for personnel entering a confined space will vary depending on the existing or potential atmospheric hazards. It is imperative that response personnel be trained for each different type of respirator that they may have to wear. In addition, fit tests administered by qualified testing facilities and technicians are required. A fit test will determine what size mask an entrant will wear in order to provide a tight seal on the face, preventing contaminants from entering into the mask.

AIR-PURIFYING RESPIRATORS

Workers who enter into a confined space identified as containing adequate oxygen but possibly toxic vapors may choose to wear air-purifying respirators. Air-purifying respirators are designed to protect the wearer from dangerous levels of toxic contaminants, gasses, and vapors by filtering out or cleaning chemical gases through canisters attached to the mask that is held against the wearer's face by adjustable straps. The canisters are designed and built to filter out specific contaminates. Another type of respiratory protection is in the form of a particulate respirator that is designed to protect the wearer from particulates such as dust. This type of respirator offers the least protection of all the air-purifying respirator types.

One of the disadvantages of the air-purifying respirator system is that it does not protect the wearer from every known contaminant nor does it protect the wearer in an oxygen-deficient atmosphere. It is very important to identify the contaminant within a space so that the correct canister may be chosen.

SELF-CONTAINED BREATHING APPARATUS

Air-supplied respirators provide air to the wearer from a supplied air source, regulating it to normal breathing pressures. This not only protects the wearer in oxygen-deficient atmospheres that can be created by displacement gasses, but it also protects the wearer from the vapors from toxic chemicals and other dangerous gasses that may not be applicable to air-purifying respirators. Air-supplied respirators can be in the form of a self-contained breathing apparatus (SCBA) or supplied-air breathing apparatus (SABA).

SCBAs are used by firefighters for structural firefighting or hazardous materials operations. This type of respirator is easily identified by the air cylinder that is attached to the frame that the user wears on his or her back. The cylinder can be made from steel, aluminum, and, most often, a carbon fiber-wrapped composite material. Their sizes vary, providing the wearer 30 to 60 minutes worth of breathable air. This time frame is dependent on the user and how quickly he breathes the air within the cylinder. The user wears a full-face mask attached to an air line connected to a regulator that converts air from the high-pressure cylinder to a lower breathable pressure. SCBAs are now designed to provide positive pressure. This system delivers pressure within the face mask that is slightly above outside ambient air. If the seal between the face piece and the user face is broken, the positive pressure will prevent contaminants from entering inside the face piece. Although an SCBA is very durable, easy to use, and offers excellent protection, its use for confined-space rescue operation is limited due to its bulkiness, excessive weight, and limited air supply.

A confined space with small passageways and obstacles makes an SCBA a dangerous option for the entrant. If the decision is made to use the SCBA as the respirator of choice, implementation of an air management plan is critical. This plan will base time in the confined space on the size of SCBA cylinder that the entry team is using. For example, if the rescue team is using a 4,500 pounds per square inch (psi) SCBA cylinder, it must be understood that the average person will have approximately 30 to 45 minutes of air. Variations are due to the physical conditioning of the entrant and the amount of stress he is under. Also, if we decide that we will set and maintain a reserve of 25 percent of the total psi for an emergency egress, this further reduces the available amount of air. This total will have to be divided among the time it takes to get to the patient; package, transfer, and remove the patient; and exit the space. This ultimately may reduce the working time in the space to approximately 10 to 15 minutes.

An **air management officer** should be assigned to keep track of the entry team's time in the space and air levels. He should request each member's air level at least every

5 minutes. When the team member with the lowest air level reaches the minimal psi, the entire team should exit the space.

SUPPLIED-AIR BREATHING APPARATUS

The supplied-air breathing apparatus (SABA) is an air-supplied respirator whose air source is kept outside of confined space, as opposed to the entrant wearing an air cylinder. The user still wears a full-face mask, but the air line attached to the mask is secured to the user's full body harness and connects into another air line that is stretched to the outside of the space and connects into the pressure-reducing regulator on a customized air cart where the air cylinders are located. The advantages of a SABA system are that the user is offered the same level of respiratory protection as a SCBA but without the bulky profile, and this allows the entrant to maneuver through extremely narrow passages and around a variety of obstacles. Like an SCBA, the SABA system has positive pressure capability. With SABA, the user has an unlimited air supply. The air cart is designed to hold various sources of air, including SCBA bottles or larger cascade bottles. When in use, only one bottle at a time is used by the entry team. Typically, an entry team consists of two persons who are breathing off a single bottle until it reaches a minimal pressure of, typically, 500 psi. At that time, the air supply officer has the ability to switch to the full bottle attached next to the one in use. Once the air supply officer conducts the switchover, he will place a full bottle into the side where the empty one was attached. The advantage of using the larger cascade bottles is that they can last much longer than the smaller SCBA cylinders.

SABA has its limitations. The maximum distance that the air lines can be stretched is 300 feet. Although the SABA creates a lesser profile for the entrant, the air lines can create an entanglement hazard for the entry team, especially when more than two members of the team are inside the confined space at the same time. In the event of a failure of the SABA system, a 10-minute escape bottle is attached to each entrant's full body harness, giving the entrant a self-contained emergency air source capable of giving him a minimal time to make a quick escape out of the confined space. This has been found to be the best option for confined-space rescue operations.

OSHA regulations require that an attendant be stationed outside the confined space when an entrant is conducting any kind of work. When the entry team enters the confined space, a backup entry team must be set up, in place, and ready to perform a rescue of the initial entry team should trouble ensue. A separate supplied-air system should be set up for the backup team to utilize. This level of redundancy ensures that if the initial entry team becomes incapacitated due to a failure of the air-supply system, the backup rescue team will not be affected.

VENTILATION EQUIPMENT

The normal concentration of oxygen in air is between 20.8 and 21 percent. Any concentration below 19.5 percent is considered an oxygen-deficient atmosphere and above 23 percent is considered an oxygen-enriched atmosphere. An oxygen-deficient atmosphere may be the result of a contaminant or inert gas pushing the oxygen out of the space. Once the atmosphere has been tested for oxygen levels, toxic contaminants, and gasses, it should be flushed with fresh air using a positive pressure blower. Electric blowers should be intrinsically safe so that there is no risk of causing an explosion if used in an explosive atmosphere. Attachments to the blower that can be dropped into the confined space, such as a large flexible air hose, can allow fresh air to flush out any potential contaminants. If the entrance to the space has a small-diameter opening, such as a manhole, the flexible hose can easily occlude the passageway, reducing the area the rescue team has for entrance and egress. To address this issue, an attachment, the Saddle Vent, connects to the flexible hose. The Saddle Vent has a narrowed center section that broadens out on both ends, allowing for connection of the flexible hose on both ends. This narrowed section connects and sits against the wall of the passageway entrance, reducing the size of the obstruction.

COMMUNICATIONS EQUIPMENT

Communications is a required component of confined-space operations. Two means of communication are required between the entry team and attendants outside of the space before an entry may occur. This redundancy allows for a backup communication plan in the event that the primary means of communication fails. A reliable communication system is required during entry into a confined space between the attendant and the entry team. The attendant should conduct a **personnel accountability report (PAR)** with the entry team every 5 to 10 minutes.

The easiest and simplest form of communication is direct line-of-sight and voice communications between the entry team and the attendants. Radios can be effective in spaces where the configuration of the space does not interfere with the radio waves. Because the entry team will, in most cases, be wearing respiratory protection in the form of SABA, clear communication is difficult, making it difficult to understand the entry team when they speak into the radio through their masks. Attachments, such as throat-mikes or mask-mike adapters that are made for such operations, can be used. Many of these attachments have hands-free options, allowing the entry team member to communicate with the other team members or the outside attendant without having to push a transmit button. Another type of device is hard-wire communications equipment. Each of the entry team personnel has his own separate communications cable that connects to his throat-mike or headset, which then links him directly to a communications hub or console outside of the confined space so that the attendant can monitor and communicate with the entry team members. Each entrant relying on a SABA system will often utilize a single protective Kevlar sheath that encloses the air line and hard-wire communications line. This serves to condense both of these lines, reducing the potential for entanglement as well as protecting the lines from damage. These cables, however, cannot be used as retrieval lines. Additional rescue ropes can act as the backup means of communications, allowing for rope signals to be used between the attendants and the rescue team. These ropes also act as the retrieval line. Further, if the rope is long enough, the rescue team can daisy chain themselves on the same rope, reducing the entanglement hazard. As part of the personnel accountability system, routine communications PAR checks should be conducted every 5 to 10 minutes in order to maintain accountability of the entry team. Failure to communicate with the team should be just cause to deploy the backup rescue team.

ACCESS AND EGRESS EQUIPMENT

There is crossover between the various types of equipment and skills used by rescue responders. For this reason, many technical rescue teams are cross-trained in different disciplines, allowing them to be proficient in using the wide range of devices available to them. An awareness-level responder does not have to possess the qualifications of an operations- or technician-level provider to be an expert at using a specific piece of equipment. However, it is important for awareness-level providers to understand when and how to prepare equipment for use, especially before it is needed.

VERTICAL RESCUE EQUIPMENT

Not every confined space has easy access. Most confined spaces require the entrant to utilize **access and egress equipment** to enter into and exit the space. This might be something as simple as a ladder. If there is not a connected ladder giving entrants a means to enter into the space, other avenues will have to be utilized, such as a tripod. A tripod is a commercially designed system that allows for attachment of both a high-point connection for lowering and a retrieval system. Tripods are constructed using steel or aluminum and can be easily assembled and placed above the entrance of the vertical confined space. A hand-crank mechanical winch is also used by attaching one of the tripod legs that will be used to lower and raise the entrants on a steel cable. A mechanical winch is not the preferred device to use in confined-space rescue operations as it can lead to additional injuries.

Another unique device that can be used to lower and raise a rescuer, as well as the victim, is a prerigged mechanical haul system. These devices utilize a 3-to-1 or a 4-to-1 mechanical advantage haul system. They can be easily constructed on site using standard vertical hardware or stored prebuilt in their storage bags until needed, reducing the time required to place them in operation at the scene of a rescue. A mechanical advantage system utilizes rope and a series of pulleys that takes the total weight (load) and divides it proportionally through the physics of the system, reducing the weight and making it more manageable to pull. These haul systems can also be adapted to pull the load horizontally through passages. (See Figure 8.10.)

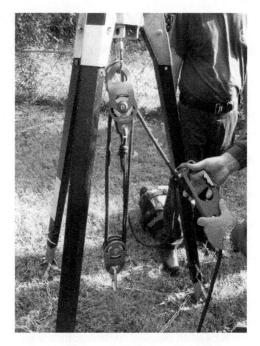

FIGURE 8.10 A prerigged mechanical haul system attached to a tripod offers an easy and safe method for lowering and raising rescuers from a vertical space. *Source: Photo courtesy of David C. Harrington.*

PATIENT PACKAGING AND EXTRICATION DEVICES

Once the victim has been located, if uninjured it may be as simple as assisting him out of the space, or **packaging** the patient prior to bring him out. If the victim is unconscious or injured, rescuers must package the patient in an extrication device. Rescue teams use three different types of extraction devices. A patient who is unconscious and has to be navigated horizontally through narrow passages will most likely be placed in a full-body extraction device. This device, similar to a full-body sleeve, cocoons the victim, reducing his profile and allowing the rescuers to slide him through extremely narrow passageways. This device has attachment points on the end toward the head of the victim, allowing for a vertical lift while maintaining the victim in an inline position.

Another packaging device is similar to the Kendrick Extrication Device (KED) or XP-1 immobilization devices used by EMS for removing patients from motor vehicle collisions. This type of device has hard attachment points built into the shoulder and chest straps, allowing for the victim to be lifted vertically using either a mechanical advantage or the cable from a tripod. Both of these devices are designed to be used in conjunction with other immobilization tools if the patient requires cervical spine protection. The KED can be used to immobilize a victim inside of a confined space. However, unlike other similar devices designed specifically for confined-space rescues, the KED does not have attachment points for vertical lift. Under ideal conditions, however, a victim who is not suffering a traumatic injury involving the cervical spine and is wearing a full-body harness can be easily removed from a space by simply attaching the retrieval line to the victim's harness, allowing him to be hoisted out.

Wristlets—wide, padded straps secured around an entrant's wrists—are not normally used unless there is no other means of extraction. The opposite ends of the straps secure to the haul system. Once attached to the haul system, the entrant can be pulled horizontally or lifted vertically through narrow passages. The use of wristlets significantly decreases an entrant's profile by bringing his arms above his head, thus reducing the likelihood of becoming entangled while being moved. Although this can significantly reduce a victim's profile, it can also injure him since it does not offer cervical spine protection and can easily dislocate the wearer's shoulders.

PATIENT CARE CONSIDERATIONS

Providing appropriate patient care within a confined space is very difficult to do. In most cases, rescue teams are not notified until things have gone really bad. If the victim has suffered a medical event due to a hazardous atmosphere, chances are likely that the victim will already be deceased by the time rescuers gain access to him. CPR under most conditions cannot be effectively performed within a confined space and should not be initiated. However, if the patient is unresponsive or not breathing, attempts should be made to open the airway and perform supportive care. If the patient has suffered a traumatic injury, care should be performed only in life-threatening conditions such as bleeding control. Cervical spine immobilization can be easily initiated in conjunction with the use of a KED or other patient extraction device, but other care for non-life-threatening conditions should be delayed until the patient has been removed. If the patient has been contaminated with any hazardous materials, decontamination should be conducted prior to moving the patient to the back of a clean ambulance.

CONFINED-SPACE PRE-RESPONSE

Like every technical rescue operation, pre-response begins with the intensive training required for that particular discipline. The NFPA-recommended and specific training for each level of response personnel also incorporates within it how a team should respond to an incident. Response to a confined-space incident begins with conducting a thorough and complete size-up. A size-up is the process of gathering accurate and relevant information about a situation that will assist response personnel to create an effective and safe incident action plan. In terms of confined space, if you have an industrial facility within your jurisdiction, the size-up should always begin with a facility orientation, which is also known as a preplan tour. This should lead into the development of a library of preplans that detail the confined spaces within the facility. Preplans offer the rescue team valuable insight as to what each facility or site has in terms of the number of permit-controlled confined spaces, configuration types, hazards, lockout/tagout requirements, and equipment needs. These preplans should be updated at least every 2 years or any time additions or changes are made to a facility or site. A rescue team should never wait until an incident occurs to become familiar with a specific facility or site. This can only lead to delays in bringing resources together, further reducing the likelihood of a would-be victim from being saved.

Best Practice

Successful Confined-Space Rescue of Public Works Sewer Worker

On September 17, 2008, in Pleasant Hills, Pennsylvania, Baldwin EMS along with the Pleasant Hills Fire Department was dispatched to a report of an unconscious worker inside of a confined space. Baldwin EMS, which is the primary technical rescue provider for Allegheny County, responded with a heavy rescue unit and medic units. On arrival, rescuers found a semiconscious male patient in a seated position in a storm sewer that was approximately 12 feet deep and just under 2 feet in diameter. Interviews with the co-workers indicated that the victim had been performing work when he came to the surface complaining of difficulty breathing. He then went unconscious and collapsed back into the space.

Rescue crews immediately initiated air monitoring of the space. Initial readings indicated an oxygen content of 20.9 percent. Even though there was also a reading of 250 to 300 ppm of carbon monoxide, no LEL atmosphere was detected. Positive-pressure ventilation blowers were placed, and the space was ventilated in an effort to decrease the carbon monoxide levels. Within a short period, the patient's level of consciousness appeared to improve significantly. As rescue crews communicated verbally with the patient, a small oxygen cylinder was lowered along with an attached oxygen administration mask. The patient was instructed to place the mask on his face. A Baldwin EMS paramedic trained in confined-space rescue operations donned a full-body harness and was lowered into the space from a positioned tripod using a 4:1 haul system. Once patient contact was made, a further assessment was conducted. With the carbon monoxide levels now down to 0 ppm, the patient had improved and was only complaining of dizziness. As a precaution, the patient was immobilized using a cervical collar and an extraction device. The patient was attached to the haul system and removed vertically from the confined space. Once removed, the patient was secured to a long spine board and transferred to the awaiting medic unit. The patient was then transported to the local ED for evaluation and treatment.

The success of this operation was due to the high quality of the response personnel and their training, giving them the ability to recognize the conditions and hazards associated with a confined space. Proper hazard mitigation was accomplished, allowing for expedient access to the patient. These actions resulted in the patient being successfully extricated from the confined space.

CONFINED-SPACE RESPONSE

Upon receipt of a possible confined-space incident, detailed information should immediately be gathered by the 9-1-1 dispatcher and disseminated to the appropriate response personnel. If the location of dispatch is not an actual address or if the scene is located in a rural area, landmarks identifying the scene should be gathered. When responding to an industrial facility, personnel should request an escort to be a guide through the facility. Many facilities can be confusing to navigate even based upon the best-drawn floor plan. In addition, facility personnel are expert on the processes and equipment as well as their associated hazards, thus creating a safer environment for response personnel. Other information should include, if known, whether the space is vertical or horizontal, additional hazards, and the number of patients both inside and outside the space.

ON-SCENE OPERATIONS

Upon arriving on the scene, discipline should be used to resist the urge to immediately enter into the actual site of the incident without properly assessing for hazards. Before committing any resources, apparent hazards around the site should be determined. As response personnel approach the site, they should also be observant of any clues that would indicate what the true emergency entails. If responding to a farm or agriculture facility, grain bins, deep wells, manure pits, or storage areas are mostly likely to be present and may be the location of the patient or, in many cases, patients. Response personnel should never be lured into approaching a confined space by the frantic nature of the situation. It should be assumed that the people who are already there may not be aware of the hazards associated with the space.

If responding to an industrial environment, there can be even more hazards. A knowledgeable facility liaison can be a good source of information pertaining to the work processes, on-site hazardous materials, and lockout/tagout needs. Remember, industrial, public works, and private sectors are required to follow state and federal regulations pertaining to confined-space entry. If an incident has occurred on one of these sites, it is likely that the event has migrated beyond the facility's ability to mitigate it with its on-site resources.

Safety should be the first consideration for any incident. The order of safety is the responder first, followed by the safety of fellow rescuers, then the safety of bystanders, and then the safety of the victim or victims. Self-discipline and effort may have to be taken to restrain bystanders, family members, and co-workers from entering into the space to effect a rescue. Security or law enforcement may have to be utilized to accomplish this task.

CONFINED-SPACE RESOURCES

As the size-up is completed, the resources that will be needed to deal with the situation should be identified. Part of preplanning should have identified what resources are available within a jurisdiction. A resource book that lists the area rescue and public work resources, their response times, and qualifications should be carried on every command vehicle. This information should include the response capabilities of the area rescue teams and how long it will take them to arrive. Many agencies may be trained only to the awareness level, allowing them to perform a rescue from outside of the confined space but preventing them from being able to make entry into the space. Others may possess an in-house technical rescue team trained to the operations or technician-level in confined space. This information is vital when making such a request. The facility itself may have an internal rescue team and is already effecting a rescue or recovery. Other resources to consider are local utilities that can isolate the electric, gas, and water lines.

A hazardous materials team will be warranted if it is suspected that a hazardous materials release has occurred. Law enforcement should also be considered in order to assist in traffic control as well as scene security. If the incident results in a fatality, law enforcement will also be required to conduct an investigation.

CONFINED-SPACE INCIDENT COMMAND

Regardless of who arrives first, command should be immediately established. Typically, the highest-ranking official is in command in accordance with **National Incident Management System (NIMS)** guidelines. Depending on the size and complexity of the overall operation, the incident commander may choose to create an operations sector under which all rescue and recovery portions of the mission will be working. Additional functions will also be under the operations sector, including medical, hazardous materials if warranted, and any other roles deemed necessary to carry out the mission.

Another vital function that must be initiated early is a staging area for incoming resources. Despite whether the situation is in an urban or rural area, the amount of resources required to mitigate this type of rescue can easily add up, challenging the best logistics officer. An apparatus staging area should be created in a parking area, freeing up the main entrance and egress of the site location. Emergency response personnel should also be staged in a safe area well away from any hazards. Equipment staging should be in an area accessible to the rescue site, but not one that blocks the entrance or egress to the space.

As equipment and personnel arrive on scene, a resource officer should begin creating an accountability list that will serve to keep track of all on-site responders. As rescuers are assigned to specific functions, this list can be modified and reflected on the NIMS incident command system forms completed by the command staff. As rescuers are released or leave the incident, it becomes important for the accountability officer to indicate this in his accountability system. Periodically, a PAR check should be conducted, confirming that all responders are accounted for.

An awareness-level provider at a confined-space incident may be faced with having to effect a rescue from outside of the confined space. As specified within NFPA 1006, awareness-level providers should be familiar with the use of retrieval systems. If a victim is still attached to a retrieval line on a tripod, it may be quite possible to remove the victim from the confined space with minimal effort. This quick action can save valuable time and quite possibly the life of the victim.

Caution should always be employed. If a hazardous material is suspected as being the culprit, do not approach the entrance of the confined space until it has been properly assessed and ventilated if needed. If the victim experienced a medical emergency while in the space, no contaminant is suspected, and the retrieval line is still attached, the victim can then be lifted out of the space to safety. If the victim is not attached to a retrieval line, this complicates matters, and in this circumstance you should not go into the space to connect anyone. If the site has a hooker pole available, this valuable device can be employed to connect a retrieval line to a connection point on the victim's harness.

A hooker pole is an extendable fiberglass pole with a self-locking carabiner connected to a distal attachment point. (See Figure 8.11.) The end of the retrieval line is attached to the carabiner on one end, and the other end of the

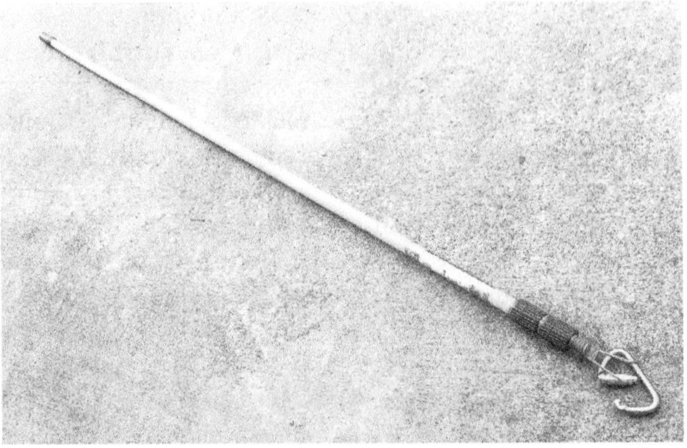

FIGURE 8.11 An extendable hooker pole with an attached carabiner can be used by a rescuer outside of the space to connect to an entrant's body harness. Prior to approaching the space, rescuers must properly test the atmosphere around and in the space to ensure that it is safe. *Source: Photo courtesy of David C. Harrington.*

retrieval line remains outside of the space and becomes part of the haul system. When attaching to a victim's body harness, it is important to make every attempt to connect into a high point on the victim, such as the connection point on the patient's shoulder or dorsal attachment point. (See Figure 8.12.) This will ensure that the victim is lifted in a more vertical fashion. A dorsal attachment point is a strap or attachment point built into the upper

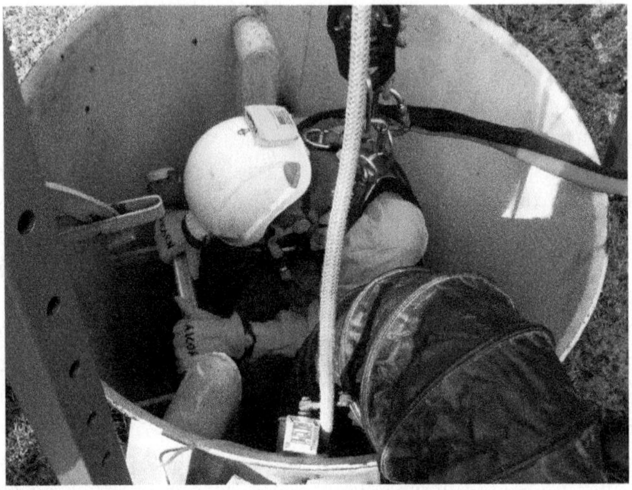

FIGURE 8.12 A rescuer wearing a full-body harness while breathing off of a supplied-air breathing system climbs into a vertical confined space. Note that the haul system is connected to the harness's dorsal attachment point. *Source: Photo courtesy of David C. Harrington.*

center of a full-body harness. Connections made toward the mid-body will only serve to cause the victim to become horizontal during the lift, adding to the complexities of trying to bring him through a small vertical opening. However, in a true emergency, go with whichever attachment point on the harness you can manage to access.

If the victim cannot be removed with the available resources, securing the victim will allow for the responding rescue team to easily complete the retrieval. It must be emphasized that if the victim came into contact with electrical lines while inside of the confined space, great caution should be taken before touching any retrieval lines, especially if they are of the cable type. This equipment may still be energized. As part of the lockout/tagout procedures, electrical energy within the space should be shut off and secured by qualified personnel prior to affecting any rescue or recovery.

Once the victims have been removed from the space and transferred to the care of EMS, the rescue team will then begin the demobilization portion of the operations. This begins with ensuring that all rescue personnel are accounted for and safe. Equipment will then be removed from the space, decontaminated if required, and placed back in the staging area. As equipment is made ready for the next response, it will be placed where it came from.

A critique should then be conducted in order to address any immediate issues pertaining directly to the operation. A more formalized critique should be scheduled for later. Lockout/tagout can be removed when the facility of site is turned back over to the owners.

In any situation involving the injury or death of a worker, the state OSHA office will conduct an investigation. Leaving evidence in place and undisturbed until the investigation concludes may be required. As response documentation is prepared, be aware that everything that occurred should be thoroughly documented. This may very well be used later on during the investigation phase conducted by the authorities.

CHAPTER REVIEW

Summary

As an awareness-level provider responding to a reported confined-space incident, the responsibility is to gather as much information as possible in order to build an accurate picture of what to expect on arrival. Rushing into the scene can only spell disaster for responders. It is important to be observant for existing and potential hazards. By understanding the limitations of awareness-level training, the rescue team may utilize what is within its capability when responding to a confined-space incident and requesting resources. Knowing what resources are available in an area and how long it will take responders to reach the situation makes it possible to create a better incident action plan that can guide the operation toward success. Furthermore, the greatest traits that any emergency responder can possess are self-control and the discipline to know when not to do something, no matter how tempting it may be. Of all fatalities involved in confined-space incidents, 60 percent are the would-be rescuers. Complacency and lack of knowledge are two key ingredients to a disastrous end to an operation.

WHAT WOULD YOU DO? Reflection

As you approach the scene, you should be observant for plume clouds or any other signs of hazardous materials. Be observant for victims in and around the scene. Attempt to identify any witnesses or workers who may be able to offer additional information about the incident. Expect the possibility of a hazardous atmosphere inside of the space—possibly carbon monoxide from the gasoline pump running inside the confined space. Electrical hazards from any faulty wiring submerged in the water could also be a risk.

Initially, the scene should be secured to prevent any additional persons from entering the confined space. A safety corridor should be established to prevent anyone from being overcome from the possible vapors exiting the space. Incident command should be established and communicated to dispatch. Additional resources should immediately be requested. A staging area should be established for incoming apparatus and personnel.

Initial response resources should include fire, EMS transport, a technician-level confined-space rescue team, hazardous materials team, public works, and law enforcement.

Review Questions

1. What are the criteria for an enclosure to be classified as a confined space?
2. What are the criteria for a confined space to be classified as a permit-controlled confined space?
3. List six types of enclosures that are identified as confined spaces.
4. Which level of responder is trained to recognize the need for confined-space rescue, identify the hazards associated with confined-space incidents, recognize the different types of confined spaces, and have the ability to only perform a non-entry rescue of a victim?
5. Which NFPA document identifies the different levels of training for responders to confined-space rescue incidents?
6. What devices may be used to effect a non-entry rescue of an entrant?
7. When responding to a reported confined-space incident, what information should be obtained that will assist responders during the size-up phase?
8. The process of deenergizing a piece of machinery by shutting it off at the circuit breaker and attaching a circuit breaker lockout along with a lockout hasp and padlock is part of what OSHA standard?
9. What are the differences between an oxygen-enriched environment and an oxygen-deficient environment?
10. List the different hazards associated with a confined space.

References

Eady, M. (2006, September). "The Rescue Technician and NFPA Standards." *Fire Engineering*.

National Fire Protection Association. (2009). "NFPA 1670: Standard on Operations and Training for Technical Search and Rescue Incidents." (Quincy, MA: National Fire Protection Agency.)

National Fire Protection Association. (2013). "NFPA 1006: Standard for Technical Rescuer Professional Qualifications, Confined Space

Rescue." (Quincy, MA: National Fire Protection Association.)

Occupational Safety & Health Administration. (2011a). OSHA CFR 1910.146: "Permit-Required Confined Spaces." See the organization website.

Occupational Safety & Health Administration. (2011b). OSHA CFR 1910.147: "The Control of Hazardous Energy (Lockout/Tagout)." See the organization website.

Key Terms

access and egress equipment The equipment utilized by confined-space rescue teams to enter into and exit from a confined space.

air management officer An attendant who is assigned to oversee and track the time in and air usage by entry personnel while operating within a confined space.

attendant Someone trained in permit-required confined-space entry and surface rescue who remains outside of the confined space and monitors the safety of the authorized entrant or entry team.

concentration Quantity of a substance dissolved in, or mixed with, a specific quantity of another substance.

engulfment An event during which a liquid or fine granular solid substance converges in surrounding and/or burying the victim.

entrant An employee or rescuer who is trained to enter a permit-required confined space.

entrapment A condition in which a victim cannot self-rescue due to being trapped by debris, soil, or other product.

flash fire A sudden, intense, but very short in duration fire caused by the ignition of a mixture of a flammable substance such as dust, a flammable or combustible vapor, or a flammable gas dispersed in air.

gate-valve lockouts Devices used to cover a control valve that denies access to unauthorized personnel preventing them from opening the valve.

immediately dangerous to life and health (IDLH) A condition that poses an immediate or delayed threat to life or that would cause irreversible adverse health effects.

lockout hasps Scissor-like lockout devices with multiple slots for padlocks; attached to a switch, panel, or other loop to prevent access by unauthorized personnel.

lower explosive limit (LEL) The minimal concentration of a gas or vapor in air capable of producing an explosion in the presence of an ignition source.

National Incident Management System (NIMS) A comprehensive, national approach to incident management that includes the incident command system, multi-agency coordination systems, and public information systems.

packaging The process of preparing a patient for removal from a confined space with the use of specially designed equipment to protects a patient's cervical spine, torso, and extremities.

parts per million (ppm) The concentration by volume of one part of a gas or vapor, or by weight of a liquid or solid, per million parts of air or liquid.

personnel accountability report (PAR) A systematic process conducted by incident command and used to account for all response personnel on the scene of an operation.

pipe blanks Disks or flanges placed on the end of or within a pipe connection that prevents liquid product from flowing through the pipe.

upper explosive limit (UEL) Highest concentration of a gas or vapor in air capable of producing an explosion in the presence of an ignition source.

ventilation The process of purging a contaminated atmosphere within a confined space with fresh air by the use of specially designed fans or blowers.

CHAPTER 9

Above-Ground and Below-Ground Rescue

Scott Chappell

Objectives

After reading this chapter, the student should be able to:

9.1 Define the priorities for incidents involving above-ground or below-ground rescues.
9.2 Describe the role of EMS in above-ground and below-ground situations.
9.3 Identify ways that initial responders could expedite patient contact in complex rescue situations.
9.4 Discuss the hazards that are unique to various above-ground and below-ground incidents.

Key Terms

anchors
caves
carabiners
excavation
fall factor
FinnForm boards
ground pads
harnesses
pulleys
Occupational Safety and Health Administration (OSHA)
Stokes baskets
trench
trench box
U.S. National Grid (USNG)
webbing

WHAT WOULD YOU DO?

An EMS agency responds to a single-vehicle collision on a remote mountain road. As units arrive on the scene, they find skid marks and evidence of a vehicle leaving the roadway and going down the hillside. Crews see a vehicle and an injured person approximately 200 feet down the 400-foot hill. Although the hill is very steep and covered with rocks and debris, the EMS personnel will be able to walk down the hill to the patient if they choose to do so. You are the EMS supervisor on the scene and in charge of the incident.

Questions

1. What hazards exist for the rescuers and the patient?
2. If the crew chooses to walk down the hill, should they package and move the patient back to the ambulance on the roadway? Why or why not?
3. What, if any, additional resources should be requested?

INTRODUCTION

Occasionally, EMS assists patients who are located above- or below-ground level. In some incidents, a patient has a medical emergency while in a precarious location, and at other times the location of the patient precipitates the emergency. In all cases, victims must be accessed, evaluated, treated, and then removed from the location. EMS agencies play a vital role in this process and must work with other first-response agencies to assist with rapid patient care and a seamless transition from the rescue crew to the EMS providers. This chapter will discuss the rescue of victims and patients who are in situations both above- and below-ground and who require specially trained rescuers with the proper equipment to remove or even access those in need of assistance.

When an emergency occurs in which a victim is above- or below-ground level and is unable to be reached or removed by conventional techniques, a specialized team of rescuers must be called in to assist. Many agencies have a special operations team that is charged with performing this type of rescue. The host agency may be a fire department, EMS agency, law enforcement, or another group, but regardless of origin the rescuers must have proper training and equipment to safely execute a rescue. National standards exist that outline the training requirements of the rescuers and standards for their equipment. In addition, rescuers must continuously train and familiarize themselves with industry best practices, including new equipment and techniques that are constantly being introduced. (See Figure 9.1.)

There are five categories of above- and below-ground rescue discussed in this chapter: high-angle rescue, low-angle rescue, trench/excavation rescue, cave/cavern rescue, and wilderness/rough terrain rescue. Although there are similarities in each rescue scenario, rescuers will find challenges unique to each category that must be addressed during the treatment and extraction of the victims or patients. Each category will be examined in terms of command considerations, hazards and safety, treatment challenges, and rescue challenges. Although responders must mitigate emergencies based on the particular situation, they must be prepared for all emergencies to support a swift and efficient operation from the time of dispatch to

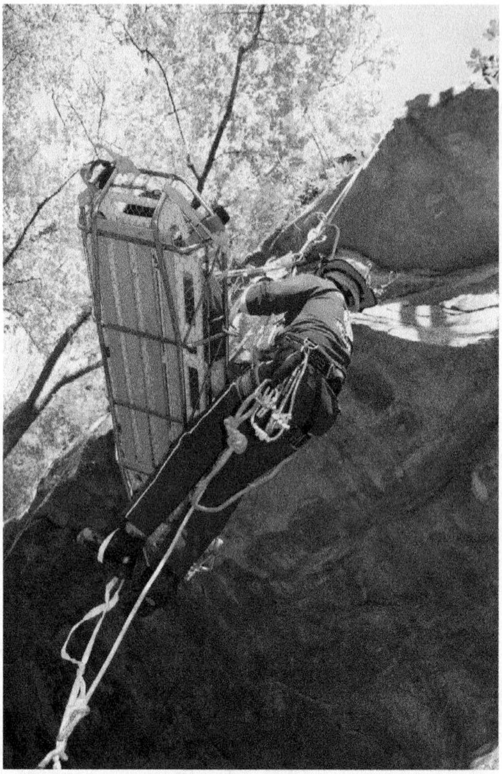

FIGURE 9.1 Above- and below-ground rescues may present hazards to both the rescuer and the patient. Specialized training and equipment are required to ensure a safe and efficient rescue.

patient contact, patient rescue, and ultimately patient transport to the most appropriate facility.

COMMAND CONSIDERATIONS FOR ABOVE- AND BELOW-GROUND RESCUE

The nature of above- and below-ground rescues places rescuers and patients in harm's way. In some cases, the patient is in no immediate distress or danger until he is attached to a rope and raised or lowered out of his situation. In other cases, the patient may be in need of immediate rescue to prevent him from falling. Both scenarios require rescuers to move from a safe area into a hazardous environment to effect a rescue. Scene management must include scene isolation and the establishment of an exclusion zone to keep civilians and well-intended rescuers from becoming victims should they attempt to work beyond their training and experience. In addition, these scenarios may include a steep and perhaps drastic change in elevation. (See Figure 9.2.)

Situations involving above- or below-ground rescue must be quickly identified and the necessary resources summoned. In some

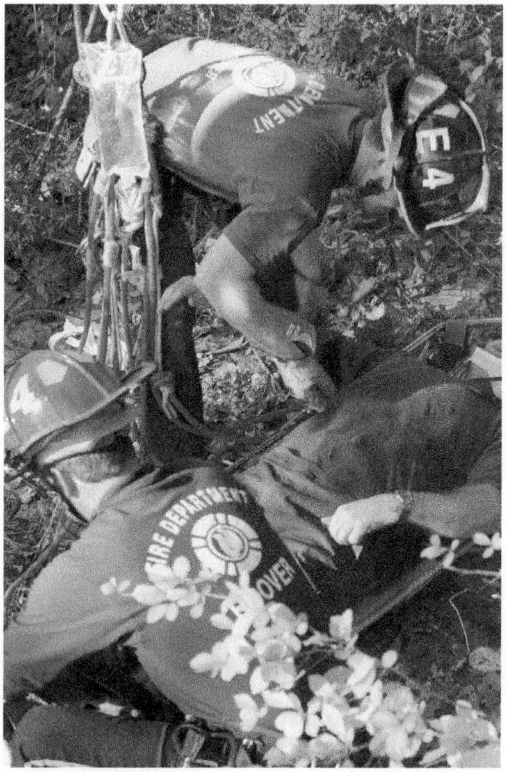

FIGURE 9.2 ■ Rescuers provide initial care while preparing their patient for a high-angle extraction.

cases, physical patient contact may not be made until qualified and equipped rescuers arrive. If that is the case, visual and verbal contact with the victim should be made whenever possible. Priorities for incident commanders managing these rescues should include scene stabilization, rapid access to the victim, immediate treatment of life-threatening injuries or conditions, patient removal/rescue, and then patient treatment and transport. To expedite the transition from the initial response crews to the specialized rescue

Side Bar

Timeline: Key Events from Response to Patient Transport

As emergency responders and supervisors, our scene management and actions must be coordinated to decrease the time delay in all areas possible, with safe and rapid patient transport to an appropriate facility being our final goal.

- Time of emergency
- Time of call for assistance
- Time of dispatch
- Response time to scene
- Time to patient contact
- Time to initiating patient care
- Patient packaged, extracted, and moved to transport truck
- Transport

crew, a work area should be cleared to allow for setup and execution of the rescue. In addition, vehicles should be appropriately positioned to allow easy access for the incoming crews.

HIGH-ANGLE RESCUE

Land-based rescues utilizing rope can be divided into two main groups: high-angle rescue and low-angle rescue. In high-angle rescue situations, the terrain is at such an angle that the rescuer and victim are unable to stand or walk to safety. High-angle rescue utilizes ropes and equipment to build systems that will get the rescuer to the victim and then enable safe removal of both the victim and rescuer. High-angle rescues are divided into two subcategories. The first category includes situations where the first responders can gain access to the patient but are unable to remove him, such as an unconscious construction worker on the roof of a building with ladders being the only access. The second category includes a situation where the first responders are unable to make contact with the victim due to his location—for example, a window washer on a high-rise building with an inoperable lift system. In both cases, the execution of proper rescue techniques is crucial to ensure patient and rescuer safety.

In scenarios like the one where a construction worker suffers from a medical emergency on a rooftop and is unable to move himself to the ground, EMS personnel may be able to quickly but safely access the patient and begin patient care while additional rescue resources are being dispatched or are responding. Once the appropriate personnel and resources are in place for the high-angle rescue to take place, the patient is passed to one of the rescuers who will likely accompany the patient in his journey from the roof to the ground, where additional personnel will assume responsibility for patient care and prepare for transport. On the other hand, in the scenario where the window washer is in need of assistance while hanging from the top of a high-rise, there may be no safe way for initial response crews to make patient contact and begin treatment until a high-angle rescue team arrives. (See Figure 9.3.)

Side Bar

High-Angle Rescue Situations

Every agency responds to areas with potential for high-angle rescue situations. Some examples include the following:

- High-rise buildings
- Structures that are under construction
- Sky cranes/elevated work platforms
- Cellular towers
- Bridges
- Mountain sides/cliffs
- Ravines

When making patient contact and beginning patient care can be safely accomplished, EMS personnel should play an active role in doing so. Necessary resources should be requested as soon as the need is anticipated, and preparations should be made for the operations on scene to transition to the incoming rescuers. EMS personnel should continue to support the rescue scene as the patient is rescued and should be ready to receive and care for the patient once the rescue is made.

SCENE SAFETY

High-angle rescue scenarios present both overhead and fall hazards for rescuers and

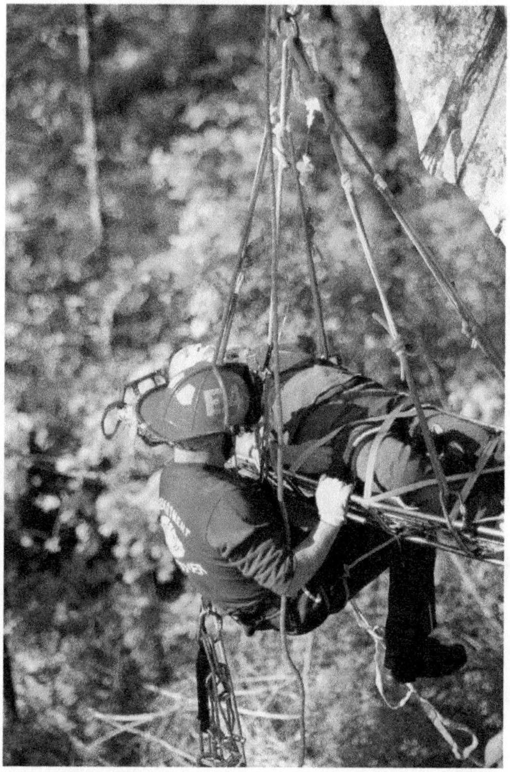

FIGURE 9.3 A rescuer tends to his patient during a high-angle rescue. Initial care and lifesaving aid should be provided while preparing a patient for a high-angle rescue. Once the patient and rescuer are ready for the ascent, a team of rescuers works to haul them to safety.

victims. In situations where rescuers approach the victim from above, fall hazards exist for all rescuers involved and for the victim. As the rescuer is lowered to the victim, consideration must be given to the fact that falling equipment or debris may cause injury or death to anyone below. Once patient contact is made, the rescuer should rapidly secure the patient to the rescue rope and ensure that the patient has a helmet and any other necessary protective equipment. In situations where the rescuers must climb to access the patient, the rescuers on the ground may not have a fall hazard to consider, but must be constantly aware of the dangers associated with falling equipment or materials.

EQUIPMENT

High-angle rescues require proper equipment and training to ensure safe execution. The National Fire Protection Association (NFPA) sets standards for both equipment and training of technical rescue personnel. The equipment needed for high-angle rescue incidents includes rope, **webbing**, **carabiners**, **pulleys**, **Stokes baskets**, and **harnesses**. NFPA sets standards that each type of equipment must meet. In general, this standard assumes that a person weighs 300 pounds and then sets a 15:1 safety factor for equipment strength. Rope being used for rescue purposes will likely have to bear the weight of both the rescuer and the victim, and therefore must be rated to have a minimum breaking strength of 9,000 pounds.

TYPES OF HIGH-ANGLE RESCUE

High-angle rescues can be broken into two basic groups: rescues in which the victim is below the location of the rescuers, and rescues in which the victim is above the location of the rescuers. A window washer stranded on the side of a high-rise is an example of a rescue in which the victim is below the rescuers: Even though the victim is high above the ground, the rescuers in this incident will assemble and set up on the roof of the high-rise and then lower rescuers to the victim. In this case, the rescue team may choose to raise the patient to safety on the roof or lower the patient to safety on the ground. On the other hand, a worker who is

Best Practice

Example of a Central Florida Rescue Team

In 2008, an urban Central Florida fire and rescue department responded to an incident where scaffolding had fallen onto and injured two construction workers. Responding to construction injuries is not uncommon, but in this case the worker was on the seventh floor of a nine-story building that was still under construction. This building was in the downtown area and, coincidentally, was next to city hall. Rescue personnel responded to the scene and found that the only way to access the patient was via a narrow and temporary construction stairway. As crews carried equipment up the narrow stairs, it was quickly recognized that additional personnel would be needed to lower this patient to the ground for transport. Although it may have been possible to move an injured patient down fourteen flights of a narrow construction stairway, it would have risked additional injury to the patient and the rescuers.

As the initial rescue crews treated and packaged the patients, additional rescuers arrived on scene to set up and execute the rope rescue that would be needed to move this patient from the seventh floor of this building to the ambulance below. The most serious patient was removed first, and as he was placed and secured into a Stokes basket, a rope-rescue lowering system was constructed. Many options for constructing this system are available and can be as simple as building an anchor system on the floor above and attaching a rope with a lowering device. In this case, the team leader chose to utilize a crane operated by an experienced crane operator to assist in lowering the patient. Both the patient and a rescuer were attached to the system and lowered to the ground floor where treatment and transport could continue. In this situation, the rescuer who was with the patient for his descent from the seventh floor acted as an attendant, keeping the patient calm, explaining the events of the rescue as they occurred, and remaining ready to protect the patient and troubleshoot complications as needed. While the first patient was being lowered, the second patient was being packaged for lowering. In all, it took about 40 minutes for both patients to be lowered to the ground for transport.

The dynamics of each incident involving above- or below-ground rescue will dictate the specific needs and actions of rescue crews. It is through training and preparation that these incidents can be safely and quickly resolved.

stranded on a cellular antenna tower is an example of a high-angle rescue where the victim is above the rescuers. In this case, the rescuers will be required to climb up to access the patient, create a rope system to lower the patient to the ground, and then execute the rescue.

LOW-ANGLE RESCUE

Low-angle rescues are similar to high-angle rescues in that virtually all of the same equipment and techniques are used. In low-angle rescues, the grade of the terrain is low enough that a rescuer is able to walk or stand. It is this fact that gives a false sense of security to many rescuers. Although the terrain may appear to be negotiable to an untrained rescuer or civilian, disaster may occur if the unprepared rescuer were to slip or fall while attempting to extract the victim. It is this hazard and its potential for catastrophic results that incident commanders must consider when planning a rescue.

Scene stabilization should be one of the first priorities in all above- and below-ground rescues. If patient contact and initial care can be safely made prior to a specialized rescue team's arrival, then it should be done. However, if the dangers are too great to move the patient up or down the steep terrain, then, as for the previous example of the construction worker on the roof, treatment should be given until it is time to transfer the patient to the rescue crew for them to safely remove the patient from harm's way. It is the hidden dangers in this steep but navigable terrain that will present challenges for well-intentioned rescuers and incident commanders. Recognizing these dangers and stabilizing the scene must be accomplished as quickly as possible by responding personnel and supervisors.

SCENE SAFETY

Low-angle rescue situations may present covert hazards that can lure rescuers into areas from which they are unable to escape. Low-angle rescues occur on slopes that are flat enough to allow someone to stand fully upright, but they may present difficulties and dangers when someone attempts to navigate. These difficulties are compounded when a rescuer has a patient in his care.

Controlling the scene and only allowing properly trained and equipped personnel into the low-angle environment are musts. Preventing access and isolating the area immediately around, below, and above the victim is a crucial part of scene stabilization. Well-intended rescuers without the proper training and equipment may injure the victim or themselves and become another victim in need of rescue.

Similar to high-angle rescues, low-angle rescues present fall hazards for both the patient and the rescuer. In addition, both the rescuers and the patient may find themselves in the path of falling debris or equipment that becomes loose from above.

EQUIPMENT

The equipment needed for low-angle rescue is essentially the same as that for high-angle rescue. Through a series of **anchors**, lowering systems, hauling systems, harnesses, and carabiners, rescuers can safely access and package the patient for removal. The same safety factors and equipment standards exist for low-angle rescues as for high-angle rescues.

TYPES OF LOW-ANGLE RESCUE

Low-angle rescues can be divided into two basic groups: rescues in which the patient is located below the rescuers, and rescues in which the patient is located above the rescuer. In both cases, patient contact and scene stabilization are the priority for rescue crews. Low-angle rescues may also involve vehicles or machinery that has drifted or fallen down a slope. In these situations, rescuers will need to be prepared to disentangle or extricate victims while in the low-angle environment. Scene and vehicle stabilization must be a priority in these cases to prevent a bad situation from becoming worse.

Rescuers who access their patient from above are "lowered" via rope as they walk down the terrain to access their patient. Once the target is reached, the rope is secured and rescuers are able to operate safely while secured from above. Any victims should be placed in harnesses and secured to the rope system to prevent any other falls. Once the rescuers are ready and the patient is properly packaged, the crew that lowered the rescuers will convert its system to a haul system and assist as the rescuers ascend. In low-angle rescues, the rescuers may walk up the slope but only as quickly as the haul rope is pulling them. This will prevent slack in the line and will reduce the **fall factor** should something go wrong.

Rescuers below the patient's location may approach the rescue slightly differently. The rescuers will need to ascend to the patient, at times climbing above their anchor point. Once patient contact is made, the victim should be stabilized to prevent a fall. Other rescuers can then climb past the first rescuer and victim, create an anchor and lowering system, and lower the rescuer and victim to safety.

TRENCH/EXCAVATION RESCUE

As with the rescue scenarios described above, **trench** and **excavation** rescues can be divided into two groups: situations where a medical emergency occurs while the patient is in a trench, and situations where an event happens in the trench or excavation that causes the victim to be in need of rescue. Although intact excavations may be entered by rescuers, the dangers associated with trenches cannot be overstated and no rescuer should enter a trench without the proper training and equipment. In addition, although the **Occupational Safety and Health Administration (OSHA)** does not have a specific standard when it comes to trench rescue, general OSHA standards apply to all workers, including rescuers, who enter trenches. Rescuers must be cognizant of the dangers associated with trenches and understand the magnitude of the repercussions if OSHA standards are not followed, especially if the rescue were to prove unsuccessful.

Personnel responding to emergencies involving trenches and excavations should park at least 200 feet away and approach the scene on foot to prevent their vehicle from disturbing the ground near the site and potentially causing a trench collapse. If the trench is intact and the patient can exit the trench under his own power or with the assistance of other workers, the patient should be instructed to do so. If the trench is intact but the patient is unable to exit the trench, appropriate resources should be requested before the rescue is initiated. The rescue of this patient can occur very quickly once the properly trained personnel arrive, the trench is examined, and entry into the trench is made.

If the emergency involves victims in a tenuous or collapsed trench, the rescue must be approached with even greater caution. If properly trained and equipped rescuers are not included in the initial dispatch, they should be requested as soon as it is recognized that a trench collapse may have occurred. Again, emergency vehicles should park at least 200 feet away and rescuers should approach the scene on foot. In the event of a trench collapse, all machinery in the area of the collapse should be shut down and left in place so as not to disturb the already unstable ground. All nonessential personnel and civilians should be kept away from the edge of the trench, and **ground pads** should be placed in the work area around the trench to distribute the weight of the rescuers in order to minimize ground disturbance and help prevent additional collapse.

Trench rescues can be very time-consuming and labor-intensive rescue situations. As rescuers enter the trench, they will use a **trench box** or properly shore the trench to protect both the rescuers and the victim from additional collapse. Once patient contact is made, the ground around the patient must be removed until the patient can be freed. It should be noted that the soil and debris that have been removed must be placed where they will not interfere with patient removal or cause additional trench collapse. All personnel on the scene should offer their assistance to the special rescue team to help expedite the rescue efforts. In addition, a transport unit should be identified, positioned for easy departure, and prepared to immediately receive any patients once they are removed from the trench.

The dangers associated with a trench rescue do not go away once the patient is removed. If anything, the trench becomes more dangerous once the shores or trench box are removed. Even though the patient has been removed, rescuers must maintain heightened situational awareness, as they will still be operating in a hazardous environment while they retrieve their equipment and prepare to leave the scene. When considering the retrieval of equipment, a risk/benefit analysis must be performed. Although placing properly trained rescuers in harm's way to rescue a patient may be acceptable, placing additional personnel in harm's way to retrieve equipment may not be.

SCENE SAFETY

Proper scene control in trench rescues is of the utmost importance. The already unstable walls of the trench can be deadly for both the victim and the rescuers. Vehicles and machinery within 200 feet of the trench should be turned off to reduce ground vibrations and disturbance. Only the personnel needed for the rescue should approach the trench, and they should walk on ground pads to help distribute their weight. Rescuers must protect themselves and the victim by constructing shores to hold the trench wall in place or by utilizing a trench box that will create a safe area as they work to free and extract the victim.

EQUIPMENT

Trench rescues can be labor intense and may require equipment and materials that will likely be used only on this type of rescue. Rescuers entering a trench must be aware of the hazards and protect themselves and the victim from any additional collapse. As such, trenches must be approached systematically and with caution. Shovels may be needed to clear the area around a trench to allow access and prevent a spoil pile from contributing to a collapse. Ground pads should be placed on any area immediately around the trench to distribute the weight of the rescuers. Rescuers must shore the walls of the trench using materials such as **FinnForm boards**, 4 × 4 lumber, 6 × 6 lumber, air shores, a trench box, and screw jacks. Some trench rescue teams may choose one approach over another, but all must take the necessary precautions to ensure the safety of all concerned.

Building the shores can be labor intense and will require teams of rescuers to measure, cut, and assist as rescuers in the trench construct the shores. Once access to the patient is made, rescuers may need to render immediate care and begin the process of freeing the victim. While ensuring that they do not injure the patient, rescuers may need to expeditiously dig by hand or with small hand tools. Some teams use vacuums and air tools to loosen the soil and remove it from the trench. Since the patient will ultimately be removed from the trench, rescuers should build their shores in a way that minimizes complications as both debris and the patient are removed.

TYPES OF TRENCH/EXCAVATION RESCUE

Trench rescues can be divided into two main groups: rescues without trench wall collapse/failure and rescues with trench wall collapse/failure. The first may involve a worker or passerby who sustained trauma or a medical event while located in a trench. If the trench rescue team evaluates the trench and determines that it is properly shored or does not require additional shoring, rescuers may enter the trench, package the patient as needed, and remove the patient. Insufficiently shored trenches will need to be shored even if no collapse has occurred. Rescues involving trench wall collapse will likely require the previously discussed precautions and the building of shores. Even though proper shoring may exist on parts of a collapsed trench, the fact a collapse occurred illustrates that whatever safety measures were taken were insufficient.

There are various types of trenches. Trenches may be a straight trench or an "L" trench, a "T" trench, or two intersecting trenches. The shape of the trench may dictate the amount and type of shoring required. In addition, four different soil types must be taken into account when working in and around trenches:

- Solid rock
- Type A cohesive soil with a compressive strength of 1.5 tons/square foot (e.g., clay)
- Type B cohesive soil with a compressive strength between 0.5 and 1.5 tons/square foot (e.g., clay with gravel)
- Type C cohesive soil with a compressive strength less than 0.5 tons/square foot (e.g., sand)

Solid rock is the most stable, and Type C soil is the least. If there is ever a doubt about the soil type, Type C soil should be assumed.

CAVE/CAVERN RESCUE

Caves and caverns can be found across the United States as part of a park or organized attraction or on private property. The obvious hazards of cave and cavern rescues include remote and difficult access, no light, rough terrain and obstacles, deep crevasses, sudden drop-offs, water hazards, and both ground and overhead obstructions. These hazards are complicated by the fact that cellular phone and radio systems do not work underground. Underground communication is done verbally or via a messenger. When all of these conditions exist, there may be a long delay from the time that an emergency occurs to the first call for assistance.

Due to these hazards, it is usually an agency's special operations team that is called to handle cave rescues. Unlike some other rescue situations, no OSHA standards apply to caves and, depending on the response agency's procedures, personnel with little or no cave experience may be utilized to assist in the cave. An organized approach with clear directional markings should be used to help ensure that rescuers do not get lost. Untrained personnel should be paired with those who

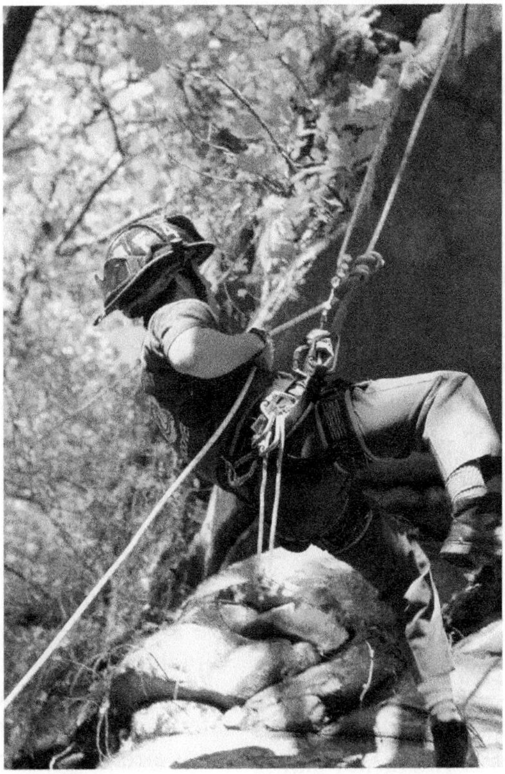

FIGURE 9.4 A rescuer descends into a cavern to find the entrance to a cave. Challenges can arise when gaining access to a cave and must be taken into account when preparing for a cave rescue.

are trained, and a system for proper personnel accountability must be maintained at all times. (See Figure 9.4.)

SCENE SAFETY

Emergency response agencies covering areas with caves should prepare for cave rescues as they would prepare for any other target hazard. Although caves are very likely stable, the potential for a collapse does exist. Situational awareness should be maintained. Hazards associated with cave rescues include unstable ground, sudden drop-offs, deep crevasses, no light, water hazards with potential drowning and hypothermia, animals/wildlife, poor communications, and rescuer/victim disorientation. Although the hazards are numerous, most can be mitigated with the proper preparation and equipment. Rescuers should be familiar with the caves in their area and train to minimize the impact of the hazards.

EQUIPMENT

Much of the equipment needed for cave rescue is the same as what is needed for the other types of rescues discussed in this chapter. In addition to the ropes and rigging equipment that may be needed to access and package the patient, rescuers should also have helmets, gloves, long sleeves, kneepads, and lights. Depending on how deep in the cave the patient may be, rescuers may need to pack provisions for food and water as exiting the cave may be burdensome. All rescuers entering the cave should be self-sufficient, and carrying extra equipment may be preferred to making multiple trips in and out of the cave to handle unanticipated needs. Since radios and cell phones will not work underground, rescuers may need to send runners to pass on information, or they may need to stage personnel at various points in the cave to pass messages and requests back to the surface.

TYPES OF CAVE/CAVERN RESCUE

Some cave rescues may be as simple as locating a lost or missing person. In these cases, locating the person and leading him to safety may be all that is required for a successful rescue. In other cases, a medical emergency may occur while a patient is exploring a cave, hindering his ability to exit. In this case, rescuers may need to assist and/or package the patient for removal. Special considerations for the terrain may also need to be considered. Full-patient packaging may need to wait until the patient is out of the cave. In some instances, a victim may become anxious or claustrophobic while in a cave and may not want to go back through a tight squeeze between his location and the exit. In other instances, a victim may have an extremity or other body part wedged in a crevasse or other tight spot, thereby preventing escape. A calm, systematic approach to extracting the victim is needed to prevent further injury and to avoid compromising the cave. This can be complicated by the fact that the victim may be stuck in an area that prevents rescuers from accessing the entrapped body part.

WILDERNESS/ROUGH TERRAIN RESCUE

The treatment and removal of patients from remote wilderness areas presents challenges that are at times easily overcome and at other times prove to be more difficult than expected. It should be noted that this section on wilderness rescue discusses scenarios where the patient location is known and is merely complicated by the remote access and perhaps rough terrain. If responders can drive their apparatus to a remote location and pick up a patient, patient care should take place as it would on any other emergency with no specialized equipment or training needed. (See Figure 9.5.)

As with the other rescue situations, rapid patient contact and initial treatment are among the scene priorities. All-terrain vehicles (ATVs) may be used to transport equipment and rescuers to the patient and later for patient removal. In addition, rotary wing aircraft may be used to bring personnel and equipment to the patient's location and then to expedite patient contact, care, and transport. If neither of these resources is available, rescuers will need to move forward on foot. Essential medical equipment should be carried to render first aid; however, it is not practical to carry all of the equipment that is usually needed for routine medical emergencies. Rescuers should either be familiar with the area and terrain or partner with someone who can lead them to the patient and back to their apparatus. Depending on the anticipated length of the rescue effort, rescuers should bring water and food for everyone involved, including the patient. If patient access or removal involves any of the previously mentioned rescue situations, then properly trained and equipped personnel should be requested. Many times, the patient will need to be

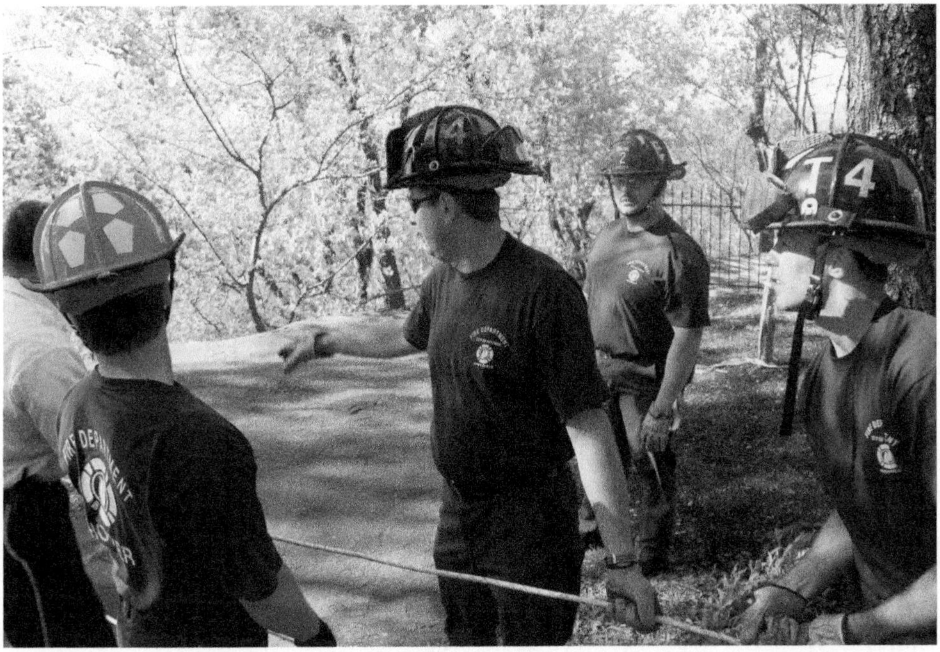

FIGURE 9.5 Rescuers prepare for the final steps of a wilderness rescue. Locating and accessing patients in the wilderness may be challenging for rescuers. In addition, rescuers may need to apply high-angle rescue, low-angle rescue, or cave/cavern rescue skills to successfully complete a wilderness rescue.

treated and carried from the scene to the awaiting transport unit.

SCENE SAFETY

Each wilderness rescue involves safety and hazard considerations that are unique to that terrain and climate. Whether it is a missing hiker or a downed airplane or something else, rescuers must be prepared to face any situation that may arise. Knowing the location of the patient is perhaps the first step to making a rescue, but successfully getting rescuers to that location and back presents both challenges and hazards. (See the sidebar for a standard that FEMA developed to describe patient locations.)

> **Side Bar**
>
> **Describing Patient Location: The U.S. National Grid**
>
> FEMA has established the **U.S. National Grid (USNG)** as the standard coordinate system to be used by all ground search-and-rescue personnel. Its coordinates are written in a format—for example, 17R LN 84003 44055—that precisely describes a location within 1 meter. This is perhaps the most versatile coordinate system and can be used to reference both points and areas with just one set of coordinates.

Agencies responsible for rescues in relatively inaccessible wilderness areas should consider them target hazards. Personnel should be prepared and trained for emergencies that may occur in these places. Safety concerns are magnified by the size of the operational area and complicated by the possibility of poor communications due to the nature of remote areas and rugged terrain. All of the hazards are too numerous to list, and they include rough terrain and steep grades, wildlife, weather, and long operational periods with no relief. Rescuers should keep in mind that they will need to overcome obstacles that their patient is unable to overcome, while treating and perhaps even carrying their patient to safety. Personnel accountability in wilderness rescue situations, although challenging, is an essential requirement.

EQUIPMENT

In addition to the equipment needed to remove a victim from a situation, rescuers must be prepared and equipped to navigate to the victim, treat and package him, and then remove him and the rescue team to safety. Navigation tools include maps, a compass, and GPS. Backup equipment should be considered to prevent the failure of a single piece of equipment from halting the rescue operation. Trucks, ATVs, and aircraft may be utilized, but rescuers often will need to travel on foot for at least part of their journey. Rescuers must be prepared for other hazards and situations that they may encounter, including an overnight stay wherever they are operating.

TYPES OF WILDERNESS/ROUGH TERRAIN RESCUE

Situations surrounding wilderness rescues can range from one extreme to another. Variables include the following:

- Events leading up to the rescue situation
- The location of the patient in the wilderness
- Climate and weather
- Altitude
- Terrain
- Time of day that the rescue attempt is started
- Patient condition
- Latitude (affects the amount of available light each day)

A wilderness rescue can involve all of the intricacies of any other rescue, but it can be further complicated by the remote location of the event.

CONSIDERATIONS FOR MANAGING A RESCUE TEAM

When commanding an above- and below-ground rescue incident, managers must quickly recognize the need for and request properly trained and equipped rescue teams. Incident priorities will vary, but all will likely include the following:

- Scene stabilization
- Patient stabilization
- Patient rescue
- Patient treatment/transport

Emergency crews must prevent anyone else from becoming a victim and then access and secure the patient to the rope rescue system. Once the victim is properly connected into the rope rescue system, the scene becomes much more stable. Rescue crews can then hoist or lower the patient to safety knowing that the patient is already much safer than he was prior to the rescuers' arrival. Once the patient is rescued and removed from harm's way, he is then transferred to the care of the EMS provider for full evaluation and transport if needed. In all cases victim, rescuer, and bystander safety should always be considered and constantly monitored.

CHAPTER REVIEW

Summary

Above- and below-ground rescue situations present unique challenges that first responders must be prepared to face. Some scenarios are unique to certain topography or terrain, whereas others can be found in any agency's first-response area. Rescue crews and supervisors must recognize the hazards and identify the resources needed to ensure responder safety and efficient patient treatment and transport. The main priorities for many rescue situations remain the same, whereas the resources needed to accomplish these priorities may vary in each situation. Supervisors should anticipate what might be needed at a developing rescue scene so that the agency will be in the best position possible to facilitate a rapid and safe rescue whenever necessary.

WHAT WOULD YOU DO? Reflection

The steep incline coupled with the potential for a 200-foot fall and the need for a 200-foot ascent to safety creates a situation that may appear benign, but it is filled with dangers. Insufficiently trained or equipped rescuers may become patients as they attempt to access and rescue the patient. They also may find that they are unable to bring the patient to safety, and although unhurt they are nonetheless a victim of the situation and also in need of rescue.

Even surefooted rescuers should recognize the additional challenges that they will face if they attempt to negotiate this terrain on foot while carrying an injured patient. If the initial rescuers are able to access the patient, patient stabilization and initial treatment may occur, but any attempt to remove the patient may place both the patient and the rescuers at unnecessary risk.

A properly trained and equipped rope rescue team should be requested to assist in this situation. Agencies and supervisors should identify these resources prior to being called to an incident where they are needed. If a need is recognized but no resource exists, supervisors and administrators may need to consider creating, training, and equipping their own team.

Review Questions

1. Name the incident priorities described in this chapter.
2. Describe the differences between high- and low-angle rescues.
3. According to OSHA, are untrained rescuers allowed to enter a trench to rescue a patient in distress?
4. List some of the challenges that rescuers may face when encountered with a cave rescue.
5. When describing patient coordinates for a land-based wilderness rescue, what coordinate system should be used?

References

National Fire Protection Association. (2009). "NFPA 1670 Standards on Operations and Training for Technical Search and Rescue Incidents." See the organization website.

Occupational Safety and Health Administration. (n.d.). "Trenching and Excavation." See the organization website.

Roop, M., T. Vines, and R. Wright. (1998). *Confined Space and Structural Rope Rescue*. St. Louis, MO: Mosby.

Key Terms

anchors A natural or manmade object that is used as part of a system to anchor the ropes and rigging devices used in a rope rescue system.

carabiners An oval or D-shaped metal, load-bearing connector with a self-closing gate, used to join components of a rope system.

caves A natural, underground space that is large enough for humans to enter.

excavation Any manmade cut, cavity, trench, or depression in an earth surface that is formed by earth removal.

fall factor A ratio used to describe the force exerted on a rope when it stops a falling person. The ratio of the total length of rope compared to the distance of the fall.

FinnForm boards A heavy-duty plywood that is generally 4 feet × 8 feet × 1 foot in dimension.

ground pads Pads that are generally made of plywood, but can be made of any material, and are used to distribute the weight of workers and equipment in the area of a trench to prevent a possible collapse.

harness A system of material that creates a belt, seat, and sometimes chest strap to be used as a tool to connect a person (rescuer or victim) into a rope system.

Occupational Safety and Health Administration (OSHA) A part of the U.S. Department of Labor that works to ensure safe and healthy working conditions for men and women by setting and enforcing standards and by providing training, outreach, education, and assistance.

pulley A tool used either to increase mechanical advantage in a rope system or to decrease friction when ropes change direction in a rope system.

Stokes basket A device used as a part of a rope system to secure sick or injured victims as they are moved through the system.

trench A narrow excavation made below the ground surface. In general, the depth is greater than its width, and the width is not greater than 15 feet.

trench box A prefabricated shoring/shielding device that is placed into a trench to protect workers from a collapse.

webbing A type of soft, flat woven material used in rope systems to secure loads.

U.S. National Grid (USNG) A ground-based gridded coordinate system designed and implemented to provide a seamless, standardized system of reference for nationwide use during times of crisis.

Safety Officer

10 CHAPTER

KEVIN SPRATLIN

JEFFREY LINDSEY

Objectives

After reading this chapter, the student should be able to:

10.1 Identify the safety officer's place in the incident command system.
10.2 Identify the major duties of the safety officer.
10.3 Define hazard and risk as they relate to the safety officer's role on the emergency scene.
10.4 Discuss the concept of risk management and its place in the safety officer's decision-making process.

Key Terms

command staff
cultures of unnecessary risk
emergency incident rehabilitation
immediately dangerous to life and health (IDLH)
risk avoidance
risk control
risk evaluation
risk identification
risk management
risk reduction
risk transfer
situational awareness
unsafe practices

WHAT WOULD YOU DO?

You are dispatched to the scene of a collapsed parking garage along with your EMS providers and other specialty rescue personnel. The initial dispatch information indicates that an aftershock from a recent earthquake has caused the structure to fail, resulting in a "lean-to" collapse. Intelligence reports from the scene indicate that there is a high probability that several victims are trapped in various voids that have been located within the rubble. As the safety officer for your agency, you will be in charge of safety operations on the scene of this technical rescue incident.

Questions

1. How will you determine the level of acceptable risk that permits your personnel to make entry into the collapsed structure in order to make contact with the victims, begin emergency medical care, and extricate them?
2. How will you work with the incident commander to establish an effective system for ensuring personnel accountability during all phases of the incident?
3. How will you ensure that a proper rehabilitation plan is put into place to ensure that all personnel are monitored and rested after participating in rescue operations?

INTRODUCTION

The safety officer is responsible for monitoring and assessing safety hazards and developing measures to ensure the safety of personnel operating on the scene of an emergency incident. (See Figure 10.1.) It is important to remember that safety is not a separate task on the emergency scene; it must be integrated into every activity and embraced by all personnel who are operating at the incident. Safety must be the top consideration of all who are involved in the mitigation of an incident involving a technical rescue.

It is important to remember that the safety officer is a member of the **command staff** and is tasked with being the eyes and ears of the incident commander (IC). The IC is ultimately responsible for the safety of all persons present at the incident; therefore, it is vitally important to have effective lines of communication between the IC and the safety officer at all times. As part of his duties, the safety officer reports directly to the IC and is often granted the authority to alter, suspend, or terminate a task or operation on an emergency scene whenever appropriate. These decisions may or may not require prior approval of the IC.

DUTIES OF THE SAFETY OFFICER

The safety officer's primary mission is to ensure safety during all aspects of the incident operation. Specifically, the safety officer is tasked with identifying any existing or potential hazards that may pose an immediate threat to the safety of the rescuers. This can be a challenging proposition considering that the technical rescue operation is part of an often hazardous or hostile environment, which contains numerous risks where providers may be injured or killed. The assigned responsibilities of the safety officer are broad and varied, so it is helpful to separate these duties into their

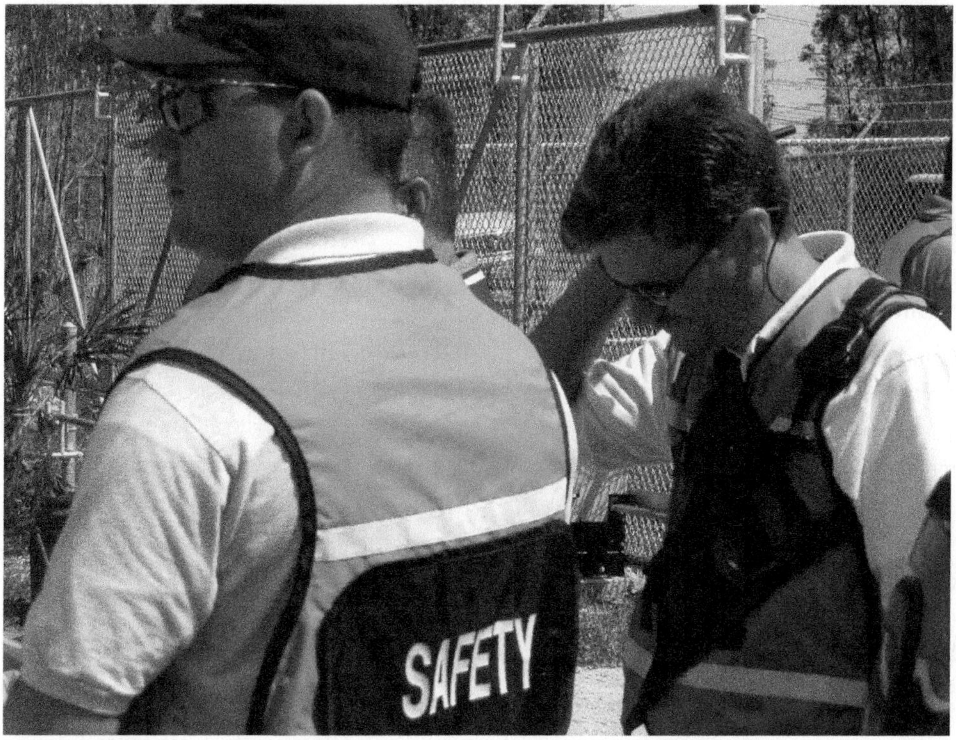

FIGURE 10.1 It is important to remember that the safety officer is a member of the command staff and is tasked with being the eyes and ears of the incident commander. *Source: Courtesy of Estero Fire Rescue.*

individual components. The following areas are not all-inclusive; they are intended to be a reminder of the myriad duties that are required of the competent safety officer and are based on training that is provided during the Urban Search and Rescue (US&R) Task Force Safety Officer Course established by the Federal Emergency Management Agency (FEMA).

Side Bar

Roles and Tasks of a Safety Officer

- Respond
- Assess personnel at incident scenes
- Identify and correct safety hazards
- Attend post-incident analysis
- Know applicable laws and regulations
- Investigate all on-the-job injuries
- Keep accurate personnel records
- Maintain inspection and service records
- Investigate emergency vehicle crashes
- Liaison to other organizations

ENSURING SAFETY

The safety officer should strive to ensure that safety precautions are taken during all facets of the operation, working to establish that injury prevention concerns are paramount in the minds of all providers. For example, the use of the appropriate personal protective equipment (PPE) is necessary whenever personnel are involved in the incident. Part of the safety officer's job is to gather information and assist with the decision as to what level of

PPE is appropriate and to ensure that the mandatory PPE is in place. Aggressive providers must often be reminded that they are no good to the victim if they become victims themselves.

Side Bar

Shift Health and the Safety Officer Vehicle Inventory

- Garage door opener
- 1—Mobile radio
- 1—Garmin navigational device (dash mounted)
- 1—Light and siren control (dash mounted)
- 1—Portable computer (mobile data computer/mobile data terminal)
- 1—Portable radio with an additional battery, battery charger, portable mic, and carrying case with strap
- 1—Camcorder/still photo camera with appropriate cords, camera bag, additional battery, and two digital video cassettes
- 2—Traffic cones, 16–18 inches
- 1—Yellow hazmat bag
- 1—Vehicle power cord and reel
- 1—Breakaway reflective vest
- 1—Plastic bin that includes the following:
  - ADC map
  - 1—emergency response guide
  - *Chem Bio Handbook*
  - Red biohazard bags
  - Employee assistance program brochures
  - 1—Box of large exam gloves
  - 2—David Clark microphone protectors
  - 1—N100 Mask
- 1—Clipboard
- 1—Accident/Injury, Property Damage Forms Manual
- 1—Folder bin that includes the following forms:
  - Insurance forms
  - Authorization for Release of Medical Records
  - Employee Statement
  - Employer's Accident Report (formerly Employer's 1st Report of Accident)
  - Exposure Report Form
  - Family and Medical Leave Act Information
  - Form to File a Claim (against the city)
  - Loss Prevention Form
  - Near-Miss Report Form
  - Physical Capabilities Statement
  - Physician Panel List
  - PMA/Genex Information
  - Property Damage Report
  - Safety Officer's Investigation Form
  - Supervisor's Investigation Form
  - Treating Physician Selection Form
  - Witness Statement
- 1—AED with two sets of adult electrode pads
- 1—O_2 bottle with adult nasal cannula and adult non-rebreather mask
- 1—Stocked EMS bag with CO detector attached
- 1—Water rescue bag with three safety light sticks, one rope throw bag, and one personal flotation device (PFD)
- 2—Accountability passports
- 2—Bottles of disinfecting wet wipes
- 2—Bottles of hand sanitizer
- 1—Flashlight
- 1—Mounted SCBA 1—Fire extinguisher
- 1—Thermal imager mounted with charging station

1—Box light in mounted charger

2—Mobile radios rear mounted with one headset

1—Jump bag (red duffel) that includes the following:

- Multi-gas monitor
- Disposable camera
- 2 rolls of yellow fire line tape
- 2 rolls of red danger tape
- 1 roll of red/white tape

1—Sharps red biohazard bin with a supply of red biohazard bags

1—Red safety officer's vest

1—Plastic storage bin that includes the following:

- 1 Box of large exam/EMS gloves
- 1 Box of medium exam/EMS gloves
- Box of safety glasses (1 dozen)
- 2 Safety goggles
- Firefighting gloves:
    - 2—Extra small
    - 2—Small
    - 2—Medium
    - 2—Large
    - 2—Extra large

1—Plastic storage bin that includes the following:

- 1 Non-breakaway reflective vest
- 2 Rolls yellow fire line tape
- 2 Rolls red/white tape
- 2 Rolls red danger tape
- Multi-gas monitor equipment (tubing and pump)
- 2 Voltage testers
- Measuring wheel
- Chalk line reel
- Binoculars
- 25-foot tape measure
- Landing zone kit
- Flares and safety light sticks
- Sound-level meter
- Volt probe

PLANNING

Since the safety and welfare of emergency providers is the number-one concern during the incident, the safety officer should be an active participant in the planning process, working to ensure that safety is well integrated into all components of the operation. Part of this ongoing process will include developing the safety portion of the incident action plan (IAP) as well as creating safety messages that will be disseminated to all personnel. These brief messages should be no more than one page in length with only a few bullet points listed. It is best to keep the safety message concise and to the point. Otherwise, some providers may not pay attention and miss the message altogether.

RISK MANAGEMENT

The safety officer is tasked with providing the IC with periodic risk assessments that will allow the IC to make prudent decisions as to the strategies and goals of the mission at hand. These strategies will be translated into the tactics employed by the operations chief, utilizing safe practices at all times. The safety officer is fundamental in determining "acceptable risk" in pursuing the goals of the mission at hand. (Risk management is described in greater detail later in this chapter.)

RECONNAISSANCE MISSION

One of the first things that a safety officer must do upon arriving at an incident is to survey the scene in order to better understand the risks and challenges that providers will face. A strong grasp of the complexities and intricacies of an incident scene will allow the safety officer to make better recommendations to the IC.

Part of this reconnaissance will be identify collapse zones and other hazards that are potentially dangerous to personnel, such as traffic hazards, fire risks, inclement weather conditions, and communication hindrances.

PERSONNEL ACCOUNTABILITY

A personnel accountability report (PAR) should be conducted on a regular basis to ensure that all responders are safe and not in need of assistance. This will also help protect against freelancing activities that can often lead to compromises in safety. As a group, emergency responders tend to be aggressive and action oriented; these attributes are commendable but may lead to situations where providers become endangered. Due to the nature of the emergency scenes where technical rescues occur, there are intrinsic risks, which unavoidably place rescuers at risk. Providers who came up through departments with entrenched **cultures of unnecessary risk** must learn to value the incorporation of safety practices into all aspects the operation.

RADIO TRAFFIC MONITORING

Listen closely to the radio traffic to ensure that proper and effective communications are occurring while also monitoring how well the incident operation is progressing. The use of 10-codes, abbreviations, and acronyms should be discouraged since these may lead to misunderstandings about the message that is being transmitted. It is also important to conduct all radio communications in plain English to avoid misunderstandings (International Fire Service Training Association [IFSTA], 2004, p. 406).

LIAISON WITH OTHER AGENCIES

Multiple agencies often perform simultaneous operations on the scene of a large-scale incident, with each having separate leadership structures that are part of the unified command. The safety officer must serve as a liaison with safety personnel from these other agencies to help maintain a common focus on the scene.

RISK MANAGEMENT AT THE EMERGENCY SCENE

Risk is intrinsic to emergency services. Many of these risks are unavoidable and must be dealt with appropriately. Others are avoidable and should be handled in a manner that allows rescuers to mitigate the emergency incident. There is no practical way to protect providers from all hazards. However, it is advisable for a safety officer to use the concepts of **risk management** to help make these decisions. Attempting to identify *acceptable* risk will aid in decision making. Safety officers who engage in ineffective risk management or choose to altogether ignore risk place providers at a higher chance of unnecessary injury or death.

It is prudent to first define the key words associated with the topic of risk management. The National Fire Protection Association (NFPA) 1500, "Standard on Fire Department Occupational Safety and Health Program," defines risk as "a measure of the probability and severity of adverse effects". (*Source: Reproduced with permission from NFPA 1500: Standard on Fire Department Occupational Safety and Health Program. Copyright © 2013 by the National Fire Protection Association.*) More succinctly, risk can be defined as an event or action that poses a threat to rescue personnel. It is important to remember that risk cannot be entirely avoided; certain risks are inherent to the EMS field, such as traffic hazards and exposure to communicable and infectious diseases that are too often present. NFPA 1521, "Standard for Fire Department Safety Officer," defines a hazard as "the potential for harm or damage to people, property, or the environment. Hazards include the characteristics of facilities, equipment systems, property, hardware or other objects and the actions and inactions of people that create such hazards". (*Source: Reproduced with permission from NFPA 1521-2008, Standard for Fire Department Safety Officer. Copyright © 2007 by the National Fire Protection Association.*)

Risk management involves four components as defined by NFPA 1500. These include risk identification, risk evaluation, risk control, and risk management and monitoring.

RISK IDENTIFICATION

Risk identification is the process through which safety officers attempt to recognize and assess potential problems. Emergency incident scenes are dynamic, ever-changing events, so the safety officer must constantly reassess his surroundings and make decisions based on these findings. This need for situational awareness and the ability to adapt to an ever-changing environment cannot be overemphasized. **Situational awareness** is the process through which rescuers grasp what is going on around them on the emergency scene, convert that information into a format that is useful for making decisions, and logically think through the consequences of the decisions that they make.

The competent safety officer recognizes that much can be learned from looking at previous incidents that were technical in nature and/or that generated multiple patients. This historical perspective affords the safety officer the opportunity to avoid some of the mistakes that may have occurred during these incidents. The adoption of best practices for safety operations during an incident can help to manage risk to acceptable levels.

Of the many aspects of an incident that must be identified, those that are **immediately dangerous to life and health (IDLH)** must take precedence over all others. The IDLH concept is familiar to many individuals, especially those who have previously undergone training in hazardous materials incident mitigation. It may take many forms—for example, those situations that require various levels of respiratory protection or even fully encapsulated entry suits with self-contained breathing apparatus (SCBA) due to hazardous environments.

The fact of the matter is that providers face risk throughout all phases of the incident, starting even before arrival on the emergency scene. These risks include training evolutions and equipment preparation all the way through lights-and-sirens response to the scene. Once on the scene, the safety officer must continually evaluate conditions that would necessitate a change in operations. (See Figure 10.2.) These might include minimizing exposure to bloodborne pathogens and other biohazardous risks, mandating a certain level of respiratory protection and other PPE, requiring periodic rest and rehabilitation periods, and rotating personnel during long-duration events.

RISK EVALUATION

Risk evaluation is the second component of risk management and involves determining

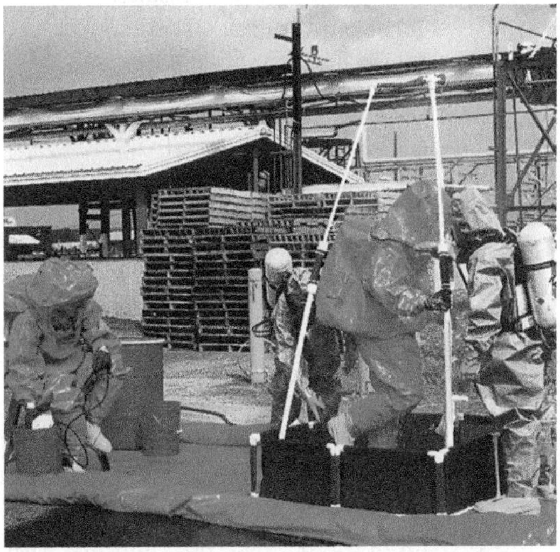

FIGURE 10.2 ■ The safety officer cannot be everywhere on the incident scene, but he enables all personnel on the scene to observe for a safe working environment.

the potential of the severity of loss and the probability of occurrence. Determining the severity of loss is the process through which the safety officer attempts to assess the degree of seriousness of the challenges that are faced during an emergency incident. Although there is no established formula for doing this, the safety officer may draw insight from a variety of sources, including historical data from similar incidents. The safety officer should attempt to determine the frequency with which something occurs so that he can properly prioritize risk. These two factors are quite helpful in allowing the safety officer to correctly evaluate risk and attempt to minimize loss, thereby limiting injury and death.

> **Side Bar**
>
> **Considerations for Special Operations Forecasting**
>
> - Incident duration will be longer than most incidents.
> - Technical experts must be consulted.
> - Responders must be properly equipped.
> - Time can be a benefit or an enemy.

RISK CONTROL

Risk control can be separated into three components: **risk avoidance**, **risk reduction**, and **risk transfer**.

Risk Avoidance

It stands to reason that the best method for minimizing risk is to avoid it. The manner in which to accomplish this is situation dependent. For example, consider the problem of EMS providers being stuck accidentally with contaminated needles. One way to avoid this risk is to embrace procedures that completely eliminate needles from the process, such as through the use of intranasal medication delivery devices to administer certain drugs to patients. Another example is the prophylactic administration of the hepatitis B vaccine (HBV) to providers. Although this does not eliminate the possibility of being exposed to HBV, it does severely reduce the risk of becoming infected. On the scene of a technical rescue incident, the safety officer may choose to not allow an EMS provider to enter a confined space or otherwise dangerous situation if the provider's safety cannot be ensured. As with other types of incidents, the safety officer and the IC are constantly performing mental risk/benefit analyses to determine what level of risk is acceptable when attempting rescue of an injured patient from a less-than-ideal situation. It is not acceptable to unnecessarily endanger a provider's life in order to attempt the recovery of a deceased victim; however, it would be considered acceptable to send a trained provider into the rubble pile to disentangle and extract a viable patient from an adversely impacted area.

Risk Reduction

Unfortunately, it is not always possible to avoid risk, so the next best tactic is to reduce risk whenever possible. One way that this can be accomplished is through the development and implementation of standard operating procedures (SOPs)/standard operating guidelines (SOG) to steer operations during an emergency incident. An SOP/SOG that addresses confined-space rescue should mandate that properly placed shoring be installed before providers make entry. Even though the providers still face the risk of injury or death in the confined space, the risk is minimized because the shoring is intended to prevent a further collapse of the structure or materials.

Risk Transfer

This primarily occurs through a couple of different mannerisms: The first is physically transferring the risk to another person or agency; the second is through the purchase of insurance to minimize loss. The practical approach to this would be considering the use of outside groups such as for-profit hazardous materials mitigation teams to handle hazmat containment issues and assume the much-needed responsibility of handling hazmat on incidents that involve these threats.

Once the safety officer has decided on one of the actions to minimize risk, he must continually monitor the operation to see that these control measures are being implemented properly and that rescuers continue to pursue the mission in a safe manner.

RISK MANAGEMENT AND MONITORING

The final component is risk management and monitoring. Risk management is an ongoing process. As a safety officer, it is your job to continually manage the risk by the methods mentioned previously. In order to do this, you need to monitor the environment and personnel on a regular basis. Risk management is a never-ending process.

RECOGNIZING UNSAFE PRACTICES

Unsafe practices can be defined as those actions, whether intentional or not, that pose either a direct or indirect threat to the physical well-being of a provider. These unsafe practices often arise when decisions are made without a full understanding of the interrelated complexities of a technical rescue incident and are often not intentional in nature. A rescuer may spontaneously attempt to perform a task or procedure that falls outside of the SOP/SOG of the particular incident without first thinking through the cascade of events that may occur secondary to their action(s). The rescuer more than likely acted in good faith but without adequate forethought. For example, a young child is at the bottom of a trench. Instead of following the standard operation procedure of shoring the wall and taking appropriate precautions, the rescuer goes down into the trench to make the rescue.

Obviously, the safety officer is not able to see everything at an incident scene at all times. Therefore, all rescuers on an incident scene must be empowered to recognize unsafe practices and speak up without fear of negative consequences from their peers or being worried about their concerns being lambasted by the safety officer and other leaders on the scene. Not only must each and every provider, regardless of rank or position, be willing to physically speak up to voice concerns over safety; they also must have been granted permission by superiors to speak up. Lower-ranking providers must be told that it is acceptable to challenge the orders of a senior provider if those orders pose an unnecessary risk to those involved in the operation.

All providers must take ownership of the safety dimensions of a technical rescue incident. More important, individual providers must be willing to take personal responsibility for their own safety and, secondarily, that of their co-workers.

INCIDENT REHABILITATION OF PROVIDERS

"For 200 years we have been providing a service at the expense of those providing the service." These words are attributed to Alan Brunacini, retired chief of the Phoenix (Arizona) Fire Department. (*Source: Quote by Alan Brunacini in Fire Department Incident Safety Officer, 2E by D. W. Dodson. Published by Cengage Learning, © 2007, p. 11.*) Chief Brunacini's statement should be a reminder to all safety officers that their ultimate concern should be the health of their providers who are regularly asked to put their lives on the line in order to help others. One

Best Practice

Ketchikan, Alaska

South Tongass Fire District, North Tongass Fire District, and Ketchikan Borough joined efforts in training and utilizing personnel for a rehab team in Ketchikan, Alaska. The three departments have an auxiliary that is comprised of spouses of the firefighters, coupled with individuals who are working to be active firefighters.

These individuals meet on a regular basis. They do a drill at least once a month to hone their skills. They respond to provide rehab services on any incident for which rehab is requested. This enables the suppression personnel to focus on firefighting, and the auxiliary can be part of the incident by providing rehab services.

The personnel are trained at various levels. Some provide EMS services. Each is trained to at least the level of Emergency Medical Responder. Therefore, they can take vital signs and provide basic emergency care to fire personnel in the rehab sector. This is an excellent example of using personnel to perform rehab responsibilities without relying on suppression personnel.

---

very important way that safety officers can aid in this is to ensure on all significant events that proper rehabilitation of personnel occurs.

Emergency incident rehabilitation is commonly referred to as rehab. The U.S. Fire Administration (2008) defines rehab as "the process of providing rest, rehydration, nourishment, and medical evaluation to responders who are involved in extended and/or extreme incident scene operations" (p. 4). The goal of rehab is to ensure that all rescuers operate to their full potential while on an emergency scene and return to service without having suffered any ill effects from the activities that occurred on an incident scene. Ultimately, rehab is intended to either return providers to action on the emergency scene or return them safely to their stations.

It is vitally important to allow for thc proper rest and rehabilitation of rescue personnel during the course of an emergency operation. It has been well established that providers who are not provided rehab and adequate rehydration during an incident are at increased risk of illness or injury. Further, those providers who are excessively physically and mentally stressed during an incident are more prone to make mistakes, compounding the built-in safety challenges that exist on virtually all emergency scenes. Overstressed or overexerted providers put the successful outcome of the incident operation in jeopardy and may jeopardize the safety of other providers on the scene.

As all experienced emergency services professionals know, emergencies can occur at any time and under all types of adverse conditions. Therefore, it is important for providers to be physically prepared to respond at all times. Unfortunately, not all personnel are as physically fit as they should be when they are suddenly called upon to exert themselves at the scene of a technical rescue. Many responders from within the fire and emergency services spend considerable amounts of downtime between calls, often leading to sedentary lifestyles. This lack of physical activity may lead to these personnel becoming overweight and/or obese. For example, consider a study conducted by the National Registry of Emergency Medical Technicians (NREMT) in 2007 (Fernandez, Studnek, and White, 2008) that drew voluntary responses from 30,560 EMS providers from throughout the United States and from a variety of types of EMS delivery systems. The self-reported heights and weights of 21,149 of these respondents were analyzed, leading researchers to find that 71.5 percent of them had what is considered to be a high body mass index (BMI). In addition, the percentage of elevated BMI levels was increased in males and in higher certification levels; specifically, among paramedics.

This excessively high incidence of overweight and obese EMS providers is far greater than that of the general population of the United States. The U.S. Centers for Disease Control and Prevention (CDC) has found that "an estimated 34.2% of U.S. adults aged 20 years and over are overweight, 33.8% are obese, and 5.7% are extremely obese" based on data collected in 2007 and 2008 (Ogden and Carroll, 2010, p. 1).

This seeming epidemic of overweight and obese providers potentially limits the EMS community's ability to safely respond to and mitigate an emergency scene. These personnel are at an elevated risk of developing a wide variety of medical conditions including hypertension, diabetes, and joint problems; they are also more prone to injuries and illnesses. More disturbingly, these disease processes and others predispose EMS providers to a higher incidence of potentially life-threatening vascular conditions, including myocardial infarction and stroke.

It is recommended that rehab be mandated on the scene of technical rescue incidents, especially those that are of longer duration or that occur in particularly stressful environments. (See Figure 10.3.) Many providers are very enthusiastic about the mission at hand and may

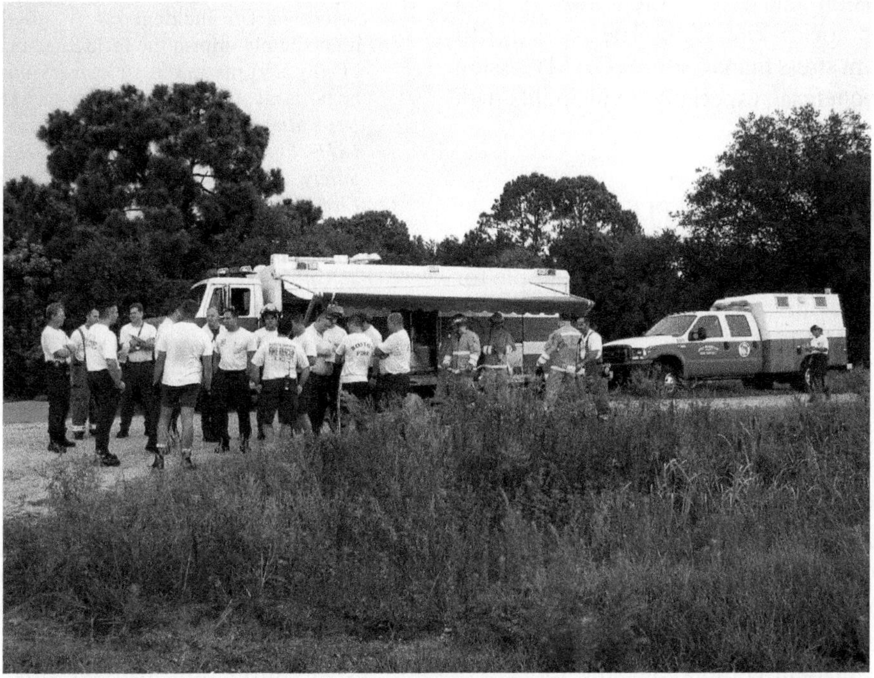

FIGURE 10.3 ■ It is recommended that rehab be mandated on the scene of technical rescue incidents, especially those that are of longer duration or that occur in particularly stressful environments. *Source: Courtesy of Jeffrey T. Lindsey, Ph.D.*

even have a sense of invincibility, convincing themselves that they can continue to persevere despite being overly stressed. In addition, young providers may not yet recognize the impending signs of exertion and may continue working until they are injured or worse. The safety officer must work with the IC and the EMS branch to ensure that formal rehab is established and the appropriate rehab protocol is followed.

In addition, the adoption of the "corpsman with a marine" model used by the U.S. Navy and U.S. Marine Corps to care for injured and ill personnel in field environments may be useful in the context of providing ongoing emergency incident rehabilitation. Assigning specific medical providers to monitor other providers on the scene will aid in looking after the well-being of all personnel on the scene. Those personnel who are directly involved in front-line patient care and rescue are often susceptible to tunnel vision and neglect their own physical and psychological limitations. The use of a critical incident stress management (CISM) session may be beneficial, especially on incidents with bad outcomes.

LEADING BY EXAMPLE

The safety officer must set a good example for all other providers to follow. It is vitally important for the safety officer to follow all safety policies and procedures at all times, to wear PPE when appropriate, and to actively and visibly support health and safety initiatives within the department. These include advocating for wellness programs that encourage personnel to get and stay in shape and generally adopt healthier lifestyles.

ALTERING, SUSPENDING, OR TERMINATING AN EVENT

According to section 2.5.1 of NFPA 1521, the safety officer is empowered to change or halt an operation when it is found to be unsafe:

> At an emergency incident where activities are judged by the incident safety officer to be unsafe or involve an imminent hazard, the incident safety officer shall have the authority to alter, suspend, or terminate those activities. The incident safety officer shall immediately inform the incident commander of any actions taken to correct imminent hazards at an emergency scene. (*Source: Reproduced with permission from NFPA 1521-2008, Standard for Fire Department Safety Officer, Copyright © 2007, National Fire Protection Association. This reprinted material is not the complete and official position of the NFPA on the referenced subject, which is represented only by the standard in its entirety.*)

CHAPTER REVIEW

Summary

EMS providers operating at technical rescue incidents where patients have been injured and/or trapped are asked to take good medicine to bad places. These situations require that the incident commander and the safety officer work together to ensure that minimal risk is assumed in facilitating the removal of these patients from often difficult circumstances while also providing optimum care. The paramount goal of any incident is making sure that all providers safely go home to their families at the end of the day. The safety officer plays an important role in this effort by enforcing safe working practices under poor conditions.

WHAT WOULD YOU DO? Reflection

As the EMS safety officer, you need to get an assessment of the scene. It is imperative to consult with the technical rescue team on the scene in order to evaluate the risks. Part of your job is to ensure that the crews working on the scene function in a safe environment. You need to confer with the incident commander and share your concerns about any safety issues you have observed. The incident commander also must be apprised of the operations from the technical rescue team, especially if the incident commander is not trained to the level of the technical rescue team. The incident commander is responsible for the operations of everyone at the incident scene, and provisions must be made to ensure the safety of all personnel and any victims on the scene of the incident. Frequent meetings are essential at each level of the process. Establishing a rehab site early on during the incident is important in providing proper safety of all personnel. Personnel tend to be adamant about continuing to work at these types of incidents. Proper rehab of personnel is essential. The incident commander should be part of the process to ensure that personnel receive the proper rehab on scene.

Review Questions

1. What are the duties of the safety officer?
2. How does the safety officer fit into the incident command system (ICS)?
3. What is the purpose of the PAR?
4. What are the four risk management components as defined by NFPA 1500?
5. What are the two ways that risks are transferred?
6. What is considered an unsafe practice?
7. In 2007 NREMT conducting a self-survey on the health of EMS personnel. What were the results of this research study?
8. Who has the authority to terminate or suspend operations on the scene of an incident?

References

Dodson, D. W. (2007). *Fire Department Incident Safety Officer*, 2nd ed. Clifton Park, NY: Delmar, Cengage Learning.

Fernandez, A. R., J. Studnek, and L. White. (2008, January). "Body Mass Index of Emergency Medical Services Professionals." Poster session presented at the annual symposium of the National Association of EMS Physicians, Phoenix, AZ.

International Fire Service Training Association. (2004). *Chief Officer*, 2nd ed. Stillwater, OK: Author.

National Fire Protection Association. (2008). "NFPA 1500: Standard on Fire Department Occupational Safety and Health Program." (See the organization website.)

National Fire Protection Association. (2013). "NFPA 1521: Standard for Fire Department Safety Officer." (See the organization website.)

Ogden, C. L., and M. D. Carroll. (2010). "Prevalence of Overweight, Obesity, and Extreme Obesity Among Adults: United States, Trends 1960–1962 Through 2007–2008." Washington, DC: Centers for Disease Control and Prevention.

U.S. Fire Administration. (2008). "Emergency Incident Rehabilitation." (Emmitsburg, MD: U.S. Fire Administration.)

Key Terms

command staff The personnel who are in charge of an incident and report directly to the incident commander.

cultures of unnecessary risk An environment that encourages participants to take on risk that is not necessary and can or does harm or kill them.

emergency incident rehabilitation The process of providing rest, rehydration, nourishment, and medical evaluation to responders who are involved in extended and/or extreme incident scene operations.

immediately dangerous to life and health (IDLH) Maximum concentration from which one could escape within 30 minutes without any escape-impairing symptoms or any irreversible health effects.

risk avoidance Not performing or doing in order to prevent an incident from occurring.

risk control A concept that is divided into risk avoidance, risk reduction, and risk transfer.

risk evaluation The act of determining the potential of the severity of loss and the probability of occurrence.

risk identification The process through which safety officers attempt to recognize and assess potential problems.

risk management A coordinated set of activities and methods that is used to direct an organization and to control the many risks that can affect its ability to achieve objectives.

risk reduction A situation in which risk is minimized because of actions taken.

risk transfer The transfer of risk to another person or agency or the purchase of insurance to reduce the cost of the risk.

situational awareness The process through which rescuers grasp what is going on around them on the emergency scene, convert that information into a format that is useful for making decisions, and logically think through the consequences of the decisions that they make.

unsafe practices Those actions, whether intentional or not, that pose either a direct or indirect threat the physical well-being of a provider.

Hazardous Materials

11 CHAPTER

Frank DeFrancesco

Jeffrey Lindsey

Objectives

After reading this chapter, the student should be able to:

11.1 Describe settings in which hazardous material incidents may occur.
11.2 Recognize indications that a hazardous material situation may exist.
11.3 Discuss the use and limitations of shipping papers, material safety data sheets, and other sources of information about hazardous materials.
11.4 Describe the different levels of hazardous material training.
11.5 State the expected functions of an EMS manager functioning at a hazardous material incident scene.
11.6 Identify patients who require decontamination prior to treatment.
11.7 Differentiate among acute, subacute, and chronic effects of hazardous materials exposure.
11.8 Recognize the effects of various categories of hazardous materials, including corrosives, pulmonary irritants, pesticides, asphyxiants, and hydrocarbons.
11.9 Describe the integration of patient care with the need for safety and patient decontamination when responding to hazardous material incidents.

Key Terms

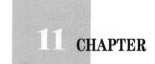

bulk
decontamination
facility containment systems
facility paperwork
Hazardous Materials Information System (HMIS)
material safety data sheets (MSDSs)
nonbulk
rinsate
shipping papers
SLUDGEM

WHAT WOULD YOU DO?

A rescue crew received a call for a man in his sixties complaining of shortness of breath. When the crew arrived, they found a man who was complaining of shortness of breath, diaphoretic, and wearing a long-sleeved shirt and long pants, both of which were wet. The crew had entered the house with all of the usual equipment and now started to conduct a patient assessment. As they were conducting the assessment, crew members smelled a pesticide, but no further thought or action was taken. The crew continued to treat the patient in the home.

As the crew began to load the patient into the ambulance for transport, the rescue crew members started to get sick. In further questioning, the patient said that he had begun to feel ill when he was just finishing the chore of spraying his house, roof, eaves, and lawn with a pesticide. The clothes the patient was wearing were the same clothes he had worn while spraying. By the time the incident was complete, the occupant and two of the four rescue personnel required medical evaluation—and all the EMS equipment that had been carried into the home, as well as the ambulance, required decontamination.

Questions

1. How could the EMS manager have handled this differently?
2. What could have prevented this from occurring?
3. What actions would you need to take?

INTRODUCTION

Hazardous materials are found during virtually every incident. However, not every incident is a hazardous material event. An EMS manager must be alert for key indicators and able to recognize hazardous material incidents. The training received in paramedic or EMT classes is merely enough to provide an awareness of hazardous materials. An EMS manager will need additional training to be able to command a hazardous materials team.

Even with training, it is necessary to have the appropriate equipment and personal protective equipment (PPE) before crews can operate at the scene of a hazardous material event. The chapter will discuss the basics required for EMS personnel to properly respond to a hazardous material (hazmat) incident. The primary source of the information contained within this section will be from National Fire Protection Agency (NFPA) standards 471, 472, and 473. The Environmental Protection Agency (EPA) and the Occupational Safety and Health Agency (OSHA) are two other sources of information that can be referenced regarding hazardous materials response.

UNDERSTANDING HAZARDOUS MATERIALS

NPFA 471 defines a hazardous material as a substance, either matter—solid, liquid, or gas—or energy, that, when released, is capable of creating harm to people, the environment, and property, including weapons of mass destruction (WMD) as defined in 18 U.S. Code Section 2332a.

Each of the terms listed at the beginning of this chapter has a specific definition written by the agency that regulates it. For example, the U.S. Department of Transportation (DOT) may define a hazardous material as a substance that is transported and regulated by the DOT as to how much and how it is transported. A specific chemical may fall into different regulatory classifications, based on the way in which the chemical is being used, stored, or transported, but the hazards of the chemical remain unchanged.

INCIDENT TYPES

Hazardous material incidents may occur anywhere, so an EMS manager must always be aware of this possibility. A chemical release can occur at a residence, during transportation, or in an industrial setting. In a residential setting, chemical incidents may occur when improperly storing or using household products. An example would be mixing a bleach agent with an agent that contains ammonia when cleaning a bathroom. Another example could occur when pool chemicals are stored in a shed or garage next to petroleum products used for the lawn mower. Chemical products are transported from the manufacturer to retail stores or directly to users via highways, railways, airways, waterways, and pipelines where spills and accidents can occur. An industry may use a variety of chemicals to create products intended for consumer use. At the manufacturing site, as a result of human error or mechanical failure, a chemical release may occur. Such releases may also occur at work sites where chemicals are stored or used. To simplify the categorization of incidents that may occur, one can classify the incident into three types: nonbulk, bulk, and facility containment systems (Trebisacci, 2008).

Nonbulk

Nonbulk packaging may hold a liquid capacity of 119 gallons (450 L) or less, a solid net mass of 882 pounds (400 kg) or less, or a gas capacity of 1,001 pounds (454 kg) or less (Hildebrand, Noll, and Yvorra 2012). The container may be in the form of bags, bottles, boxes, cylinders, or drums. Each type of container has its own potential hazards.

Bulk

Bulk packaging may hold a liquid capacity greater than 119 gallons (450 liters), a solid net mass greater than 882 pounds (400 kg), or a gas capacity greater than 1,001 pounds (454 kg) (Hildebrand, Noll, and Yvorra 2012). The packaging may include portable bins, intermodal containers, cargo containers, and tank cars.

Facility

Facility containment systems are packaging, containers, and containment systems that are part of a fixed facility's operation. These types of systems include atmospheric-pressure storage tanks, low-pressure storage tanks, and high-pressure storage tanks.

IDENTIFICATION

Five factors can help a crew determine whether a hazardous material may be involved: location, container shape, placards/labels/markings, on-site paperwork, and using one's senses.

Location

Knowing the business name and the business type could provide clues to the potential presence of any hazardous materials at a business location. For example, a plating company may have acids, bases, or poisons on site that are used for etching metals. There may be specific locations throughout the community known for the manufacture, use, storage, or disposal of chemicals. Preplanning by preparing a list and/or map of businesses in the area that have chemicals on site, as well as information about the hazards associated with the different types of chemicals, will help crews identify and deal with potential hazards in the area they serve.

Container Shape

Chemicals are stored and shipped in packages that are compatible with one another. The packaging must be capable of containing its product both by its physical characteristics (e.g., liquid or gas under atmospheric, low, or high pressure) and by its chemical characteristics (e.g., corrosives or oxidizers). The packaging of chemicals must meet the DOT's packaging requirements. In transportation, chemicals must be compatible to be transported with each other. DOT's packaging and transportation requirements are detailed in the Code of Federal Regulations, Title 49, subpart 171.

The shape of transportation vehicles and fixed storage containers may assist in the identification of the hazard type of the chemical stored within. For example, a trailer that looks like a large thermos bottle carries cryogenic materials; a rail car that has all the valves contained within a single dome is carrying products under pressure; a spherical container holds products under high pressure.

Placards/Labels/Markings

The method used for marking hazardous materials in transit is the DOT Labeling and Placarding System. Code of Federal Regulations, Title 49, subpart 171, defines the layout of the labels and the placards that must be displayed. One part of the label and placard identifies the hazard class of the chemical. The number of the hazard class is identified on the bottom of the placard, see Table 11.1.

TABLE 11.1 ■ The Nine U.S. DOT Hazard Classes

Class 1	Explosives
Class 2	Compressed gases
Class 3	Flammable liquids
Class 4	Flammable solids
Class 5	Oxidizers
Class 6	Poisons
Class 7	Radioactive materials
Class 8	Corrosive liquids
Class 9	Miscellaneous

Each substance being transported will be issued either a North America (NA) number or a United Nations (UN) number. Chemicals assigned NA numbers are substances being transported between the United States, Mexico, and Canada. Chemicals assigned UN numbers are substances being transported internationally. The numbers are usually four digits located either in the middle of a placard or in black letters on an orange rectangle field. The latter is primarily used on shipments over the railway. Placards usually show both the hazard class and the four-digit NA or UN number. In contrast, labels usually list just the primary hazard class and not the UN or NA number.

Placards are in the shape of a diamond and placed on the container. Placards and labels both have a symbol on the top corner of the diamond. The symbol is a pictorial representation of the possible hazards of the chemical. For example, the symbol for a flammable substance is a flame; the symbol for a poison is a skull and crossbones.

The last part of the label or placard a responder should be aware of is the color of the background. This is probably the most useful part of the label and placard because it can be identified quickly from a distance. For example, orange indicates an explosive, blue means that it is water reactive, and red means that it is flammable. (See Figure 11.1.)

Another form of markings is the NFPA 704 system, a voluntary compliance system designed to identify hazardous materials that are used, handled, or stored within a facility. The label is divided into four color-coded sections. (See Figure 11.2.) The first section is red,

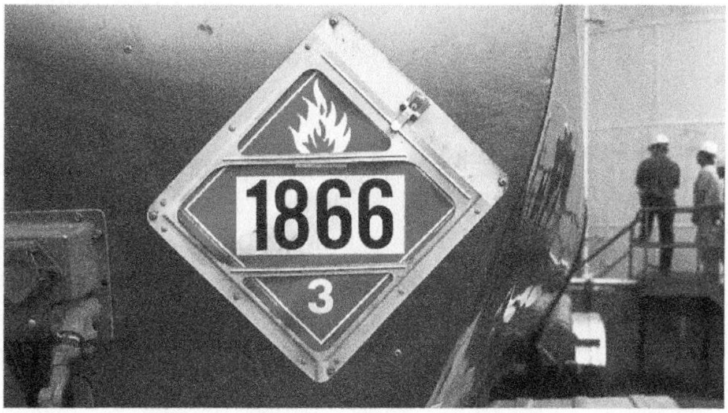

FIGURE 11.1 ■ The color background on placards identifies the contents or precautions for the content being transported or stored.

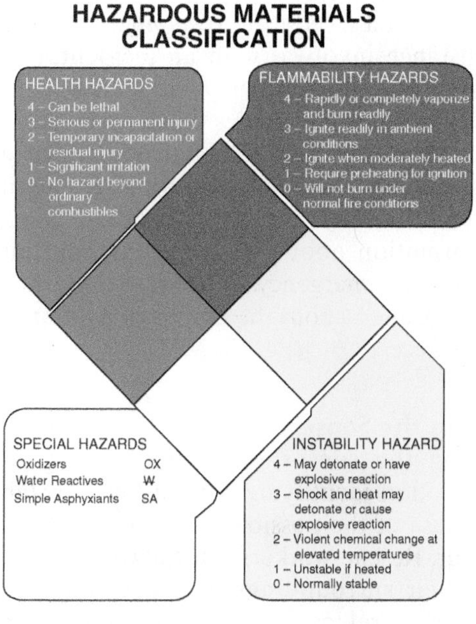

FIGURE 11.2 ■ The NFPA diamond is divided into four color-coded sections. (*Source: Reprinted with permission from NFPA 704-2012, System for the Identification of the Hazards of Materials for Emergency Response. Copyright © 2011, National Fire Protection Association. This reprinted material is not the complete and official position of the NFPA on the referenced subject, which is represented solely by the standard in its entirety. The classification of any particular material within this system is the sole responsibility of the user and not the NFPA. NFPA bears no responsibility for any determinations of any values for any particular material classified or represented using this system.*)

representing flammability. The next is yellow, representing reactivity. The third section is blue, for health. Fourth, white is for special hazards. The first three sections use a rating system from 0 to 4, with 0 being no hazard and 4 being a very high hazard. The white section identifies any special hazards, such as radioactivity or water reactivity.

A system that uses some of the same references as the NFPA 704 system is the **Hazardous Materials Information System (HMIS)**. Companies have used this system to comply with OSHA 1910.1000, Hazard Communication Regulation, and with state and local regulations that deal with the employee right-to-know standards. The system is designed to place a simple label on individual containers. The first three sections—flammability, reactivity, and health—are the same as in the NFPA 704 system. However, the white section is used for special precautions as determined by the facility that is labeling the container. The HMIS is designed for facilities to properly label containers in order to satisfy OSHA regulations. (See Figure 11.3.)

On-Site Paperwork

Another method for identifying a hazardous material is on-site paperwork, including shipping papers, facility paperwork, and material safety data sheets.

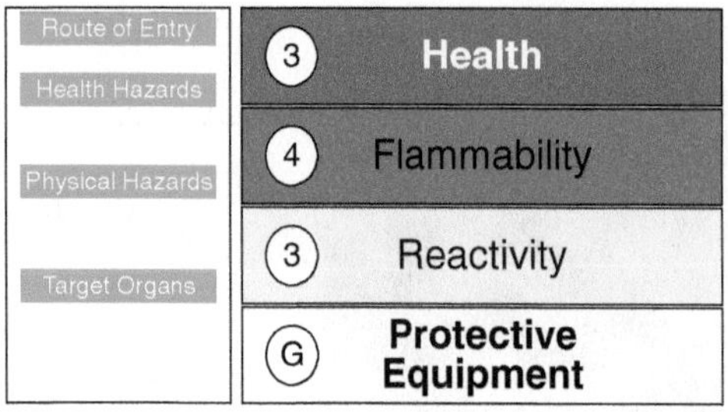

FIGURE 11.3 The HMIS label is used to comply with OSHA 1910.1000, Hazard Communication Regulation.

When chemicals are transported, proper documentation must accompany the shipment. That documentation is known as the **shipping papers**. The DOT, under Title 49 of the Code of Federal Regulations, has specific guidelines as to the layout and information required on the documentation. The chemical is listed on the documentation by its proper shipping name, which is not necessarily the trade name or chemical name. For example, a solvent commonly known as mineral spirits has a proper shipping name of petroleum naphtha. Also on the documentation, the quantity within the shipment is recorded by weight. Because most responders probably understand volume in terms of gallons or liters, shipments must be converted from the recorded weight in pounds to gallons/liters.

Facilities that handle or store chemicals are required to have contingency plans, which is a part of **facility paperwork**. These plans must document facility layouts, emergency contact information, chemical data, and any planning necessary for handling facility emergencies. In addition to becoming familiar with facility contingency plans, rescue personnel should consult the local fire departments about any prefire plans. Prefire plans will also identify hazards and necessary operations for emergency response personnel. The local emergency management office or the local emergency planning committee may also be resources for facility data.

Facilities that create, handle, or store hazardous materials are required to provide access to **material safety data sheets (MSDSs)**. The information contained in an MSDS document includes the name, address, and phone number of the manufacturer, the chemical name of the substance and any synonyms, the chemical and physical properties of the substance, PPE necessary for contact with the substance, any potential health effects if an exposure occurs, and any handling, disposal, and storing procedures.

The MSDS is an excellent initial source of information to educate responders about the substance involved with an incident, but it should be considered only one source of information. Some companies that have created an MSDS may not have documented all potential hazards involved with a particular substance or may not have included enough information about handling the substance during an emergency. Other resources should be consulted about the details of a hazardous substance.

Using the Senses

Using the senses is the most dangerous method of identifying a hazardous substance because of the possible exposures that could occur. Rescue workers must always stay alert to their surroundings. The advantage to a chemical release—if ever it could be said there is one—is that a chemical release will allow responders to either see, feel, taste, or hear the release.

ESTABLISHING A HAZMAT SCENE

When rescue personnel report to work, the size-up process begins. Size-up is the process used by responders to analyze a situation in order to determine the potential hazards. The day of the year, day of the week, and the time of day may all be used to determine potential issues. In addition, the response personnel will evaluate resources available to respond during their shift. The resources include vehicles, equipment, and staff. Depending on the day or time of day, resources may or may not be available to respond without a delay.

When an incident occurs, the size-up will continue. Dispatch must ask as many questions about the incident as possible in order to give responders a clear picture of the potential situation. EMS managers will analyze the information to determine whether the proper resources are responding. As dispatch is relaying information, weather conditions must be evaluated to determine wind direction, humidity levels, and the potential for precipitation. In a possible hazmat situation, responders should respond uphill and upwind to avoid exposure.

Once on the scene, EMS managers will evaluate the site as they approach, evaluating building construction, evacuation, smoke or gas/vapor clouds, and means of egress. In situations involving potentially hazardous materials, vehicle position is important. The emergency response vehicle should be staged in a way to allow for a quick exit if necessary. In addition, the vehicle must be placed in a way to allow for additional resources to access the scene as necessary.

Once on the scene, the rescue personnel will continue to size up the situation by asking questions of the bystanders and occupants. Information received from the occupants must be evaluated for plausibility and validity. Consider the source of the information and ask the following questions:

- Was the person directly involved with the situation?
- What is the position of the occupant within the organization?
- Where was the person when the incident occurred?
- To further evaluate the situation, ask what happened.
- Where within the facility is the problem?
- What chemicals are involved?
- What are the physical and chemical properties of the chemicals involved?
- Were any occupants exposed?
- How many people were exposed?
- Where are the exposed personnel now? Are they isolated? Have they been decontaminated?

The most important fact that an EMS manager must understand is that all information gathered should be validated. This process continues throughout the response.

TRAINING OF EMS

EMS personnel are generally trained to the awareness- or operations-level for hazmat responders and will function at the hazmat scene primarily by treating a patient—who has already been decontaminated—for airway, breathing, and circulation (ABC) and transport to a hospital. Some EMS personnel may be trained to participate in decontamination, but usually not in a hazmat rescue itself. When a hazardous material is involved in a residential call, some simple decontamination may be performed, such as removing contaminated clothing, brushing away powders, or irrigation of exposed skin or eyes, again with basic ABC care and transport. The following discussion is about hazmat incidents in general, including guidelines for rescuers, rather than about the specific role of EMS personnel.

LEVELS OF TRAINING

In 2008, the National Fire Protection Agency revised NFPA 472, Standard for Competence of Responders to Hazardous Materials/Weapons of Mass Destruction Incidents (National Fire Protection Association, 2008a), and

NFPA 473, Competencies for EMS Personnel Responding to Hazardous Materials/Weapons of Mass Destruction Incidents (National Fire Protection Association, 2008b). These documents clearly identify the core competencies required for each level of training. In NFPA 472, four levels of responders are identified: awareness-level, operations-level, technician-level, and specialist-level.

Awareness-level personnel are those who, through the normal course of their duties, may be the first to encounter a hazardous material or WMD incident. Personnel at this level primarily learn how to identify that an incident is occurring and how to avoid contamination and activate the emergency notification system. Awareness-level personnel are not viewed as hazmat emergency responders.

Operations-level responders are personnel who are dispatched to a hazardous materials or WMD incident and are expected to take action to protect life, property, or the environment. NFPA 472 states that operations personnel need to receive training in five core competencies. Response agencies, based on their determination of the level of response these personnel will be called on to perform, may train them further in any of a variety of mission-specific competencies, such as PPE and product control.

Hazardous material technicians are personnel who respond to a hazardous material or WMD incident and are expected to perform technical-level skills. These personnel receive training in addition to operations-level training to include the application of product control techniques that may be situation specific—for example, thc application of a chlorine kit to a leaking chlorine container.

Specialist-level personnel respond only to a specific location, primarily a specific occupancy with a specific type of hazard. For example, a specialist-level employee may work at an anhydrous ammonia facility. This person would be trained on emergency response only to anhydrous ammonia.

NFPA 472 also identifies training competencies for incident commanders and for hazardous materials officers. Hazardous materials and WMD incidents pose situations that an emergency response officer may not normally encounter. These competencies allow officers to learn about and identify issues that would require action during an incident.

FUNCTIONING AT THE SCENE

NFPA 473 acknowledges that there are various levels of response across the county for EMS. In this document, NFPA defines a basic life support (BLS) response and an advanced life support (ALS) response. Whether personnel are capable of providing ALS or BLS, NFPA has established basic core competencies. Responders who may be responsible for performing a rescue must demonstrate the use of PPE, perform decontamination, perform air monitoring, and perform victim rescue and removal. The authority having jurisdiction will determine the level of care beyond the core competencies. It is the EMS manager's responsibility to make sure his personnel perform within the scope of their training and equipment.

The goal of NFPA 473 for a BLS responder is that the rescuer will have the ability to analyze the situation, determine the potential hazards, perform a rescue, and deliver appropriate BLS treatment to the exposed victim. The goal of NFPA 473 for an ALS responder is that the paramedic will have the ability to analyze the situation, determine the potential hazards, perform a rescue, and deliver the appropriate ALS treatment to the exposed victim. This typically is the extent of responsibilities for the paramedic at a hazmat scene, unless he has additional training and is part of a hazmat team or special response team.

Best Practice

EMS Special Operations in South Carolina

Charleston (South Carolina) EMS has a number of special operations teams. One of the divisions is an EMS hazmat team that is specially equipped with trained paramedics. The mission of the team is to respond with other agencies in the community to provide specialized treatment to contaminated victims.

Other EMS agencies provide similar services. Pittsburgh (Pennsylvania) EMS, for example, provides hazmat services through the city EMS agency. These agencies demonstrate the best practices of EMS agencies who commit to providing hazmat response to incident scenes.

HAZMAT MEDICINE

Hazardous materials have characteristics that will have an impact on the kind of medical care that may be required for a patient who is contaminated or who has suffered exposure to hazmat.

CHARACTERISTICS OF HAZARDOUS MATERIALS

Hazardous materials come in three basic forms: solid, liquid, and gas. Each form has inherent properties. Solids are rigid and formed into their own particular shape and size; at a given temperature and pressure, a solid will occupy a specific volume. Liquids take the shape of their container but, like solids, liquids at a given temperature and pressure will occupy a specific volume. Gases, however, do not have a definite shape or volume. Gases will conform to their container and, depending on temperature and pressure, the volume of a gas will vary.

CONTAMINATION AND EXPOSURE

A substance may enter the body through inhalation, absorption, ingestion, and/or injection. The chemical may enter via one or more methods. For example, a person inhales a substance. The substance then mixes with the saliva and is swallowed. The primary exposure is inhalation, and the secondary exposure is ingestion.

What is the difference between contamination and exposure? Take the example of a plant worker who comes into contact with a hazardous powder. The worker's clothing contains some of the product. Was the worker contaminated, and was the worker exposed to the substance? The worker's clothing was contaminated with the substance. However, the worker has the potential to be exposed. A question must be asked: Did the worker inhale, absorb, ingest, or inject the substance? If none of these occurred, the worker was contaminated but not exposed to the substance. For this example, the EMS manager must realize that simple decontamination must occur and that, if properly performed, the worker may not be exposed, thus not requiring medical treatment.

Different levels of exposure exist as well. A person who is exposed to a hazardous substance may have an acute exposure, a subacute exposure, or chronic effects. An acute exposure occurs when a person is exposed to a substance and adverse health effects occur immediately. An example would be a person who inhales chlorine gas, resulting in immediate shortness of breath, along with burning of the mouth and pharynx.

Some substances do not cause adverse health effects immediately, but adverse effects occur within 24 to 36 hours after the exposure;

this is known as a subacute exposure. An example would be someone who receives a low dosage of phosgene. Shortness of breath and pulmonary edema may occur 24 hours after the inhalation exposure.

Chronic effects occur after a person has received a high dosage of a substance over a short period of time or low dosages over a long period of time. The end result could be cancer, leukemia, or emphysema, among other effects.

TREATMENT REGIMES

Treatment for chemical exposures varies according to the type of chemical involved. Some of the major chemical types are corrosives, pulmonary irritants, pesticides, asphyxiants, and hydrocarbons.

Corrosives

OSHA 29 CFR 1910.1200, Appendix A (Occupational Safety & Health Administration, 2012), defines a corrosive as "A chemical that causes visible destruction of, or irreversible alterations in, living tissue by chemical action at the site of contact. For example, a chemical is considered to be corrosive if, when tested on the intact skin of albino rabbits by the method described by the U.S. Department of Transportation in appendix A to 49 CFR part 173, it destroys or changes irreversibly the structure of the tissue at the site of contact following an exposure period of four hours. This term shall not refer to action on inanimate surfaces."

Corrosives can be classified as acids or bases. When the skin comes into contact with an acid, the skin will start to burn. Burning will continue until either the acid is removed from the skin through a decontamination process or the acid is neutralized. If the corrosive is a solid, dry particles should be brushed off and then the area flushed with water. Decontamination with the use of copious amounts of water is the preferred method to prevent further tissue damage. Neutralization uses chemical substances to counteract the acid. In neutralization, however, a chemical reaction occurs, which creates the possibility of further tissue damage. Tincture of green soap may help in decontamination. Eye injuries should be irrigated with water. Some medical directors will approve the use of tetracaine as a topical ophthalmic anesthetic to reduce eye discomfort. Vomiting should not be induced if the patient swallowed a corrosive.

When a base contacts the skin, the chemical reacts with the tissue, causing the tissue to "melt away" as bases cause degradation of fatty cells and the outer layers of the skin. This may cause a person to have the sensation of softer skin. Bases also react with many organic materials. The use of sodium hydroxide (lye or Drano) to open clogged drains is an example. The chemical causes the organic material to decay. A base such as lye can cause devastating damage to skin or mucous membranes.

Pulmonary Irritants

According to the NFPA 471, "An irritant is a chemical that causes a reversible inflammatory effect on living tissue by chemical action at the site of contact." (*Source: Reproduced with permission from NFPA 471-2002, Recommended Practice for Responding to Hazardous Materials Incidents. Copyright © 2002 by the National Fire Protection Association.*) A pulmonary irritant is one that targets the respiratory tract and causes irritation. An example of an irritant would be low levels of bleach or ammonia. This combination of chemicals is known as chloramines. Low levels of these chemicals could cause coughing and shortness of breath.

Primary respiratory exposure cannot be decontaminated. However, the patient's clothing should be removed to allow any trapped gases to be released. Decontamination with copious amounts of water is the preferred method to prevent further tissue damage. Eye injuries should be irrigated with water. Some medical directors will approve the use of tetracaine as a topical ophthalmic anesthetic to reduce eye discomfort.

Pesticides

Pesticides are chemicals designed to kill insects and other pests. Most are measured in mg/kg, with the dosage calculated to kill the target pest. Pesticides primarily include carbamates and organophosphates. The exposure can occur by inhalation, absorption, ingestion, or injection. The substances can act to block acetylcholinesterase (AChE). Organophosphate pesticides target the nervous system by activating the nerve impulses rather than shutting them down. Living organisms experiencing organophosphate poisoning will experience a series of effects represented by the mnemonic **SLUDGEM**: *s*alivation, *l*acrimation, *u*rination, *d*efecation, *g*astrointestinal problems, *e*mesis, and *m*iosis (contracted pupils). The treatment for organophosphate poisoning is atropine and 2-Pam. If the chemical is a carbamate, pralidoxine is not recommended. Do not induce vomiting if the patient ingested the chemical.

Asphyxiants

NFPA 471 states, "An asphyxiant is a substance that can cause unconsciousness or death by suffocation." (*Source: Reproduced with permission from NFPA 471-2002, Recommended Practice for Responding to Hazardous Materials Incidents. Copyright © 2002 by the National Fire Protection Association.*). The two types of asphyxiants are simple and chemical. A simple asphyxiant is one that causes suffocation through the displacement of oxygen. For example, if large quantities of nitrogen or carbon dioxide are released in a room, eventually the oxygen will be displaced. A person in that room will suffocate from lack of oxygen. A chemical asphyxiant is a chemical that will absorb into the bloodstream and prevent the red blood cells from carrying oxygen, causing vital organs to fail from oxygen starvation. An example of a chemical asphyxiant is cyanide. The Cyanokit is available as a prepackaged antidote kit for cyanide poisoning. The Cyanokit contains hydroxocobalamin to reverse the effects. Hydroxocobalamin is a precursor to cyanocobalamin (vitamin B_{12}). It works by binding cyanide from cytochrome oxidase and forms cyanocobalamin. Excess cyanocobalamin is excreted from the body via the kidneys. The prepackaged cyanide kit contains amyl nitrate, sodium nitrite, and sodium thiosulfide. The paramedic must read and follow manufacturers' recommendations, as well as those of the medical director, as to the order and drug dosages of each medication.

Hydrocarbons

Hydrocarbons are chemicals with a hydrogen and carbon base. Hydrocarbons are used mostly as fuels. The size of the hydrocarbon molecule determines the fuel type. For example, methane, a highly flammable gas, is composed of one carbon atom connected to four hydrogen atoms. Octane is an eight-carbon chain connected to eighteen hydrogen atoms. Hydrocarbon derivatives are chemicals with a hydrocarbon base attached to radicals. Radicals are molecules made up of atoms capable of combining with the hydrocarbon derivatives to form new chemical compounds. For example, benzene is an aromatic hydrocarbon. If a methane radical, known as a methyl group, attaches to the benzene, the new substance is known as toluene. Toluene is used as a solvent, has a fruity odor, and is highly flammable. Patients who are exposed to toluene should be decontaminated with large volumes of water. If ingested, vomiting should not be induced. The ABCs should be supported for patients who have inhaled a chemical.

DECONTAMINATION

NFPA 471 defines **decontamination** as "the physical and/or chemical process of reducing and preventing the spread of contamination from people, animals, the environment, or equipment." (*Source: Reproduced with*

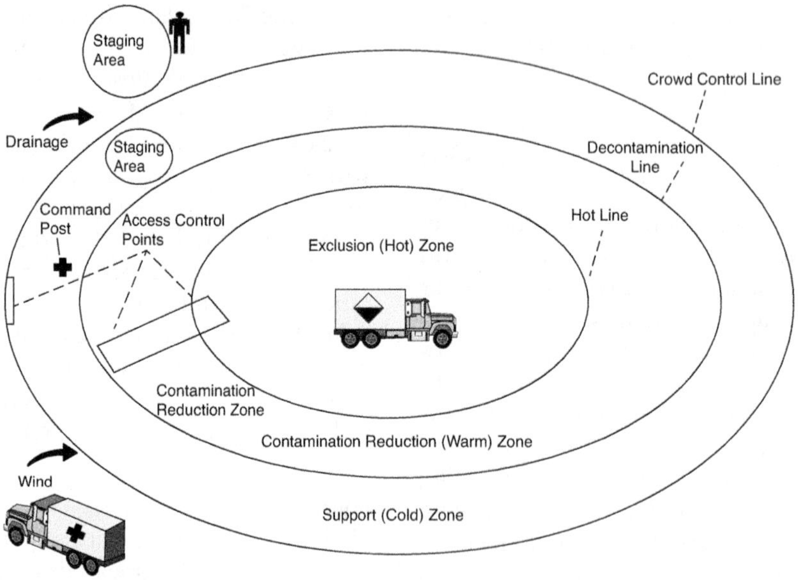

FIGURE 11.4 ■ NIOSH/OSHA/USCG/EPA/Recommended Zones.

permission from NFPA 471-2002, Recommended Practice for Responding to Hazardous Materials Incidents. Copyright © 2002, National Fire Protection Association. This reprinted material is not the complete and official position of the NFPA on the referenced subject, which is represented only by the standard in its entirety.). The agency having jurisdiction defines the levels of decontamination and how the agency will perform such actions.

NIOSH, OSHA, the U.S. Coast Guard, and the EPA recommend dividing the hazmat incident into three zones, establishing access control points, and delineating a contamination reduction corridor. The exclusion zone (hot zone) should encompass all known or suspected hazmat contamination. The respective radius of the contamination reduction zone (warm zone) is determined by the length of the decontamination corridor, containing all the needed "decon" stations. The support zone (cold zone) should be "clean"—free of hazmat contamination of all kinds, including discarded protective clothing and respiratory equipment. The command post and staging areas for necessary support equipment should be located upwind and uphill of the exclusion zone in the support area. Equipment that may eventually be needed should be kept in staging areas beyond the crowd control line. Access to the different zones should be tightly controlled and limited to as few locations as possible. (See Figure 11.4.)

Side Bar

Essential Requirements for Any Decontamination Task

- A safe area to keep a patient while undergoing decontamination
- A method for washing contaminants off a patient
- A means of containing the **rinsate**
- Adequate protection for personnel treating the patient
- Disposable or cleanable medical equipment to treat the patient

Primary assessment can be undertaken while simultaneously performing gross decontamination in the outer edge of the exclusion zone or in the contamination reduction zone. Treat any life-threatening emergencies that compromise the ABCs. Once life-threatening injuries or illness have been addressed, continue with a more thorough decontamination and secondary assessment. Appropriately trained personnel with the proper PPE should be the only individuals conducting the decontamination.

Decontamination consists of cutting away and removing all potentially contaminated clothing, including jewelry. All items must be double-bagged in plastic, sealed, and labeled. Any obvious chemicals should be brushed off the patient. In most cases, it is important to flush the patient with copious amounts of water for at least 15 minutes. You want to get the patient as clean as possible. This is accomplished by using soap and water in an organized and thorough manner. If the patient cannot be effectively decontaminated, then it is appropriate to wrap the patient loosely with a sheet in a cocoon-like fashion prior to transfer to the support zone.

Pediatric Decontamination Considerations

The PPE used by responders can be very intimidating and frightening to children. Whenever possible, children and parents or other people known to them should remain together during decontamination, treatment, and transport to the hospital.

Mass Population Decontamination

The reality of large numbers of patients following a hazmat incident, and resulting from potential exposure to a chemical agent, continues to be a threat. In this scenario, triage must be implemented to determine the entry into the decontamination process. In some cases, additional decontamination options will be needed to accommodate the number of patients.

Side Bar

Basic Decontamination Procedure

- Make sure all clothing is removed.
- Brush or vacuum particulate matter off skin.
- Decontaminate systematically from the head down with water:
    - Wash contaminated area gently under a stream of water and scrub with a soft brush or surgical sponge along with soap.
    - Limit mechanical or chemical irritation of the skin by overzealous scrubbing or forceful water flow.
    - Use warm, never hot, water.
    - Decontaminate exposed wounds and eyes before intact skin areas.
    - Cover wounds with waterproof dressings after decontamination.
    - Take care not to introduce contaminants into open wounds.
    - Remember the back, under skin folds, and genitalia.
    - Watch for any changes in the patient's condition.
- Remove contaminants to the point where they are no longer a threat to the patient or response personnel, or as far as the situation or the patient's clinical condition allow.
- Isolate the patient from the environment by wrapping him in a blanket or sheet to prevent the spread of any remaining contaminants.
- If possible, contain all runoff from decontamination procedures for proper disposal.
- Ensure that all potentially contaminated patient clothing and belongings have been bagged and tagged:
    - Properly label the bags that contain clothing or other potentially contaminated articles.
    - Consult with proper officials (e.g., safety officer, hazmat officer) regarding disposition of bags containing contaminated articles.

Establishing control of patients in these scenarios is critical to prevent contamination of other individuals and to prevent those who are contaminated from going to the hospital without proper decontamination. Large volumes of water can be used from fire equipment to quickly rinse a large number of individuals. Typically, fire departments will coordinate such an effort along with the hazmat team for your location.

Decontamination of EMS Personnel

EMS personnel and other responders will need to be decontaminated after they are finished in the exclusion zone. Personnel should remove protective clothing in the following sequence:

1. Remove tape securing gloves to suit.
2. Remove outer gloves, turning them inside out as they are removed.
3. Remove suit, turning it inside out and avoiding shaking.
4. Remove plastic shoe cover from one foot and step over the "clean line." Remove other shoe cover and put that foot over the line.
5. Remove mask. The last staff member removing his mask may want to wash all masks with soapy water before removing his suit and gloves. Place masks in a plastic bag and hand them over the clean line. Place the masks in a second bag held by another member of the staff. Send for decontamination.
6. Remove inner gloves and discard them in a drum inside the dirty area.
7. Close off the dirty area until the level of contamination is established and the area is properly cleaned.
8. Move to a shower area, remove scrub suit, and place it in a plastic bag.
9. Shower, then redress in normal working attire.

Note: Double-bag clothing and label appropriately.

CHAPTER REVIEW

Summary

Hazardous material incidents are not uncommon. An EMS manager is responsible to ensure that personnel in an agency have the proper level of training and that they understand how to function at a hazmat incident. It is essential to understand the components of the hazmat scene. The EMS manager must know the principles of identifying hazardous materials, managing a hazmat incident, and performing proper decontamination. It is essential that personnel have the proper training and equipment to function at a hazmat incident scene.

WHAT WOULD YOU DO? Reflection

As the EMS manager, it is your responsibility to ensure the proper training is in place. EMS crews must be trained on all abilities related to hazardous materials certification level and the equipment available. In this situation, the crew members did not utilize their training in scene safety. They also did not have the equipment necessary to enter the scene.

The dangerous situation could have been prevented if the crews had recognized the unsafe environment. Once they recognized that, they should have called for additional resources, more particularly hazardous material crews trained and equipped to handle such an incident. In addition, if proper decontamination of the patients had occurred, it would have reduced the risk to the providers of cross-contaminations.

After such an incident, the first priority should be to ensure that the crew is treated for exposure. Then at some point, the crew should be counseled on how to handle such incidents in the future. In addition, this is a good time to review the agency's operating guidelines and do an in-service training for all personnel as a refresher on scene safety and also hazmat incident scenes.

Review Questions

1. How do you determine whether or not a patient needs decontamination?
2. How do acute, subacute, and chronic effects of a hazardous materials exposure differ?
3. How do you integrate patient care with the need for safety and patient decontamination when responding to hazmat incidents?
4. What indicators would provide you with information that a hazmat event has occurred?
5. For what purposes would you use the shipping papers, material safety data sheets, and other sources of information in reference to a hazmat event? What are the limitations of each, and how would you overcome these limitations?
6. What are the different levels of hazmat training?
7. What role would you play as an EMS manager at the scene of a hazmat incident?

References

Agency for Toxic Substances and Disease Registry. (1992). "Medical Management Guidelines for Acute Chemical Exposures." See the CDC WONDER website.

Agency for Toxic Substances and Disease Registry. (2001). "Managing Hazardous Materials Incidents (MHMIs)." (Atlanta, GA: U.S. Department of Health and Human Services, Public Health Service)

Hildebrand, M., G. Noll, and J. Yvorra. (2012). *Hazardous Materials: Managing the Incident*, 4th ed. Burlington, MA: Jones & Bartlett.

National Fire Protection Association. (2002). "NFPA 471: Recommended Practice for Responding to Hazardous Materials Incidents." Quincy, MA: Author.

National Fire Protection Association. (2008a). "NFPA 472: Standard for Competence of Responders to Hazardous Materials/Weapons of Mass Destruction Incidents." Quincy, MA: Author.

National Fire Protection Association. (2008b). "NFPA 473: Standard for Competencies for EMS Personnel Responding to Hazardous Materials/Weapons of Mass Destruction Incidents". Quincy, MA: Author.

National Fire Protection Association. (2009). "NFPA 450: Guide for Emergency Medical Services and Systems." Quincy, MA: Author.

Occupational Safety & Health Administration. (2012). "OSHA 29 CFR 1910.1200." See the organization website.

Trebisacci, D. (2008). *Hazardous Materials/Weapons of Mass Destruction Response Handbook.* Quincy, MA: National Fire Protection Association.

University of Arizona. (2003). *Advanced Hazmat Life Support Provider Manual*, 3rd ed. Tucson: University of Arizona Emergency Medical Research Center, American Academy of Clinical Toxicology.

Key Terms

bulk A type of packaging that may hold a liquid capacity greater than 119 gallons (450 liters), a solid net mass greater than 882 pounds (400 kg), or a gas capacity greater than 1,001 pounds (454 kg).

decontamination The physical and/or chemical process of reducing and preventing the spread of contamination from people, animals, the environment, or equipment.

facility containment systems The packaging, containers, and containment systems that are part of a fixed facility's operation.

facility paperwork Plans that document facility layouts, emergency contact information, chemical data, and any planning necessary for handling facility emergencies.

Hazardous Materials Information System (HMIS) A methodology designed to place a simple label on individual containers.

material safety data sheets (MSDSs) The document that includes the name, address, and phone number of the manufacturer, the chemical name of the substance and any synonyms, the chemical and physical properties of the substance, personal protective equipment necessary for contact with the substance, any potential health effects if an exposure occurs, and any handling, disposal, and storing procedures.

nonbulk A type of packaging that may hold a liquid capacity of 119 gallons (450 liters) or less, a solid net mass of 882 pounds (400 kg) or less, or a gas capacity of 1,001 pounds (454 kg) or less.

rinsate A type of water, containing low concentrations of contaminants, that results from the cleaning of containers.

shipping papers The proper documentation that must accompany the shipment when chemicals are transported.

SLUDGEM A mnemonic for the signs of organophosphate poisoning: *s*alivation, *l*acrimation, *u*rination, *d*efecation, *g*astrointestinal problems, *e*mesis, and *m*iosis (contracted pupils).

Water Rescue and Dive Special Operations

12 CHAPTER

Sam Bradley

Objectives

After reading this chapter, the student should be able to:

12.1 Justify the need for a water rescue unit.
12.2 Explain the types of water rescue team configuration options.
12.3 Examine the risks and liabilities for divers and water rescuers.
12.4 Discuss the advantages of having a water rescue and dive team.
12.5 Explain the training requirements for divers and water rescuers.
12.6 Discuss funding considerations for creating a water rescue and dive team.

Key Terms

blackwater diving
Community Emergency Response Team (CERT)
ice rescue
Medical Reserve Corps (MRC)
swiftwater (or whitewater) rescue
water rescue

WHAT WOULD YOU DO?

A small island located just offshore in a large lake has its own fire department and EMS division, but it also relies on adjacent departments for help on larger incidents. On Memorial Day weekend, an incident occurred that would have long-term consequences for this department. A 50-year-old man, allegedly wishing to commit suicide, walked into the cold water of the lake. The fire department responded, but firefighters stood at the shore, apparently refusing to go into the water. Needless to say, this created a political and social nightmare when the victim succumbed to hypothermia an hour later. To make matters worse, police had also declined to attempt a rescue because they believed the man in the water could have been armed. The Coast Guard responded as well, but the boat used could not navigate the shallow water.

The fire department became the target for public criticism. To the public, there did not seem to be any justification for the firefighters not attempting a rescue. This was not the case. The department had previously hosted a comprehensive water rescue program that utilized shore-based and surface-based rescue techniques, but budget issues forced the program to be abandoned. Firefighters and paramedics on shore that day were following a department policy dated 3 years earlier that prohibited personnel from performing water rescues due to lack to training and certification. Not surprisingly, the family filed a civil claim against the city and county stating that first responders were negligent and breached their mandatory duty.

Drowning in negative publicity and facing political repercussions, the existing policy was changed to give incident commanders more discretion on utilizing personnel and equipment based on specific circumstances. Wisely, the department's training division reimplemented water rescue training, and shallow water rescue boats were put into service. But the damage to the department's reputation in the community will take a long time to repair. As well, department personnel who were not able to respond may suffer the effects of critical incident stress.

Questions

1. If you were the EMS chief on duty that day, how would you have managed this incident?
2. Are your policies set in concrete, or are there guidelines that could change based on the situation?
3. As an EMS manager, would you allow your incident commanders to make decisions that may go outside policy if someone's life depends on it?

INTRODUCTION

The decision to engage in a **water rescue** team as a special operations team is only relevant if a jurisdiction has water-related incidents. Incidents can be as simple an individual near-drowning, or as complex as diving accidents, swiftwater rescues, disaster responses secondary to a flood, or the need to assist law enforcement with a body recovery. This chapter will look at information an EMS manager must consider prior to engaging in a proprietary or collaborative water/dive rescue unit.

DETERMINE THE NEED FOR A WATER RESCUE UNIT

Before a water rescue unit is established there needs to be an identified need for such resources. Sometimes a tragedy is what makes a community aware of how important it is to have a water rescue unit available, and other times community members can realize that this unit should be developed, especially in flood prone areas. Due to the cost to create and maintain a water rescue unit, the EMS manager must spend time identifying necessary questions that need to be answered in advance and to think about the goals and objectives that the unit will try to address.

THE PITTSBURGH CHALLENGE

On August 19, 2011, a flash flood trapped a number of vehicles in up to 9 feet of water near the Allegheny River in Pittsburgh, Pennsylvania. Four people died in that incident, including two children. Communities in this area experience flooding every year, but the deaths heightened concerns. This incident also illuminated the risk to public safety personnel. Police, with no training or proper equipment, were faced with the decision to try and save a child's life. Only months later, life vests and rescue ropes were placed in every police cruiser. An inflatable boat was placed at one of the police stations, and forty paramedics had been trained for water rescues.

Allegheny County then went a step further and created a water response team. Members include volunteer firefighters and EMS personnel from a number of communities in the county. The justification was simple: The county has three rivers and a consistent history of heavy rain that causes flash flooding annually. There are further plans to offer 2,000 police officers, firefighters, and paramedics a basic 8-hour water survival course and to create swiftwater rescue specialty teams.

The ongoing plan is to equip all police and fire units with personal flotation devices and rescue throw bags. The city also plans to purchase eleven motorized swiftwater boats and store them on trailers at fire and EMS stations in flood-prone areas. Two hundred swiftwater team members will have an additional 48 hours of training. Those who excel will be assigned to one of two 28-member elite teams who will handle complex assignments and could also be available to other communities.

To manage this system, Allegheny County envisions a "tiered level of capability" that requires a cooperative effort for police, fire, and EMS. Unlike many systems, water rescues have traditionally been the responsibility of the EMS bureau. The hope is that this combined effort will foster a better relationship between firefighters and EMS personnel as firefighters are brought into the program. Both unions support the program that would provide enhanced safety to their members.

QUESTIONS TO ASK

Before creating or becoming part of a water rescue team, it is important to consider the need, the scope, and the type of team. The following questions will help to address this:

- What type of waterways are in place? Do the waterways host water recreation such as boating, use of personal watercraft, or sport diving?
- What are the statistics on injuries and deaths specific to water-related incidents?
- How effectively is the current system meeting the needs of mitigating water-related incidents?
- Is it possible to combine efforts with other agencies that may or may not have an established water rescue program?
- What are the current resources in terms of trained personnel, accessible marinas and bridges, or rescue equipment such as specialized watercraft?
- Is the EMS team volunteer, paid, or a combination?

- Are the personnel motivated to take on this new responsibility? Do the employee unions need to agree to this?
- Is funding coming from the public? If so, will you be able to sell the community on the benefits of the team during normal water recreation as well as in disaster situations and how the team provides service to the community?

GOALS AND OBJECTIVES

After making the decision, determining the goals and objectives for the team is the next step. As seen in the Pittsburgh example, the safety of responders as well as the public is an easily justifiable goal. A set of policies and procedures also will be needed in order to comply with occupational health and safety requirements (Bauder, 2011; Smido, 2011).

POOLS, LAKES, RIVERS, AND OCEANS

Pools, lakes, rivers, oceans, and even streams present unique challenges for a water rescue team. Swimming pool rescues can occur anywhere and require a rescuer who can swim and who knows how to safely approach a panicked victim and efficiently extricate him from the pool.

Lakes and oceans are similar as they are larger bodies of water that create dangers for people who cannot swim well, go out too far, and become too tired to return to shore on their own, or become victims of marine animal bites and stings. Large lakes and oceans have the added issues of dangerous shore breaks, strong currents and undertows, high surf, and other hazards. Lakes and oceans are attractive to sport divers who may or may not be certified, or do not practice safe diving techniques. Drivers who are impaired, unaware, or engage in risky behavior add to the hazards of boats and personal watercraft. A water rescue team must be trained and equipped to manage all types of incidents.

Rivers and large streams are also attractive to watercraft and recreational swimmers, which creates an environment for accidents and drownings. Rivers are especially dangerous because of strong currents that may push a swimmer past his capacity or force watercraft into rocks. Water rescue team members must have intense training in swiftwater rescue techniques and equipment. (See Figure 12.1.)

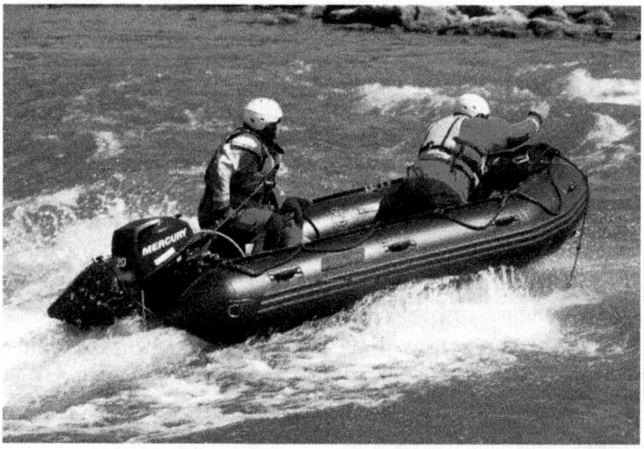

FIGURE 12.1 Rivers can be dangerous because of strong currents that may push a swimmer past his capacity or force him into rocks. *Source:* © *Specialized Fire and Rescue.*

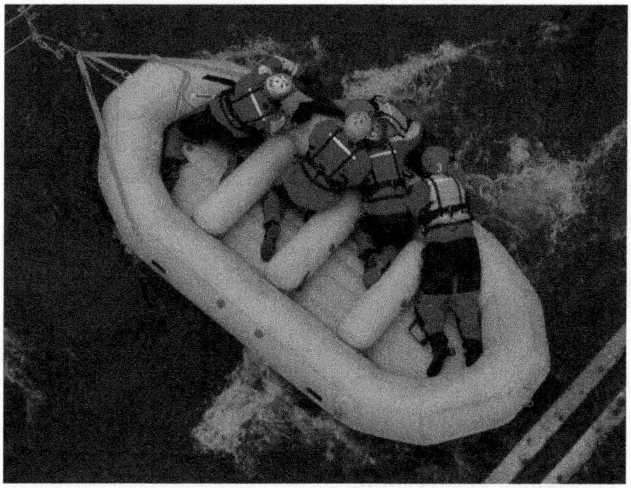

FIGURE 12.2 Flooding and swiftwater rescue requires specialized training in managing currents as well as the use of ropes and mechanical advantage systems to deflect the water's current. *Source: © Specialized Fire and Rescue.*

WEATHER-RELATED ISSUES

Flooding can create a swiftwater or whitewater rescue scenario and requires a high level of technical rescue training. Floods can develop quickly and catch people off guard, creating a number of complex and time-sensitive rescue situations. In some scenarios, first responders, untrained and unequipped for these conditions, will try to render aid and become victims themselves. People tend to underestimate the pressure and speed of moving water. They will try to drive through a flooded portion of road and will get stuck. There is also danger from floating debris. Flooding and swiftwater rescue requires specialized training in managing currents, and the use of ropes and mechanical advantage systems to deflect the water's current. (See Figure 12.2.)

Water that freezes in lakes and ponds in winter becomes an attractive playground. Especially in spring, people underestimate the strength of the ice and often fall through into frigid water. This is another situation where untrained bystanders will attempt to render assistance and often become secondary victims. These are time-sensitive emergencies as hypothermia can quickly overcome and kill a victim. Ice rescue requires specialized suits that protect the rescuer from immersion hypothermia. Rescuing a victim in these cases is not as technical as swiftwater rescue and may only require ropes, flotation devices, and perhaps a patient movement device to help bring a victim to shore. The most important skill is the ability to deploy rapidly as these are life-threatening situations.

WATER RESCUE TEAM CONFIGURATIONS

A water rescue team can be the primary responsibility of the fire, police, or EMS, depending on the needs of the area and the capabilities of each service. No matter which agency has the primary responsibility, there are requirements that each water rescue team must meet.

TYPICAL CONFIGURATIONS

Teams can be the primary responsibility of fire, police, and sometimes EMS. Many dive teams are hosted by sheriff or police agencies because of the sensitivity of recovering bodies or evidence. Law enforcement agencies may also be charged with homeland security mitigation when it involves the underwater portions of bridges or ships. Search and rescue missions typically fall to fire departments, although in some jurisdictions police may take the lead. Pittsburgh is an example of a system in which EMS is the lead agency. Some teams are joint configurations in which EMS may be included with fire. Joint teams are becoming more popular, and team members may be volunteer or career.

LEVELS OF TEAMS

Some teams collaborate with federally recognized Search and Rescue Teams. In 2005, the Federal Emergency Management Agency (FEMA) created the "Typed Resource Definitions—Search and Rescue Resources." The following is the breakdown of these requirements should a team want to qualify as a federal resource (Federal Emergency Management Agency, 2005). Regardless of which agency has primary responsibility, team configurations will have similar components. For example, a dive team is not just a cache of trained divers. Each operation requires a number of support personnel. In addition to the primary diver, necessary personnel include a primary tender, a fully deployable backup diver, a backup tender, and, potentially, a third backup diver. (See Figure 12.3.)

All teams must (minimum for Type IV):

1. Have a minimum three-member team including a squad leader.
2. Have a minimum of BLS–Advanced First Aid and CPR (probably Emergency Medical Technician) and at least one EMT-B.
3. Have Swiftwater Rescue Technician certification.
4. Have class 3 paddle skills, contact and self-rescue skills.
5. Be certified in HAZMAT and ICS.
6. Have the minimum safety equipment required for each rescuer and a BLS medical kit.
7. Be capable of supporting 18-hour operations.
8. Have portable radios and cell phones.
9. Capabilities would include low-risk land–based operations.

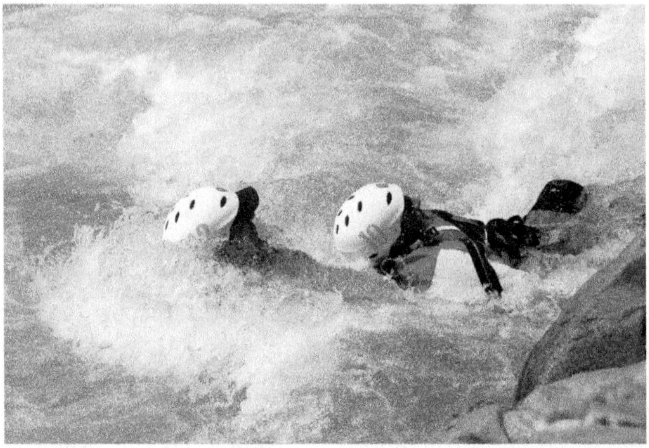

FIGURE 12.3 Water rescues are dangerous and should only be performed by trained personnel. *Source:* © *Specialized Fire and Rescue.*

To be considered Type III, a team must (in addition to Team IV requirements):

1. Have four members, including one squad leader. One member must be certified in technical animal rescue and two must be SCUBA trained and equipped. Divers must have 60 hours of formal public safety diver training.
2. Operations would add assisting in search operations with non-powered watercraft, animal rescue, in-water contact rescue and dive rescue.
3. Communication equipment must include headsets, and minimum SCUBA gear.
4. Medical equipment must include a litter.
5. Team must have one non-powered four-person vehicle.

To be considered Type II, a team must (in addition to Type III requirements):

1. Have six members, including one squad leader.
2. Two must be certified in helicopter/ aquatic rescue operations, two must be powered boat operators.
3. Be capable of supporting 24-hour operations.
4. Operations would add managing search operations, power vessel operations, and helicopter rescue.
5. Must be certified in technical rope systems and helicopter operations awareness.
6. Communications equipment must include aircraft radio.
7. Medical equipment must include a spineboard.
8. Rescue equipment must include life vests, HEED and PFD.
9. Vehicle must be one fuel-powered boat.

To be considered Type I, a team must (in addition to Type III requirements):

1. Have 14 members, including two EMT-Ps.
2. Add capabilities of ALS, communications, and logistics.
3. Divers must have 80 hours of formal public safety diver training.
4. Equipment must include an equipment trailer and personal support vehicle.
5. Must have two fuel-powered vehicles.
6. Medical equipment must include ALS and blankets. (Federal Emergency Management Agency, 2005, pp. 30–32)

SPECIAL WATER RESCUE OPERATIONS

A number of subspecialties in public safety diving require specific training and equipment that may or not be relevant to your area.

In **blackwater diving**, the diver is in conditions with little or no visibility, may be dealing with contaminated water, and must rely on senses other than sight for ensuring safety and meeting the goals of the mission. This kind of diving requires specialized equipment and training and a tender.

Swiftwater (or whitewater) rescue is necessary in areas that have rivers with swiftly moving water. This can also be needed during flood conditions. Swiftly moving water adds a layer of danger for the rescuer, the need for specialized watercraft, ropes and mechanical advantage systems, and, of course, advanced training.

Ice rescue is needed in colder climates where bodies of water ice over in winter. Victims may underestimate the thickness of the ice and fall into frigid water, predisposing them to hypothermia. Secondary victims who are untrained and trying to perform a rescue are common. This type of response requires quick action and specialized PPE, rescue equipment, and watercraft.

RISKS AND LIABILITIES

A community that has a water rescue team will see many benefits, but there are also complexities of a water rescue program that can create challenges. These include risks to team members and the need for liability protection, management of interagency issues, costs of training and equipment, and the potential effects on crews after an unsuccessful rescue.

RISKS TO DIVERS AND WATER RESCUERS

Clearly there are risks for EMS and public safety divers performing surface and subsurface operations as well as water rescue in general:

1. Not having guidelines, policies, and procedures in place to ensure safety

    If guidelines, policies, and procedures are not in writing and communicated clearly to the team, the potential for freelancing is higher. A team member may make choices that create safety issues for themselves, other team members, or victims they may be trying to save. This is inclusive of decisions to go into unsafe environments, like floodwaters, when undertrained or underequipped for the circumstances, and running the risk of becoming another victim. Guidelines, policies, and procedures go along with good training, which will reduce the likelihood of freelancing, especially early in an event before the appropriate team members and equipment are available to perform a safe rescue operation.

    Police, firefighters, and paramedics have a tendency to want to rush in to help someone in need, regardless of the hazards. Occasionally, the requirements to be successful in a rescue go outside their expertise. Even an established member of a water rescue team may not have specific expertise in blackwater diving or specific training for flood scenarios. Team training must be inclusive of all the types of situations that may occur in a given area, and should include at least awareness-level training of all public safety personnel.

2. Decisions made by company officers that do not have the expertise to make appropriate and safe decisions

    Occasionally, company officers may function as the incident commander on an event where they do not share the expertise of the team for which they are responsible. A fire officer may be great on a four-alarm fire or a hazardous material incident, but he may not be as familiar with the intricacies of a water rescue. This can be mitigated by ensuring that anyone running a water rescue has the same level of training as the team members as well as a clear operations guide to follow if unsure how to manage a specific situation. Incident commanders should also be able to rely on experienced team members to assist in decisions that may need to be made in unusual situations. The properly trained technical rescue teams must be in charge of the rescue. Personnel who do not have the expertise gained from training may cause injuries and deaths of victims and responders. More cooperation in services, sharing duties, and command are needed to effect appropriate and safe operations.

3. Not having the right team configuration to ensure team safety or not following safety standards

    Even though national safety standards are still being considered, each water rescue team needs to form and approve its own standards, put them into policy, communicate them, and train on them. Different types of rescues will require different types of expertise and different numbers of personnel. Contingencies are also needed for longer-term situations when personnel must be relieved frequently.

4. Not having appropriate, updated, and safe equipment

    Water rescue equipment, from personal safety and dive gear to boats and ropes, has limits on safety and effectiveness, especially equipment exposed to saltwater. A team must know the usable life of equipment, provide good maintenance, and replace equipment when necessary. Certain types of rescue scenarios call for specific types of equipment for a safe operation. The team should also look for updated items that may provide improved safety and effectiveness for the team. (See Figure 12.4.)

5. Not accommodating for extreme heat or cold

    People and equipment are affected by extremes of temperature, which also has a bearing on the types of incidents a team may face, such as flooding and ice rescue. More than just having appropriate safety equipment and mission-specific equipment, the effect of temperature on the team must be carefully monitored and mitigated.

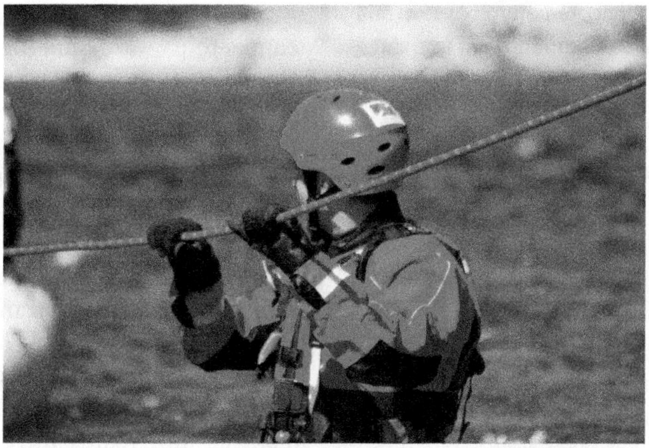

FIGURE 12.4 It is important to have the appropriate equipment when responding to a water rescue. Ropes are often used during water rescues and should be maintained properly and replaced when necessary. *Source: © Specialized Fire and Rescue.*

Hypothermia, for example, can be quickly life threatening in a water rescue situation.

6. Environmental issues such as marine animals and biohazards

   Divers and water rescuers are sometimes required to go into water contaminated by hazardous materials, including sewage. This is especially the case in a flood scenario. Floods also add the danger of quickly moving debris. Ocean situations come with the risk of bites and stings from jellyfish, rays, and even sharks. Some areas may harbor anemones, stinging coral, or poisonous starfish.

7. Risk of drowning and barotraumas

   Any time a swimmer or diver enters the water, drowning is a risk. Swimmers waiting to be rescued may panic and try to push down the rescuer. Seaweed and debris can create hazards where swimmers or divers may get caught and be unable to surface, so divers should always carry a dive knife.

   Barotraumas can occur especially with untrained or unprepared divers. The pathophysiology of this problem is the effect that pressure has on the various gases in the diver's body. The cause can be as relatively simple as unequal pressure in their ears, or it can be due to rapid ascent, which can lead to decompression sickness or the bends. Increased amounts of gases, such as nitrogen, may form bubbles in the tissues and block small blood vessels, shutting off circulation distally and resulting in hypoxia. Nitrogen may also cause nitrogen narcosis, which causes an alteration in consciousness similar to alcohol intoxication. Most well-trained divers do not suffer from these problems, but they are often called to rescue those who do.

8. Hazards specific to high-risk operations, such as blackwater rescue, swiftwater rescue, and ice rescue

   Team members involved with these specialty dive and rescue situations must have intense training and experience. Blackwater diving is done in zero or very low visibility, which eliminates the safety of relying on a dive buddy and also subjects the diver to unseen physical hazards and disorientation.

   Swiftwater rescue, whether in a river or flood, poses hazards from the swiftly moving current and the dangers of quickly moving debris and rocks. The biggest danger to the rescuer and the victim in an ice rescue situation is hypothermia. It also poses a dangerous situation when ice is unstable and people can fall in or be trapped underneath. It is not uncommon to have several victims in an ice rescue situation when untrained individuals have tried to assist and failed.

Side Bar

Risks to Water Rescue Team Members

1. Not having guidelines, policies, and procedures in place to ensure safety
2. Lack of expertise and proper training
3. Decisions made by company officers who do not have the expertise to make appropriate and safe decisions
4. Not having the right team configuration to ensure team safety or not following safety standards
5. Not having appropriate, updated, and safe equipment
6. Not accommodating for extreme heat or cold
7. Environmental issues such as hazardous materials, marine animals, and other biohazards
8. Risk of drowning and barotraumas
9. Hazards specific to high-risk operations such as blackwater rescue, swiftwater rescue, and ice diving

MITIGATION OF LIABILITIES

Most of the liability issues faced by water rescuers can be mitigated with proper planning, training, and common sense. Nonetheless, agencies hosting a dive or water rescue team must ensure that they have adequate liability and workers' compensation coverage for their personnel.

CREATION OF STANDARDS

Ensure that the team composition is adequate to meet safety standards and that team members mentor and advise more inexperienced team members. Confirm that those who make decisions and give orders in a rescue operation have the expertise to make safe decisions. Ensure that team equipment is appropriate, safe, and adequate for the working environment.

Another means of ensuring safety for the team is to provide time for members to update and maintain their skills. Technology, equipment, and techniques are consistently changing, and to stay cutting edge and safe the team must be provided with continuing education and training.

Ironically, in this ever-changing arena, nationally accepted standards for public safety divers have not been created. Public safety diving is partially exempt from requirements of the Occupational Safety and Health Administration (OSHA), and National Fire Protection Agency (NFPA) standards are not mandatory. Training agencies and teams have created their own standards with varying degrees of accountability. Without a set of clear operational standards, incident commanders who may not have complete clarity on procedures and safety issues may unintentionally make requests of their teams that are unsafe. Team members, with the goal of saving lives, may put themselves at risk. Especially in a multi-agency response, lack of clarity on fire, police, and EMS roles and responsibilities can also lead to poor accountability.

There is progress on the issue of standards. According to an article in *Fire Engineering* magazine, seven public safety diving training agencies have come together to form the Water Response Training Council (WRTC). Their goal is to develop minimum training standards to improve safety for public safety divers and mitigate the diversity in criteria for certifying instructors (Zaferes, 2012).

Although these standards are expected to be more global than specific, it is a move in the right direction. Until these standards are completed and accepted, each agency or team must have a solid and enforced set of local policies and procedures.

AGENCY INTERACTION ISSUES

When entering into a collaborative agreement with other agencies, disagreement is likely regarding who is in charge and which roles and responsibilities will be delegated to each agency. This is an especially sensitive issue if the relationship between the agencies was challenged prior to this collaboration. Some decisions will be driven by the type of team needed and the interaction required of each agency based on its expertise. Another factor may be which agency will be hosting the training and/or providing the bulk of the funding. A collaborative team has clear advantages in terms of having enhanced expertise on rescue, legal, and EMS issues; more available resources; and expanded options for equipment and funding; but the initial agreement may be a challenging task.

ADVANTAGES TO THE AGENCY AND THE COMMUNITY

In order for a team to be approved and funded, there must be solid evidence of how it benefits the agency, the community, and the stakeholders.

SAVING LIVES AND POSITIVE CHALLENGE

The main advantage of having a public safety-based or integrated water rescue/dive team is having the ability to mitigate or prevent disability or death from water-related incidents. The challenge of specialized roles and advanced training also provides motivation to employees and the potential satisfaction that comes with saving a life. Water rescue/dive team members will have a higher motivation to stay physically fit and psychologically sound. Raising the level of expertise for them also provides opportunity for advanced training for other agency employees.

Whether or not a collaborative team exists, water rescue incidents generally call for the expertise of fire and EMS, and often law enforcement. A cooperative effort with other EMS and public safety agencies lends itself to better communication and cooperation with those agencies on all levels.

COMMUNITY EXPECTATIONS AND SUPPORT

A program that is seen as beneficial to the community will foster opportunities for public monies and grant funding opportunities. However, when a community experiences disaster like floods, weather-related hazards like ice rescues, or incidents from swiftwater and aquatic recreational events, the expectation is that EMS and public safety will be trained and prepared to manage these incidents. A program that is inclusive of public education on drowning prevention would be better for everybody.

TRAINING AND EQUIPMENT REQUIREMENTS

The scope of a public-safety water rescue team is not just about water or dive rescue. The team is expected to have knowledge of evidence and body recovery methods and procedures and an understanding of the chain of custody. If a crime has taken place, law enforcement takes the lead. If officers are not part of the water rescue team, strict rules and extra training will be required of team members who are not part of law enforcement in order to ensure processes that can lead to conviction.

Personal skills include interpersonal communications. A task that typically falls to police but could include fire or EMS team members is death notification to families and mental health support for the family and the team, which both require specialized training.

Basic training should include self-contained underwater breathing apparatus (SCUBA), when appropriate; search and rescue techniques; hazardous materials recognition and management; surface-supplied air operations; and management of lift devices, cables, and ropes. Specialty training in blackwater, swiftwater, or ice rescue may also be relevant. Team members also must learn personal safety

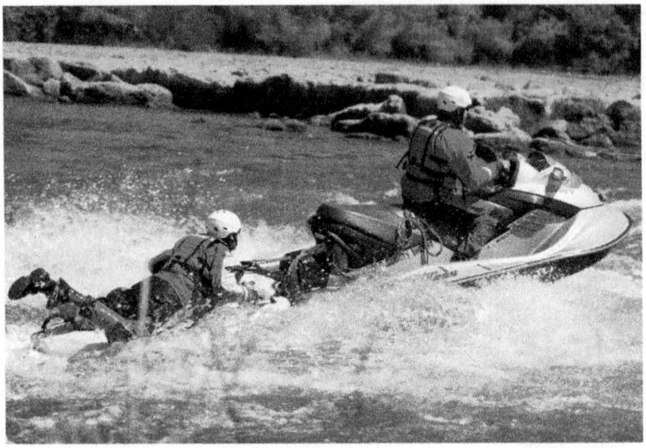

FIGURE 12.5 A watercraft is considered a type of basic equipment needed for water rescues. *Source: © Specialized Fire and Rescue.*

mitigation, including disentanglement methods and heat and cold management.

Agencies should work with disaster organizations such as the American Red Cross, **Community Emergency Response Teams (CERT)**, or **Medical Reserve Corps (MRC)** to enhance their understanding of drowning and water hazards. Discussions about how the water rescue team will fold into the local disaster management plan are important. Exercises done in conjunction with local disaster agencies will prove valuable during actual rescues.

Even basic equipment can be expensive, and it may need to be updated or replaced often. The type and amount of equipment are specific to the type of rescue work in which the team may engage. A basic list includes the following:

- Dry suits and peripherals
- Buoyancy compensators that meet specific specifications

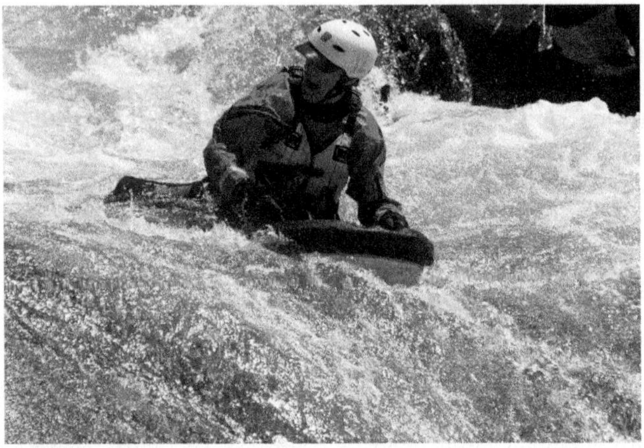

FIGURE 12.6 Rescue boards are used by water rescue teams to search for victims. *Source: © Specialized Fire and Rescue.*

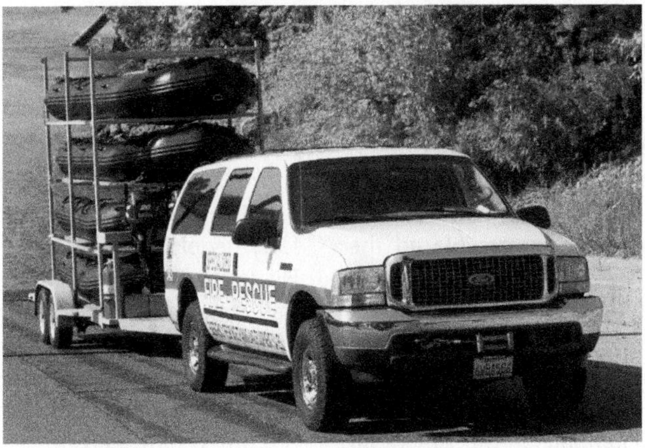

FIGURE 12.7 It is important to have the necessary equipment on scene at a water rescue to ensure that the rescuers can be safe when completing their tasks. *Source: © Specialized Fire and Rescue.*

- Cutting tools for personal safety
- Regulators
- Backup bottles (pony bottles)
- Fins, goggles, masks, gloves, carabiners, and weight belts
- Air tanks
- Chest harness for tethered diving
- Tender equipment
- Boats and other watercraft to transport team (See Figures 12.5, 12.6, and 12.7.)
- Diver's logbook

FUNDING

The advantage to a collaborative water rescue/dive team is the enhanced potential for grant funding through fire or law enforcement grants. Some grants may provide used equipment from the military or other federal agencies. The equipment may not be new, but it will be functional and enough to help get your team started. Other options are fundraisers and tapping into resources such as local dive shops that can benefit by the tax write-off and positive publicity.

If funding is coming from the community, it is important to sell the community on the benefits of the team and how the team provides service to the community. Provide training for the community and allow people to engage in the program. Interact with high schools to develop water rescue and drowning prevention programs.

Best Practice

The Advantages of Collaboration

The Willow Grove Volunteer Fire Company from Willow Grove, Pennsylvania, has served its community since 1907. Two stations are staffed by a total of seventy volunteers and career firefighters. Willow Grove engages with the "box system," which is a collaborative network of area fire companies who came together to form a task force. The incentive was the threat of Hurricane Irene in August 2011. Water rescues would be a given, and the task force arrangement allowed augmentation of resources, equipment, and personnel.

This group, which included the Hatboro Enterprise Fire Company, was called to assist an individual stuck in his vehicle in the floodwater. Speculation was that he ignored police barricades. It was clear to the firefighters that this would be a swiftwater rescue. Three firefighters placed the swift boat in service. Due to limited visibility, an underwater obstruction tipped the boat, flipping it up. The water rescue team reacted quickly and appropriately, but the firefighters on land perceived that the boat was going to capsize and triggered a mayday call. Firefighters from Abington, Roslyn, Warminster, and Fort Washington fire companies, as well as a water rescue crew from Allegheny County, responded. It turned out to be a good call.

The Hatboro water rescue team was able to locate the individual in trouble, but the strong current made a rescue effort dangerous and complex. Fort Washington's military surplus vehicle positioned itself to diminish the current and gave the crew the advantage needed to complete the rescue.

The man's bad decision required more than forty people to endanger themselves to save him. His rescue would not have happened if these small departments had not seen the wisdom of combining equipment and resources to create a united front against that which is bigger than all of them: inclement weather. The initial team of firefighters could also have perished if the boat had capsized and no other resources were available to assist them. There are advantages to collaboration, especially for smaller companies or agencies with limited personnel and resources.

CHAPTER REVIEW

Summary

Creation of, or collaboration with, other agencies on a water rescue team can have a number of benefits to an agency. A collaborative team provides opportunity for enhanced communication among agencies, offers increased expertise, and provides ancillary resources such as personnel and water rescue equipment. An EMS manager must ask a series of questions to justify the need for a water rescue team. Liability issues must be understood and addressed as water rescue, blackwater diving, swiftwater rescue, and ice rescue are not without risk to personnel.

Considerable cost is associated with a water rescue team in terms of equipment and training. Sharing of resources among multiple agencies, grant funding, and fund-raising are viable options in mitigating this cost. Adding a water rescue team as a special operation should not be done without studying all the facts, but it can help to save lives and provide an invaluable benefit to the community.

WHAT WOULD YOU DO? Reflection

There is no right answer to how you would address the situation. Nonetheless, going against the perceived "policy" would have produced risk for the incident commander and the crew members, but it may have resulted in the preservation of the victim's life and elimination of the negative consequences experienced by the fire department and its personnel.

Incident commanders responsible for the health and safety of their crews and the public must have the flexibility to look at a situation and make decisions relevant to that specific scenario. This is not to suggest that sending untrained individuals into the water would have been the appropriate decision, but boots-on-the-ground management should have the ability to measure and weigh all the facts in a given situation and the decision accordingly. As an EMS manager with overhead responsibility, you will have to decide if you can trust your incident commander to make the right decisions about whether sticking to established policy is relevant and appropriate to the incident.

Guidelines establish a set of logical or accepted processes and are not mandatory. Policies are compulsory and subject an employee to disciplinary action if not followed as written. Policies are most necessary when bad decisions could affect the safety of responders and/or patients. They also cover a company or department when failure to comply by an employee creates negative publicity or fosters a lawsuit. Often, situations found in the prehospital care arena are not always by the book. An EMS manager needs to think about the situation and determine what is the best approach to take based on the agency's policies and guidelines.

Review Questions

1. What are some important questions to ask when considering integration into, or creation of, a water rescue team?
2. What are some different types of water rescue specialties?
3. What types of issues are related to the risks and liabilities of water rescue teams?
4. What kinds of liabilities can occur without acceptable or enforced policies and procedures?
5. What are the advantages of an agency hosting or collaborating in a water rescue team?
6. What elements are required in the basic training of water rescue team members?
7. What resources are available for water rescue funding?
8. What types of support personnel are required for each water rescue dive operation?

References

Bauder, B. (2011, December 13). "Pittsburgh to Create Water Rescuers." See the Pittsburg Tribune-Review website.

Dungan, G. (2011, August 31). "Multiple Fire Departments Collaborate in Davisville Road Water Rescue." See the Upper Moreland-Wilow Grove Patch website.

Federal Emergency Management Agency (FEMA). (2005, November). "Typed Resource Definitions: Search and Rescue Resources." FEMA 508-8. Washington DC: Author.

Kariya, M. (2005, May 20). "How to Start a Dive Team." See the PoliceOne website.

Rothchild, F. (2008, January 27). "Starting a Dive Rescue/Recovery Team v.1." See the Team Lifeguard Systems, Inc. website.

Smydo, J. (2011, December 13). Water-Rescue Training Nears for City Crews." *Pittsburgh Post-Gazette.* See the organization website.

Zaferes, A. (2012, May 02). "Council's Goal Is to Safeguard Safety Standards for Divers." See the Fire Engineering website.

Key Terms

blackwater diving The act of diving in low visibility conditions.

Community Emergency Response Team (CERT) A community-level program administered by the Federal Emergency Management Agency that trains citizens to understand their responsibility in preparing for and responding to disaster.

ice rescue The rescue of victims having fallen through or stranded on ice.

Medical Reserve Corps (MRC) A federally established, community-based, organized group of volunteers (medical and non-medical) intended to supplement existing community medical and emergency response systems.

swiftwater rescue A type of rescue in environments with fast currents, such as rivers or floods.

water rescue A type of rescue of victims in a water-related situation.

Land-Based Search and Rescue

13 CHAPTER

David Harrington

Objectives

After reading this chapter, the student should be able to:

13.1 Identify the need for a land-based search and rescue (SAR) response.
13.2 Identify and describe the different environments where a land-based SAR emergency might occur.
13.3 Identify the hazards associated with a land-based SAR operation and what methods can be employed to reduce risk.
13.4 Identify what additional emergency response personnel may be required and their responsibilities in the overall SAR mission.
13.5 Describe the process for response planning and incident management and how it relates to a SAR operation.
13.6 Describe the initial actions that a rescue team should take to prepare for a SAR operation.
13.7 Identify and describe the different types of search methods and when they should be utilized.
13.8 Describe the various methods for transporting a subject from a wilderness environment.

Key Terms

accountability system
AMBER Alert Program
base of operation (BoO)
bastard search
choke point search
confinement area
containment area
despondent
emergency management agency (EMA)
grid search

hasty search
last known point (LKP)
National Search and Rescue Committee (NSARC)
National Search and Rescue Plan (NSP)
point last seen (PLS)
public information officer (PIO)
search area
search and rescue (SAR) incident
unified incident command

WHAT WOULD YOU DO?

You have been dispatched to the report of a missing elderly gentleman at a residence located in a rural mountainous area. You arrive on scene where you are met by the distressed family members who have been looking around the property, which adjoins a national park. The terrain is densely wooded with moderate to steep elevation changes that sit among occasional creeks and waterfalls. It is approaching late afternoon on what was a beautiful fall day, with a weather forecast of occasional rain showers throughout the night with temperatures in the lower 50s. The family tells you that the subject, their father, has lived in this house for more than 70 years and occasionally takes afternoon walks on trails that he had built when he was younger. This is the first time he has been gone this long.

Questions

1. What additional information would you want to know about the elderly gentleman?
2. What additional resources would you consider requesting?
3. What type of search would you initiate factoring in the current information?

INTRODUCTION

A **search and rescue (SAR) incident** is the process of locating a missing or lost person. If the person is in distress, the operation may also involve performing a rescue and providing medical aid. The discipline of SAR includes several different categories, based on the type of environment in which the incident occurs. This can include wilderness SAR, urban SAR, and air–sea SAR. For the purpose of this chapter, we will be covering the topic of wilderness SAR.

An EMS manager must possess a basic understanding of SAR theory as well as the steps involved in initiating and conducting SAR operations. These types of events, although not common in the routine day of an EMS provider, are certainly considered a true emergency and should be treated with a sense of urgency. Like all the different technical rescue disciplines, wilderness SAR possesses its own unique challenges based on human behavior patterns, environmental elements, associated hazards, and techniques gained from experience in the field.

SAR operations for lost or missing people occur in every location and in every environment. Urban environments include areas around population centers, such as downtown and commercial districts, residential neighborhoods, and other developed communities. Rural environments can be found bordering the urban regions, such as farming communities, rural residential communities, and other less populated areas. A wilderness region is defined as an area that is untouched or has not been developed by humans. This includes large wooded forests, mountainous areas, swamps and wetlands, and deserts. (See Figures 13.1 and 13.2.)

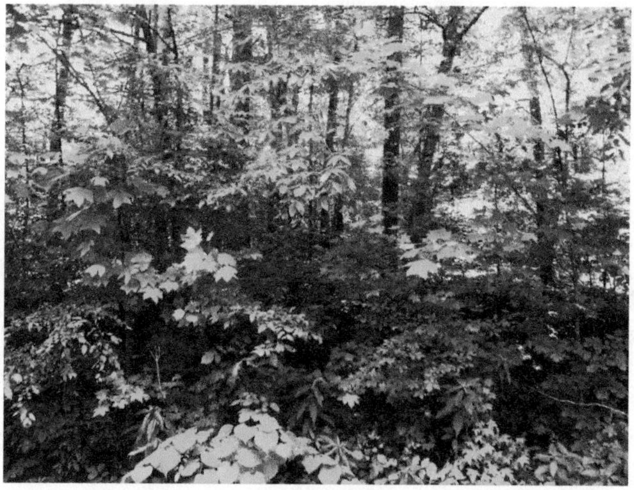

Figure 13.1 Heavily wooded areas can be dense, making them difficult to navigate as well as to visually locate a lost person. *Source: David C. Harrington.*

AGENCIES RESPONSIBLE FOR CONDUCTING SAR OPERATIONS—

The responsibility for conducting SAR operations is based upon the location of the event. In some cases, jurisdictions may overlap if it is suspected that the incident may cross specific geographic or governmental boundaries. For this reason, strong relationships between the different response organizations are a must and can make the difference between the success or failure of an operation.

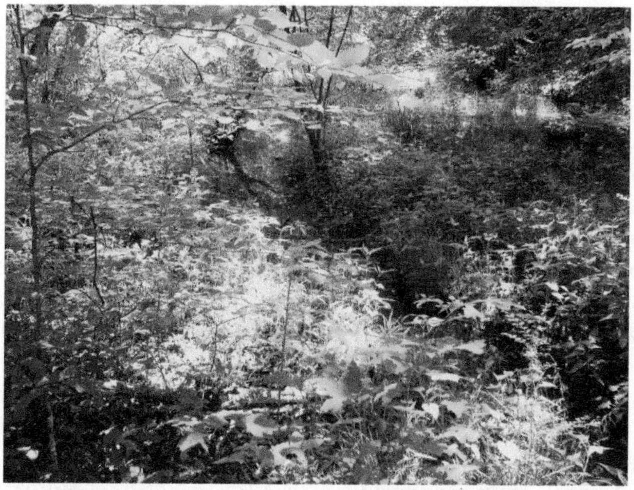

Figure 13.2 Swamp areas posses water hazards, slippery surfaces, and many hiding places for dangerous wildlife. *Source: David C. Harrington.*

Best Practice

SAR Operations in Pennsylvania

The town of White Oak, located in Allegheny County, Pennsylvania, is home to White Oak EMS. Recognized by the Pennsylvania Search and Rescue Council, White Oak EMS operates a Level 1 SAR Team. White Oak Search and Rescue (WOSAR) along with this wilderness SAR element offers a variety of SAR resources, including a dive team and an ATV/snowmobile team. The crew members of WOSAR are made up of both career and volunteer health care professionals who volunteer their efforts and talents to the nonprofit organization. Working alongside other response agencies such as the Pennsylvania State Police, law enforcement, Civil Air Patrol, and other SAR agencies, WOSAR responds to mutual aid requests anywhere within a 4-hour driving distance of Pittsburgh, Pennsylvania.

The **National Search and Rescue Plan (NSP)** was originally developed by the **National Search and Rescue Committee (NSARC)** more than 50 years ago. Today the NSARC is made up federal agencies including the Department of Homeland Security (DHS), Department of the Interior (DOI), Department of Commerce (DOC), Department of Defense (DOD), Department of Transportation (DOT), National Aeronautics and Space Administration (NASA), and Federal Communications Commission (FCC). The purpose of this plan is to achieve a commitment from the different agencies responsible for conducting SAR operations to continually improve interagency coordination when conducting a SAR operation regardless of where the incident occurs. The NSP is an excellent source of guidance to responders when conducting land-based SAR operations.

SAR operations involving maritime and waterways are typically the responsibility of the U.S. Coast Guard (USCG), whereas the national parks are the responsibility of the Department of the Interior. Likewise, the Department of Agriculture is responsible for U.S. forest land, and the Bureau of Land Management oversees all other U.S.-owned land. Events occurring within local boundaries are the responsibility of the local authorities, such as law enforcement, fire department, EMS, or other designated rescue agency. In cases where the event occurs in the wilderness area, however, mutual aid agreements with the governmental authority having jurisdiction (AHJ) use the local agencies to conduct these operations (National Search and Rescue Committee, 2013). It is in these situations that participating agencies rely on using a **unified incident command**.

DIFFERENT LEVELS OF TRAINING

Many standards define the limitations of response personnel. NFPA 1670 was prepared by the Technical Committee on Technical Rescue and is entitled "Standard on Operations and Training for Technical Search and Rescue Operations" (National Fire Protection Association, 2009). This standard identifies and establishes the different levels of functional capability for rescue personnel who conduct SAR operations. Emergency responders—regardless of whether they are representing law enforcement, EMS, fire, an **emergency**

management agency (EMA), or an independent response agency—should make every effort to meet the minimal requirements within this standard. The purpose of NFPA 1670 is to give guidance to the AHJ in the following areas:

1. Assessing a technical search and rescue hazard within the response area
2. Identifying the level of operational capability
3. Establishing operational criteria

Awareness level represents the minimum baseline of capabilities for an organization that provides response services to a technical SAR event. An operations capability allows for a response agency to properly identify associated hazards, utilize equipment, and implement specific techniques on a limited basis while conducting a technical SAR operation. Technician-level capabilities allow for the response organization to not only identify hazards and utilize equipment but also to use advanced techniques in order to coordinate, perform, and supervise the technical SAR incident. This chapter will primarily address the criteria for the awareness level provider (National Fire Protection Administration, 2009).

WILDERNESS SEARCH AND RESCUE HAZARDS

As with any technical rescue discipline, rescuers should be aware of multiple hazards and prepare for them prior to conducting an operation. Three general categories of hazards are associated with wilderness SAR (Pruitt, 2008).

ENVIRONMENTAL HAZARDS

Environmental hazards can include extreme heat or cold conditions. Rescuers should properly prepare their protective gear for not only the season but also sudden changes in temperature. Proper protective clothing that is insulated and waterproof will protect the rescuer from exposure during cold weather. Lighter-weight garments that are breathable will reduce the likelihood of heat-related injuries. Sunscreen should be worn to protect the responder from UV light from sun exposure.

Responders should be alert for extreme weather, such as thunderstorms since lightning strikes can occur as far as 30 miles from the source of the storm. (See Figure 13.3.) Responders should find low points in the terrain away from trees (which can attract

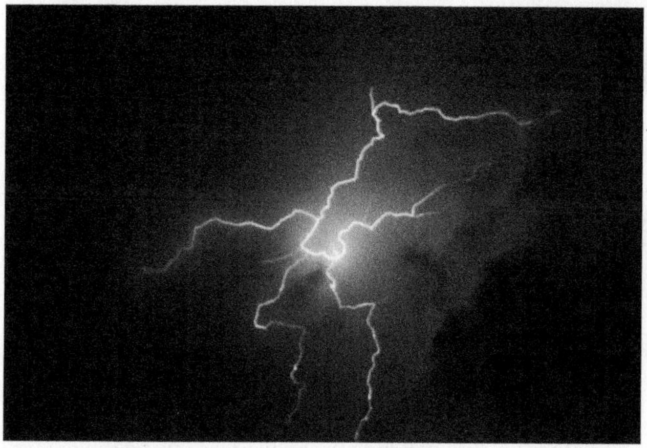

FIGURE 13.3 Lightning can strike a person up to 30 miles from the storm. *Source: Sean Waugh/FEMA.*

lightning). In addition, torrential rains from thunderstorms can result in flash flooding. During the winter, ice can become a major safety hazard. Heavy-duty nonslip ice treads or cleats can fit over a rescuer's hiking boots to reduce the risk of slips and falls.

In a wilderness environment, emergency responders are just as susceptible to the same injuries as the persons for whom they are searching. Rescuers participating in a wilderness SAR operation require a certain level of physical conditioning and stamina. In addition, they need to prepare for conditions that can potentially lead to injuries.

Despite the environment in which a wilderness SAR operation occurs, the physical activity required to conduct a search mandates that responders remain hydrated. Dehydration can occur through the loss of water due to heavy sweating. In arid climates, a rescuer may lose water even without sweating due to low humidity and dry winds evaporating the moisture in their skin. Rescuers should drink at least one liter of water per hour to combat dehydration. Other hazards associated with the environment are from stinging or biting insects, such as bees, hornets, wasps, ants, and other assorted insects. Mosquitoes can also be a hazard for their disease-carrying ability. Insect repellent should be used during the entire operation. Insect ointments to be used in the event of a sting or bite should be stocked in the responder's personal packs.

Animal and reptile bites can be even more dangerous. The wilderness is filled with many different species of creatures that can harm unsuspecting responders. To avoid snakes, try to avoid walking through high grass or around large rocks where snakes tend to hide. Walking with deliberate steps will decrease the chances of getting bitten. Snakes have the ability to feel vibrations that are transferred through the ground. This should allow time for them to detect an approaching rescuer and hide. (See Figure 13.4.)

To avoid predators, begin by avoiding surprising animals. Always make noise and remain aware of your surroundings. If confronted by a predator, remain calm, do not make any sudden movements, and do not run.

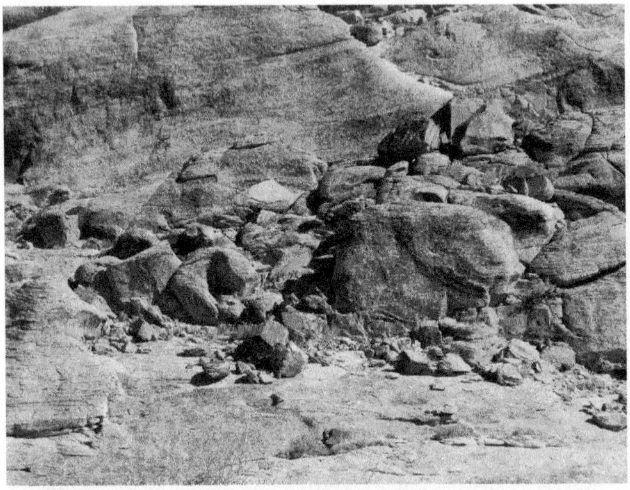

FIGURE 13.4 Snakes and other wildlife will hide in shady areas during the daytime. Rescuers should always looks carefully as they walk in those areas. *Source: David C. Harrington.*

Rapid movements may stimulate a predator's hunting instinct, causing it to chase and attack. Throwing something onto the ground may distract the predator, allowing for an escape.

TERRAIN HAZARDS

The wilderness possesses many of the world's most beautiful terrain features. However, like the wildlife that lives in the wilderness, the many features of the terrain must be respected. Mountainous areas exhibit steep cliffs, creating the potential for life-threatening falls. Overhangs may possess the risk of falling rocks and other objects. When working in these areas, it always makes good practice to wear protective helmets. Some terrain may have ponds, lakes, and creeks that can create slippery surfaces. If the environment is extremely cold, ice may have formed on the water. Responders should never attempt to walk across an ice-covered pond unless it has been confirmed that the ice is thick enough to support the weight of the responders and equipment. In mountainous areas with heavy snowfall, consideration should be given to deep snow and the potential for avalanches. (See Figure 13.5.)

Rescuers should also be prepared for a great amount of hiking, especially over uneven and rough terrain. Properly fitted boots that possess good ankle support will assist in reducing the chances of a twisted ankle. If the boots are too large or the rescuer's socks have become wet from either sweating or walking in water, blisters can easily form. This can later lead to open sores and infection. Changing socks when they become wet as well as using foot powder to reduce sweat buildup can assist with blister prevention. As a rescuer is navigating over rough terrain, caution should be taken with every move not to step on loose rocks or uneven surfaces that may cause a slip or fall and result in cuts, scrapes, and possibly musculoskeletal injuries.

Other terrain features that can be found in nearly every environment or rural community are wells, caves, and old abandoned mines. These present numerous hazards, including the potential of a responder falling into one.

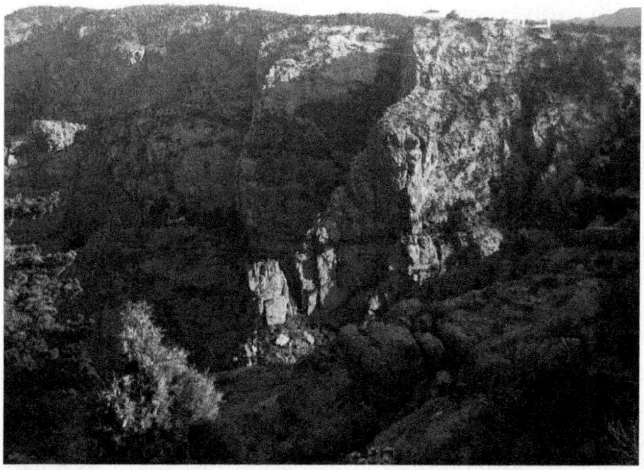

FIGURE 13.5 ■ Mountainous terrain can have many hazards including steep bluffs, loose rocks, and a variety of wildlife. *Source: David C. Harrington.*

MANMADE HAZARDS

Manmade disasters can consist of hazardous material dump sites, clandestine drug labs, illegal stills, booby traps, attack dogs, and suspects with weapons. Care should be taken to avoid trespassing upon private property. Responders should always be on the alert for illegal still or drug labs that may be booby-trapped or guarded by attack dogs or armed individuals. If a search is to be conducted in an area of question, law enforcement elements should be attached to the search team for protection.

LAND-BASED SEARCH AND RESCUE EMERGENCY

A land-based SAR incident that occurs in a wilderness area may include a hunter who got lost and overwhelmed by an unexpected change in the weather conditions. In an urban setting this type of search may involve a friend or family member who does not arrive at home or show up to work at the expected time, or an automobile accident that occurred on a stretch of roadway where the vehicle drove off into a heavily wooded area and is unseen by passersby. These are just a few of the many examples that would warrant declaring an emergency requiring a SAR response. Additional factors must also be considered when assessing a potential SAR response.

DELAY IN ALERTING RESPONSE PERSONNEL

Delays in notification can occur for a variety of reasons. A person who does not have local or close family members could easily go missing, with no one realizing it until several days later when co-workers wonder why the person has failed to show up for work on Monday. Family members may also assume that a loved one is delayed or off doing other activities before becoming concerned when he does not come home by a certain hour. If a child is missing, especially in the outdoors, family members will tend to conduct their own search for several hours before calling for help. For whatever reason the delay occurs, it leads to further delays in SAR operations commencing.

SUBJECT'S SURVIVAL PROFILE

Statistics indicate that 50 percent of survivors are located within the first 24 hours and more than 75 percent are located within the first 2 days (United States Homeland Emergency Response Organization, 2006). The potential for a subject to suffer an injury or a medical condition while lost in the wilderness is extremely high. Another factor that drives the urgency of the event is the subject's survival awareness and knowledge of the outdoors. All too often, ill-prepared hikers travel into the backcountry without the proper equipment or knowledge for dealing with sudden changes in the environment.

When evaluating the urgency of a SAR response, answers to critical questions should be quickly gathered by response. Despite when a SAR callout is conducted, it is important to ascertain how much daylight is left, the forecasted weather conditions, and how long the subject has been missing. Although subjects may stay put and not travel at night, trying to organize a SAR operation in the dark can become quite complex. The total number of subjects missing is also important. This can lead to confusion, especially when the missing group separates into smaller groups. The age of the subject will allow for the rescue team to predict human behavior patterns and potential medical issues that may affect the person's ability to adapt to harsh environments. Subjects with known medical conditions or who take any prescribed medications are increasingly vulnerable to extreme weather elements. Both the very young and very old may also lack the knowledge and resources to deal with surviving the elements. If a subject is missing in a wilderness area, important information to gather should include whether or not the subject possesses the adequate knowledge, skills, and experience to recognize the inherent dangers associated with a wilderness environment. Just as important, knowing what, if any, survival equipment the subject is carrying is another factor to consider when determining the urgency of the search. Interviewing individuals who are familiar with the search area may provide some information (United States Homeland Emergency Response Organization, 2006).

These important facts should be obtained as early as possible using a systematic approach. Ideally, the 9-1-1 dispatch center would follow a standardized procedure that assists in gathering much of this information. If this is not possible, the caller's name and a callback phone number should be obtained, allowing for the SAR team leader or representative to call the family member, friend, or witness back to begin the interview process. As this information is assessed, the SAR team leaders will begin to conduct the risk/benefit analysis. The priority of the response is then decided, which in turn dictates the level of response.

POTENTIAL SUBJECTS

Potential subjects can be missing children, individuals with mental retardation, the elderly, despondent individuals, subjects suffering from Alzheimer's or other mental disorders, subjects affected by drugs, hikers, climbers, subjects of disasters, victims of criminal abduction, and fugitives from law enforcement. Each of these subjects possesses specific behavioral patterns that dictate the urgency of the response as well as the search tactics (Pruitt, 2008).

CHILDREN AGES 1 TO 12 YEARS

A missing child strikes a chord with anyone who has or cares about children and immediately increases the stress of any operation. Children between ages 1 and 3 years, for obvious reasons, lack the natural sense of direction allowing for navigational skills. These children will not be aware of being lost and tend to wander aimlessly without any specific direction. As they begin to tire, they will attempt to find a convenient location, such as under a park bench or table, under a large bush, under an overhanging rock, or inside of a hollowed-out log.

As children reach age 3 to 6 years, they will tend to travel farther than younger children. Because of their age, they will exhibit more independence, allowing themselves to be drawn away by their natural tendency to explore. Children of this age can also be easily drawn toward animals and other children. As a child gets older, he possesses more awareness of being lost and may attempt to return to a familiar area. Like younger children, when they begin to tire, these children will attempt to find a spot to sleep. Often children are taught to stay away from strangers; however, this can work against rescuers as they may not answer or talk to rescuers even when called by name.

Children ages 6 to 12 years are even more independent and have a lot of the same fears and issues that adults have; however, they lack the knowledge and maturity to make sound decisions. Children of this age group possess a more developed sense of direction and navigational skills, allowing them to be more oriented to their surroundings. These older children may intentionally run away to escape punishment. The need to gain attention or to sulk may also drive them to run away. A tendency toward immaturity may result in the child not answering when called. As darkness falls and a sense of hopelessness sets in, this unique group will tend to accept help and be found.

THE ELDERLY

The elderly age group begins at age 65. Although most of the population that makes up this age group is fully functional, a certain portion, especially those who have extensive declining health issues, requires different levels of supervision. Medical conditions, such as dementia or Alzheimer's, often can result in these subjects walking away from their homes or health care facilities. Subjects suffering from these conditions often live in the past as opposed to the present and will attempt to relive a past routine, such as waiting at the bus stop to go to a job they may have retired from many years before. These individuals may require the same supervision as would a child.

The vast majority of the elderly population is very active and still retains full mental faculties. However, the elderly can easily overextend themselves, which can potentially lead to exhaustion resulting in sudden high-acuity events. Because of declining health, many people of this age group will have different health conditions and may be taking many different medications that can make them susceptible to, and not able to compensate for, extreme environmental conditions.

INDIVIDUALS WITH INTELLECTUAL DISABILITIES

Persons with intellectual disabilities will often have the same behavior and habits as children who are age 6 to 12 years. They may not necessarily have any physical impairment; however, they may not recognize the need to do what may help them survive. In some cases, these individuals may be shy or scared and reluctant to respond to rescuers. They may instead remain hidden from view while they try to protect themselves from the environment.

DESPONDENT INDIVIDUALS

The term **despondent** is used to describe someone who seeks solitude, usually due to a stressful event or severe depression. Subjects suffering from this condition may seek an area that is away from people but still within sight and sound of population. Despondent individuals will tend to go to prominent locations, such as scenic lakes or overlooks. Most often, they will find a secluded location there that provides an elevated position from which to see. Generally despondents do not want to be found and will not respond to rescuers as they are regarded as intrusions to their desired solitude.

HIKERS

Areas both within and around national and state parks possess recreational areas that attract hikers. Unfortunately, many of these individuals are amateur hikers and are not experienced with harsh environmental extremes. However, even experienced hikers can fall into trouble when unexpected events occur. Typically, the vast majority of hikers will stay on the trails, with a destination in mind when they begin. It is when hikers stray off the trail, or are forced to navigate a trail that has not been properly maintained or has been covered with moderate to deep snow, that they begin to get into trouble. It is always recommended that people hike in groups. Even then, if the hiking party is made up of different levels of experience and conditioning, it is not uncommon for the group to be divided, with one or two of the less experienced hikers falling behind, becoming disoriented, and becoming lost. As the seasons change, hikers of all levels can become subject to sudden unexpected weather changes, such as early- or late-season snowstorms, torrential rain, and thunderstorms. If hikers expected mild weather, they may have only packed minimal, if any, survival equipment.

HUNTERS AND FISHERS

Hunters often fall into the same category as hikers. There are many different levels of ability. Some hunt in groups, whereas many choose to hunt in solitude. Like hikers, many will underestimate the weather changes, not dressing or packing properly for extreme weather changes or for having to stay outdoors overnight. Most often, hunters tend to get in trouble by failing to maintain situational awareness. This occurs when hunters totally concentrate on their prey and not on navigation.

Fishers fall into the same classification as hunters. Even though fishers may be more aware of their location, they tend to fall victim to environmental conditions from either slipping or falling into the water or experiencing a boating accident. If fishers fall into swiftwater, they can easily be swept downstream or downriver some distance from where the fall occurred. If they happen to survive and are able to self-rescue from the water, they then become susceptible to hypothermia.

GROUND SEARCH AND RESCUE MISSION ACTIVATION

A notification for a wilderness SAR operation may result from any number of events, including transportation accidents. Downed aircraft, train derailments, and maritime accidents all occur in wilderness regions. Once the initial call is placed, there may be only a small window of opportunity to obtain critical information and build up the proper resources for initiating a successful mission. Whether the mission results in finding the lost individual alive or recovering the body of a loved one for the family so they may have closure, every step of the process is important.

THE INITIAL CALL

The rescue team will most likely receive the initial call from a local 9-1-1 center, the local law enforcement agency, or some other emergency response agency. In some cases, the rescue team responsible for conducting the land-based SAR operations may receive the initial call from the actual victim.

When a call is received, it is important to always treat the situation with the utmost urgency by obtaining reliable information. This starts with the caller's name, callback phone number, and call location. Reliable information is extremely important so that the appropriate resources are utilized and not misdirected to wrong locations. Every piece of information should be written down and the answers repeated to the caller to confirm accuracy. This portion of the process should not be rushed. It is important that the caller be given a contact number to use in order to provide any additional information. As an awareness-level provider, it is important to recognize the need for a land-based SAR operation in a wilderness environment. The acquisition of vital information is just as important as everything else and should be forwarded as soon as possible to a more highly trained rescue team.

ADDITIONAL NOTIFICATIONS

Early within the operation, quick notification of SAR response teams should be the priority. Information gained during the initial call should be directly relayed to resources responsible for conducting the SAR operation. Vital information should include details about the potential subject, location of the caller, and reliable contact information. It pays for rescuers to be knowledgeable of the primary SAR organizations within their own jurisdiction and how to make contact with them. This information should be part of an agency's standard operation procedure for land-based wilderness SAR responses.

SITE/SCENE ORGANIZATION AND CONTROL

Whether the rescue team is the first agency to arrive on scene or is called in as a resource, every effort should be made by the first-arriving unit to gain control of the scene and prevent any potential evidence from being damaged and witnesses from leaving. Incident command should be established with a command post announced to all incoming units and visibly marked for easy recognition. A flag or a green flashing beacon should be used to mark the command post. Once command has been established, the incident commander (IC) will assign a scribe who will generate a logbook to document every event and decision that is made throughout the operation.

It is very important as a rescue team arrives on the scene to create an atmosphere of cooperation as members integrate into an operation that has already started. Every conversation should begin by the leader of the rescue team introducing himself and asking "What can we do to help you?" Experience has shown that initiating a conversation with the lead agency and its IC early can go far toward building mutual trust and respect that will assist the operation tremendously. Any negative or aggressive attitude on the part of the rescue team can easily result in the team being asked to leave. Despite the emergent nature of the situation, etiquette plays a big role in the success of any mission.

Some communities will have SAR teams through their local law enforcement, rescue squad, fire department, or EMS agency that has already taken the initial steps, committed resources, and begun carrying out the search. These teams may only be in need of additional trained personnel to assist with the search. Other communities may not have any organized rescue infrastructure and are relying on an outside rescue team to tell them what needs to be done. If the arriving rescue team is being integrated into the existing command structure or is being given command, it may help with the future logistics of the operation to request that the lead agency's IC remain in the command post and convert the incident command into more of a shared unified incident command. As the face-to-face briefing is conducted, it is important to find out from the first-arriving agencies what has already been done, and if personnel already conducted a search of the immediate area. It is also important to know if witnesses have been interviewed.

As in any other technical rescue operation, the safety of responders should be the biggest priority of any SAR operation. This process should begin with the accountability of all rescuers on scene. An **accountability system** should be initiated early to keep track of all resources in real time. An accountability officer should be assigned to this task for the entire duration of the operation. His job will be to ensure that response personnel, as they arrive on scene, are signed in and directed to the appropriate staging area. As individuals are assigned to a search team or other position, the accountability officer will make appropriate adjustments to the accountability board that is used to track the location of all personnel. Once the team or responder has completed his assignment and has returned to the **base of operation (BoO)**, this will be reflected on the accountability board. Periodically, personnel accountability reports may be requested by the IC to ensure that all personnel in the field are accounted for. If at any time during an operation a responder is not accounted for, the operation will be temporarily halted until the responder is located. All responders should remain in the accountability system until they are demobilized and released from the scene.

Another immediate consideration is the plan for staging all arriving apparatus and equipment. Without this important detail addressed, mass chaos will ensue as dozens of vehicles and personnel flood the scene, blocking all access and egress. This will also lead to bombarding the operation with unneeded resources, thus setting the stage for freelancing. To reduce this, a staging area should be established in a location where resources can arrive and be kept until they are needed. In addition, keeping a clear path for arriving and departing vehicles is important so that the most critical resources can be utilized exactly when they are needed and not held up by a gridlock of vehicles that prevents anything from moving. Many organizations have adopted a system that issues a well-guarded password to only the agencies that are requested by the IC. When agencies or responders arrive on scene and attempt to gain access without the proper password, they are turned away or directed to an off-site staging area until proper identification or arrangements are made. This system has been proven to reduce the incidence of freelancing and self-dispatching.

If the operation is determined to span several work cycles, arrangements must be made to accommodate the rescuers who will be occupying the BoO. These accommodations include food, latrines, shelter, fuel, electrical power, lighting, heat or cold, clean water, specialized equipment, and anything else that is determined to be a necessity for the operation. In most cases, larger teams are self-sufficient and bring their own equipment, supplies, and facilities with them. In other cases, the logistics specialist will obtain whatever equipment and supplies are needed from local vendors.

Nearly every SAR operation will catch the attention of the local media and, in some cases, national media outlets. For this reason, a **public information officer (PIO)** should be assigned to deal directly with the media. In many areas, the PIO may be associated with the local government. If the rescue team has its own PIO, he should work closely with the host agency's PIO to carefully release information pertaining to the operation. The privacy of the individual and his family should always be respected. It also should be understood that if there is any speculation that the operation may be related to a criminal investigation, information should only be released after consent of the lead investigative law enforcement agency. The media will want information to release in order to meet their own deadlines. If this is neglected, the media will seek it wherever they can, regardless of accuracy. By working with the media, the agency can prevent a future public relations disaster.

In certain situations, however, the news media can be utilized to get vital information distributed to the public to assist in locating the subject. Similar to the nationwide **AMBER Alert program**, information such as releasing a physical and clothing description, age, name, last known location, other pertinent information, and a phone number that people may call to report any sightings can create leads for locating the subject.

When a member of the community, especially a child, goes missing, emotions of family members, as well as the community, will be running high. In many cases, family and community members have begun their own search for the subject. These unorganized searches can lead to the destruction of evidence that could lead to a delay in finding the subject. For this reason, it is imperative that a liaison be placed with the family to answer any questions and continually brief the family on progress in the operation. Department chaplains serve this purpose very well and can offer support as needed.

INTERVIEWING WITNESSES

Witnesses can be the most important element in locating a missing person. It is key to gather every piece of information possible before witnesses leave the scene. Witnesses include neighbors, bystanders, service station attendants, park service workers, other hikers, campers, or climbers, and any other person who may have seen or come in contact with the subject. As individual interviews are conducted, contact information should be obtained that will allow the individual to be contacted later if required. Information collection is one of the most important steps in the SAR process and should be done thoroughly and completely the first time since there may only be one chance. It is important to look and act professional and treat witnesses with respect while conducting interviews. If possible, interviews should be conducted in locations that offer a quiet, comfortable, and private setting that reduces distractions.

The person conducting the interview should begin by introducing himself, the agency he is affiliated with, and the purpose of the interview. Questions should be carefully asked in a manner that does not talk down to or above the individual. It is important to ask open-ended questions. While being careful not to disclose any related details of the operation, the interviewee should be allowed to answer all questions with his own words and without interruption. If the interviewee has issues remembering specific points in time or certain details, a minimum of details about the situation should be offered, just those that will assist the person in remembering. Providing too much information can only serve to allow the witness to exaggerate the facts.

As an interview is conducted, remember to remain patient and not rush the interview process; otherwise, important information may be left out. Projection of a calm attitude can create an environment of trust, allowing for the person to feel free to be open with information. It is important for the interviewer to listen carefully to every word that the interviewee has to say. Having a scribe present to write down answers supports this intention.

Other than where and when the subject was last seen, typical questions should address the following information: the subject's physical description, any medical conditions including medications, personality habits, and clothing last seen wearing. If the subject is on a camping or hiking trip, what is his experience level, trip plans and schedule, and camping or survival equipment? If the subject is a child, it is important to establish what training the child has had on what to do if he gets lost. Does the child talk to strangers? Is the child afraid of the dark or of certain animals?

Once the interview has concluded, the person conducting the interview should offer the interviewee his contact information and ask for a callback if additional information comes to mind. All information should be compiled and evaluated for accuracy based upon other information that has been gathered.

INITIATING THE SEARCH

The most pressing question is where to start looking. Obviously, this question may be answered based upon the information that has already been gathered through interviews, assessment of the clues from the scene, and the vital information gathered from the subject and scene profile. Once the search begins, it must have a logical approach. The **last known point (LKP)** is the location where evidence indicates that the subject was last known to be. This can be ascertained by key indicators, such as the subject's parked car, an article of clothing or some belonging found along the trail or at a makeshift campsite, footprints, and disturbed vegetation. Additional indicators might be phone records or receipts for fuel or other items providing a specific location where the subject might have been.

If the subject was identified by a witness as having been at a specific location, this would be considered a **point last seen (PLS)**. The LKP and the PLS may be the same; however, it is important to continue to update this information with any additional information that may come in throughout the search. As these clues are found, it remains important to protect their locations until all the potential clues are identified and gathered. If items of interest are found, they should be left where they are found until they are photographed and documented. Resist the urge to touch or handle any clues that are found. Items such as articles of clothing could later be used by canines for scent. The areas around the LKP and PLS should also be secured to prevent freelancing searchers from going into the terrain around the sites. Doing so could create confusing signs and scents for search teams and canines.

Once the subject and other pertinent information have been established, the rescue team will make a decision on a specific area to begin the search. This decision is based on the probabilities of where a subject may be found. Rescue teams will look at the subject profile, terrain features, LKP, and PLS to formulate these probabilities. If the information is credible and the probabilities are high, this will allow for the rescue team to confine the **search area** to a much smaller, more manageable area. This will later assist in what type of search to conduct (United States Homeland Emergency Response Organization, 2006).

TYPES OF SEARCHES

The unique conditions of the incident, including the environment, terrain features, subject profile, and available resources, will dictate the type of search that will be conducted. There are several different search tactics employed. They include land field searches, canine searches, and vehicle searches.

Land Field Searches

When a person goes missing, whether it is in the wilderness or confined areas of the suburbs, rescue teams may choose to employ a search that focuses on the use of trained rescuers who utilize organized search tactics. The different types of searches include bastard search, containment and confinement search, hasty search, grid search, and choke point search. The choice of search tactics depends upon the urgency of the search, the size of the search area, and terrain. The search area will be predetermined by the probabilities and defined on the map using grids or lines. These lines form grids that divide the map into search areas typically labeled with an A, B, C, D, and such, or with 1, 2, 3, 4, and so on. Search teams will be assigned a specific grid in which to search. Once the search area is cleared, the team will be assigned another search area to clear. (See Figure 13.6.)

Bastard Search

For a **bastard search**, rescuers look in obvious places while assuming that the person was not really lost. In many cases, the person being searched for either has found his own way out or has gone home without telling anyone. This type of search is conducted by first gathering reliable information about a subject's habits, plans prior to going missing, names and locations of friends, and hangouts. A quick search of probable locations where the individual normally goes can eliminate the implementation of a larger, more complex, and unnecessary search. It should never be assumed that this is always the case. A thorough and complete investigation should be conducted before jumping to any conclusions. If the subject is not found after conducting this type of search, the operation can be upgraded.

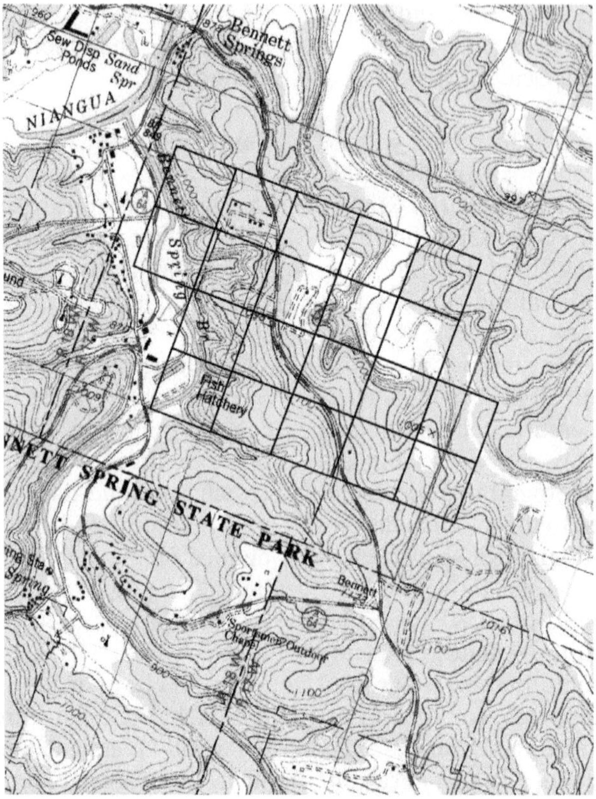

FIGURE 13.6 Topographical maps are used by rescuers to prepare search areas. *Source: Reproduced with permission from David C. Harrington, City of Oak Ridge, Tennessee, Fire Department.*

Containment and Confinement Search

After a rescue team has conducted its initial interviews and established a PLS, it can make a determination of a probable area that the subject could have traveled. This **containment area** is based upon when and where the individual was last seen or known to be, age, and the theory that a person can reasonably walk a determined distance per hour. Once the approximate distance has been determined, field teams are sent to the outer boundaries of the **confinement area** and positioned to wait for the subject at roadways, bridges, creeks, open fields, and other potential pathways that the individual may cross. The confinement tactic can employ search team members who are not necessarily trained in SAR operations. While the confinement area is monitored, trained search teams continue to search other locations within the containment area. The most important element to keep in mind is not to let the subject leave the containment area.

Hasty Search

For purposes of bringing an end to a search, many well-trained teams will conduct a **hasty search**. This tactic employs a ten- to twelve-

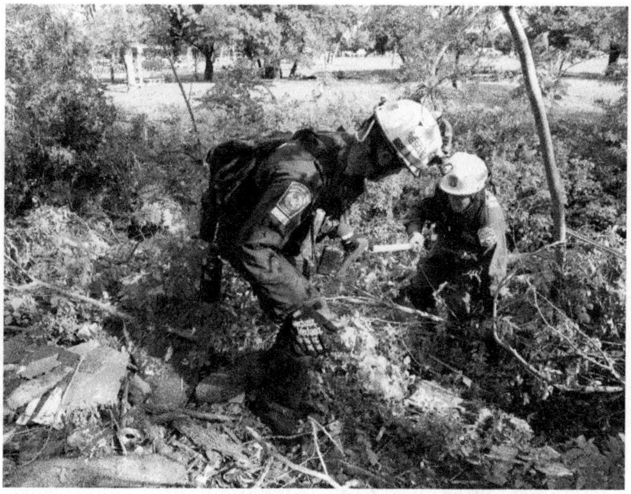

FIGURE 13.7 During hasty searches, rescuers will search in structures, caves, ditches, drains, wells, cliffs, and other locations that might have created an entanglement in which a lost person may be trapped. *Source: Jocelyn Augustino/FEMA.*

person team of highly trained searchers. They are inserted into an area of high probability and allowed to quickly search through the most obvious places that a subject is likely to be. These places include empty structures, caves, ditches, drains, wells, cliffs, and any other location that might be an entanglement. There is no organized pattern to this type of search, but more of a free movement throughout the area of interest. The search may also be used to find additional clues that might have been left behind by the subject if he had crossed through the area, such as footprints and disturbed foliage. Statistically, if the subject is in the immediate area where the hasty search is being conducted, chances are likely that he will be found. (See Figure 13.7.)

Grid Search

SAR teams will typically use a **grid search** as a last resort. These types of searches are slow to conduct, require large numbers of trained and well-disciplined searchers, and can only cover small areas at a time. A grid search requires the trained members to line up at a designated distance apart from each other in a horizontal line. They then will walk side by side in a slow and deliberate manner while looking for the subject or clues that might have been left behind. (See Figure 13.8.) The discipline portion comes into play by requiring the grid searchers to maintain an even spacing and not take the path of least resistance, meaning that they must go directly through any patch of foliage as opposed to going around it. Lost people, especially children traveling in the dark, can easily get caught in these entanglements.

Choke Point Search

A tactic used by experienced search teams is the **choke point search**. This method is also based upon the behavior of subjects and the theory that if they are in a specific area of high probability, they will tend to follow the natural terrain, such as valleys and waterways. Rescue teams who use this tactic will position rescuers at choke points near the base of valleys, waterways, bridges, and so on. Like the

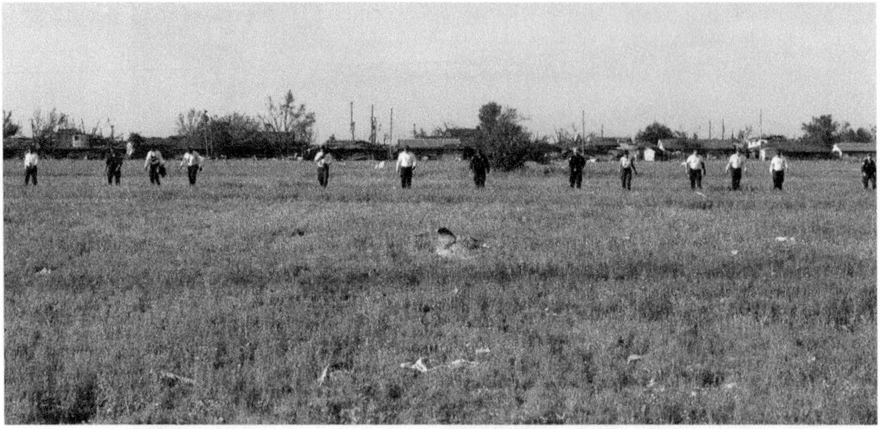

FIGURE 13.8 A grid search requires rescuers to walk side by side in a slow deliberate manner while looking for the missing person or clues to their whereabouts. *Source: Jocelyn Augustino/ FEMA.*

containment tactic, the goal is to not let subjects get past the rescuers.

Use of Canines

A very successful method of searching for a subject is with canine search teams. Canine teams are made up of highly trained air-scent search dogs that specialize in locating subjects in a variety of different situations. Specialties include underwater, avalanche, and cadaver searches. However, air-scent dogs are also trained to locate live subjects. Canines are trained specifically to employ three different tactics when searching for subjects: air-scenting, tracking, and trailing. (See Figure 13.9.)

Air-scent dogs work a search area by being deployed downwind and allowed to detect and follow a scent that has been left by a human or carried by the wind. Canines that specialize in tracking are trained to follow a specific scent left by a specific person. A person naturally leaves scent nearly everywhere he goes by the natural means of losing dead skin cells as new ones are created. If an article of clothing of the subject is acquired, the dog

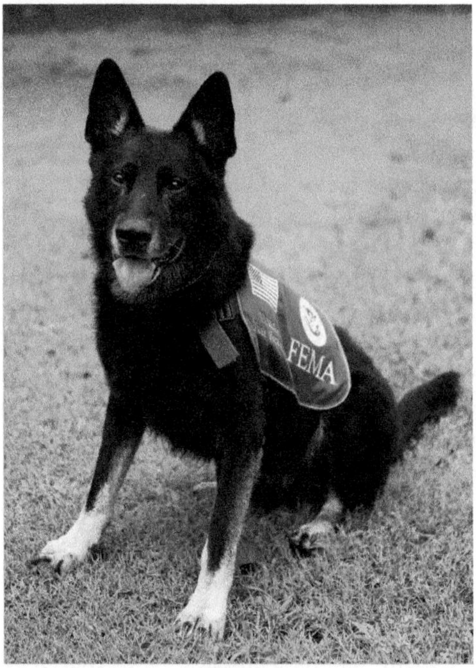

FIGURE 13.9 Canines are highly successful in locating lost persons when used early in the search operation. *Source: David Fine/ FEMA.*

can pick up the scent, and from the LKP the canine can potentially track the scent through the variety of terrain and environments. Remember, though, that it is important for canines to be brought in early during a search. As time goes by, the scent can begin to fade, causing broken tracks that can confuse the canine. Canines can also be confused by additional scents that mask the target scent left from multiple people who have contaminated the scene. For this reason, it is important to secure the area around the LKP or PLS to prevent this cross-contamination. To further prevent confusing the search canine, it is important to clear the upwind area of all search personnel as well as to keep the search team as far behind the canine search team as possible. Dogs that specialize in trailing use a lot of the same principles of tracking dogs; however, they have the ability to continue to pick up scent that originates in addition to the original track. Additional tracks are caused by the subject leaving a trail of dead skin cells on leaves and limbs against which they brushed.

When using a canine search team, it is important that all actions are coordinated with the dog handlers and that their instructions are followed. These animals are highly trained, but any outside interactions can negatively affect their abilities. While in the BoO, it is very important that all personnel keep away from the search dogs unless permission is given by the handler.

Vehicle Searches

Vehicle searches can be used early in a SAR operation, especially when employing the hasty search tactic. Search teams can quickly cover the roadways in the search area while attempting to locate the subject or vital clues. This tactic works well during natural disaster events not only to search for subjects but also to assess and report damage to the command post. When using this method, it is important for the searchers to keep their eyes scanning from left to right, right to left, near to far, and far to near. Multiple persons in the same vehicle will only scan a quadrant or sector. Any actions taken should not distract the driver, who should be concentrating on driving.

RESCUE OPERATIONS

Once the subject has been found, the stabilization phase of the operation should be conducted. This is the rescue portion of the operation where the subject has been located and now his disposition is assessed by the on-scene resources. If the subject is unhurt and ambulatory, he may simply be assisted out of the area by rescuers. A subject injured or suffering from a medical condition should be given medical treatment in an effort to stabilize prior to transport. If the subject is not easily accessible, the situation must be assessed for risk/benefit as to what degree of danger the rescuers will face. If the subject is alive, then obviously the benefit is greater and allows the rescue team to take a slightly higher risk to perform a complex rescue. If the subject has expired, then the benefit is much less, reducing the amount of risk that should be taken to achieve a recovery. In such a situation, more attention will be given to carefully planning out the recovery operation to further reduce the amount of risk that the rescuer will have to be placed under while conducting this portion of the operation. For example, in cases where the subject is trapped on the side of a cliff or trapped in the middle of a swiftly moving waterway, resources specializing in these specific situations should immediately be called in to perform these highly technical operations.

MEDICAL CARE

The subject should be assessed for any life-threatening conditions. A wide variety of hazards are found in both wilderness and urban environments that can inflict traumatic injuries compounded by heat and cold. Prehospital care providers must be prepared to provide immediate and, in some cases, ongoing care until the patient has been transported out of the environment and delivered into the hands of more advanced care providers. Depending on the location of the patient, response vehicle that carry all the required EMS and transport equipment may not be able to just drive up. If the subject is in the backcountry, rescuers will most likely be carrying in all the EMS equipment that will be needed to provide this care, including the equipment required to package and carry out the patient.

Most often, response personnel will encounter climbers, extreme hikers, and water enthusiasts who have sustained musculoskeletal injuries as well as traumatic head and internal injuries. Environmental afflictions can include heat exhaustion or heat stroke, hypothermia, frostbite, and, in the extreme case, altitude sickness. The subject may also be suffering from insect stings or bites, rashes, and animal scratches and bites. An insect sting or bite has the potential to become serious if venom was injected into the subject's skin, resulting in poisoning or an allergic reaction. Likewise, animal bites can cause serious traumatic injuries and lead to infections. The EMS responder should be thorough when assessing these patients. All of these mechanisms can easily mask or be masked by other medical conditions or injuries.

Just like prehospital care in the urban setting, the approach to patient care should be a systematic process. Personal safety of the rescuers is always foremost, with the scene being assessed for any existing or potential hazards. The patient should be removed from any immediate danger and protected from further injury. This might be as simple as placing a helmet on the patient's head if there is a risk of overhead falling objects. If the subject is dangerously near or on the side of a bluff, a makeshift harness from webbing or a rescue harness should be placed on the subject and then secured to a lifeline. The patient's responsiveness should be assessed using the AVPU scale: A-Alert, V-Verbal, P-Painful, U-Unresponsive. Any level of responsiveness less than alert should be considered potentially serious. The pulse should be assessed immediately, keeping in mind that if the patient is suffering from hypothermia, the pulse might be extremely slow and difficult to find. The responder should attempt to feel for a carotid pulse for no less than 1 minute. If a pulse cannot be found, the downtime of the subject should be assessed. If it appears that the subject has been without vital signs for a long time, then it may be decided that CPR should not be initiated. Performing CPR in a wilderness setting is difficult at best, with little more than a dismal patient outcome. In many cases, responders have conducted CPR for several hours while carrying the patient out of the wilderness area. If it is determined that there will be a lengthy delay before the subject can be delivered to definitive care, the decision may be made to begin a trial of CPR. If no spontaneous circulation returns after 20 minutes, then efforts may be stopped. If a patient has sustained injuries that are incompatible with life, then resuscitation efforts should not be attempted.

During the initial assessment, if a pulse is found, the patient's airway should then be assessed, opened, and cleared of any obstructions while attempting to protect the cervical spine. Assessment of the patient's respiratory function should be next. Any required assistance should be provided, including supplemental oxygen administration.

If the patient is wearing heavy bulky clothing and other gear, exposing potential injuries such as lacerations, hematomas, and fractures should be carefully done so as to prevent the patient from further loss of body heat. Determining the mechanism of injury of a patient can be difficult if there are no witnesses. The rescuer must rely on clues around the patient, such as fallen rocks, broken limbs, or an impact point on which the patient may have fallen from an elevated position. Despite the lack of diagnostic resources available to responders in the backcountry, patient care should not be delayed. It is important in a mild to cold environment that the patient's body heat be preserved in the event the patient is suffering from shock or hypothermia. Heat packs, emergency blankets, and the patient's own clothing, if dry, can easily be used to accomplish this.

Treatment guidelines in the wilderness setting are obviously different from those in urban areas. Because of the long transport times that can last for hours and even days, it is recommended that open wounds initially be thoroughly scrubbed, irrigated, and cleaned prior to dressing. In a humid environment, wounds are very prone to infection and should also be constantly monitored. The use of waterproof dressings is not recommended in these cases as they prevent air circulation, which can increase the likelihood of an anaerobic infection. It is recommended that the rescuer instead cleanse the site with soap and water, or another antimicrobial solution, and replace the dressings often.

Another difference between care provided in the urban setting and care provided in the wilderness setting is how fractures and dislocations are treated. In the urban setting, most treatment guidelines follow the concept of securing musculoskeletal injuries in place and then transporting the patient. In the wilderness setting, many wilderness EMS treatment guidelines recommend, if possible, to reduce dislocations in the field. By reducing the dislocation, distal limb ischemia with associated damage may be prevented. Reducing the dislocation can also assist in lessening the pain for the subject, in turn making the evacuation for subject and rescuer easier. This treatment should not be performed unless the EMS provider is properly trained and authorized by his protocols to provide such care.

As the patient is transported out of the wilderness, the responder should recheck all bandages and dressings and be prepared to change them several times throughout the trip. As when placing a dressing for the first time, distal pulses along with sensation and movement should be checked periodically to ensure that circulation is not interrupted. If splints have been put in place, distal circulation should also be monitored on a regular basis.

As the patient is prepared for transport, cervical spine immobilization should not be neglected. Transporting a fully immobilized subject out of the wilderness is manpower-intensive and slows down the transport process significantly. If the patient is fully responsive with no complaints of midline neck tenderness, no focal neurological deficit, and no major painful injuries that will limit the neck assessment, cervical spine immobilization may not be warranted based solely on mechanism of injury or injuries above the clavicle. Prior to immobilizing a subject, rescuers must weigh the risks of a cervical spine injury versus the benefits of not immobilizing the subject. While cervical spines should not be cleared by SAR responders, selective C-spine immobilization may be required.

Any treatment guidelines or protocols should be reviewed and approved by each agency's medical director. In addition, response personnel should be thoroughly trained in the administration of wilderness EMS.

EVACUATION

Once the patient has been assessed and injuries and medical conditions have been addressed, the patient must be evacuated. If the subject is in an urban or semirural environment, simply transferring the patient to a waiting ambulance will allow for the subject to be transported to a hospital. However, if the subject is located in the wilderness, some special equipment and resources will be needed, as well as a sizable force of trained rescuers. An evacuation plan should consider the equipment and appropriate measures necessary to safely and quickly move the subject to definitive care. Once a subject has been located, and before committing to an evacuation plan, the SAR team will evaluate his ability to communicate with outside resources, availability and distance to the closest advanced health care facility or provider, current and forecast weather conditions, terrain conditions, and nature of the subject's injuries. All of these conditions play a role in assessing the risk—not only for the patient but also for the rescue team—of susceptibility to the harsh environment. Some conditions may require that the rescue team set up a bivouac or camp where the patient was found rather than attempting to move the patient out on foot. Ultimately, every rescue team understands that there must be a certain expectation of uncertainty that will drive the team to have to adapt to ever-changing conditions, forcing them to change their plan of action. Depending on these factors, the rescue team may elect to evacuate the patient by air, ground, or water. All three approaches come with their own complex issues that again require the assessing the risk/benefit matrix.

Search and Rescue by Air

Using aircraft to conduct search and rescue is a very complex and potentially dangerous option if not conducted appropriately. Aircraft inherently have their limitations and should only be used when the conditions are suitable. If a rescue team is on the ground and with the subject, they should be in constant communication with the aircraft, assisting with coordination of the rescue.

The two types of aircraft are fixed wing and rotary wing. Unless there is an approved airstrip nearby, fixed wing aircraft should not be used. However, fixed winged aircraft can play a highly important role in directing ground resources to a known subject as well as dropping beacons, flares, survival radios, and other survival equipment to survivors when the terrain allows. Rotary wing aircraft, or helicopters, offer much more versatility and are very suitable as a resource. Helicopters can easily maneuver and get into smaller, harder-to-reach areas. Depending on the type and size of the helicopter, the onboard equipment such as a hoist, and—most importantly—the training and experience of the flight crew, rescue teams can be inserted directly into the location of a known subject. In addition, once the subject has been appropriately packaged, he can be hoisted out by the wench on a rated cable. Once the subject is in the helicopter, more medical care can be administered while he is transported to the hospital.

Helicopters do have limitations and certain disadvantages that must be considered during an operation. Weather is something that is constantly changing, especially in mountainous areas. A mission may be underway during excellent weather with clear visibility and within a very short time can deteriorate, requiring the flight crew to abort the mission because of rain, low visibility, heavy turbulent winds, downdrafts, and possible icing depending on the temperature. The summer not only brings the likelihood of sudden development of thunderstorms but also high humidity. Heavy humidity, especially at higher altitudes, decreases the helicopter's lift ability, in turn reducing its weight payload capability. Once a helicopter has arrived at the location of a subject, the rescue team on the ground must be prepared for the possibility of high turbulent winds and noise from the rotary wash. The noise can easily interrupt verbal communications between the helicopter and the ground team, requiring the use of hand signals. Time over the rescue site may also be limited by insufficient fuel reserves.

Because of this, every effort should be made to have everything ready to extract the patient from the site (National Search and Rescue Committee, 2013).

If the rescue team is fortunate enough be near an open area such as a field, a landing zone (LZ) could possibly be established. When selecting an LZ, several parameters have to be met in order to meet with most safety guidelines. The LZ has to be large enough to accommodate the helicopter. Most recommendations are for the LZ to be at least 100 feet by 100 feet. This may change, depending upon the size of the helicopter as well as the preferences of the pilot. There should be no obstructions that could endanger the helicopter, such as trees, power lines, fences, light or telephone poles, buildings, vehicles, and so on. Everyone should closely monitor the area for wildlife or livestock that could unexpectedly enter into the LZ. Prior to the helicopter approaching the LZ, the rescue team should perform a foreign object debris (FOD) walk through the area. Any object that could potentially be caught up in the rotary wash and thrown up into the rotary blades of the helicopter or sent through the air as a projectile should be removed. Ultimately, the pilot has the final say about taking a mission and the use of any landing zone.

If the decision is made to use a hoist to lift a nonambulatory subject, the subject should be secured in a rescue litter even if he is already on a long spine board. In addition, the subject should be placed in a secondary harness and tied in directly to rails of the rescue litter. Even with the regular straps from the rescue litter in place, the tendency for the rescue litter is to begin spinning during the lift. This spin can easily develop so much centrifugal force that the patient, even though secured to the long spine board, can be ejected midair from the rescue litter, board and all. The same applies for a patient who is not fully immobilized and is just placed in a rescue litter. It is very important that extensive training with a designated aeromedical provider should be conducted continually in order to maintain safe operational performance.

Transport by Water

In situations where the subject is located near a large body of water, such as a lake or river, rescue teams may decide that it is easier to bring in a suitable watercraft, such as a Zodiac inflatable or other rescue boat, to take the patient back to a launch. If this option is used, care must be taken to keep the patient dry and warm. If possible, a rescue litter that has floatable rail guards should be used in the event of the patient accidently going into the water. This will allow for the rescue litter to float, keeping the patient from sinking in the water.

Transport by Ground

Transporting a subject out of the backcountry by ground still remains one of the most common and undesirable methods. This method is very time consuming and places the rescuers at much greater risk. A team of fifteen to twenty rescuers can only move a subject in a rescue litter at a speed of approximately 1 mile per hour, depending upon the terrain they have to navigate. In severe cold environments, this can lead the patient to an increased risk of hypothermia, as well as frostbite. If the subject is already suffering from acute hypothermia, the constant rough movement from being carried can lead to ventricular fibrillation due to the patient's ventricular threshold being reduced from the hypothermic condition. All patients suffering from acute hypothermia should be treated gently. In addition, all exposed body parts should be covered if the temperature is below freezing.

Ground Transport Devices

The use of a litter wheel is an excellent alternative to having to physically carry the weight of the rescue litter with the subject in it. The litter wheel is a single, large, air-filled all-terrain wheel within a frame that is attached directly to the rescue litter. This lets the weight of the subject and litter be supported by the device, allowing for a minimum of four rescuers who only have to balance the rescue litter as they walk. This greatly reduces physical stress on the rescuers as well as the subject.

CHAPTER REVIEW

Summary

Wilderness rescue is an extremely complex and challenging discipline requiring SAR teams to constantly train in many different environments and terrain. The hostile conditions and hazards associated with wilderness rescues should never be underestimated. Rescuers can easily become subjects themselves. Understanding and respecting these hazards can allow for response personnel to safely perform a wilderness rescue. In addition, response personnel who participate in SAR operations should be familiar with the behavior patterns of all the different age and personality groups. These traits will assist rescuers in possibly predicting the location of a potential subject or the direction in which a subject might be heading.

Like many of the different technical rescue disciplines, medical treatments may be slightly different from what responders will encounter in the urban setting. This will require responders to adapt, in some cases, what they may have originally been taught. Ultimately, most rescuers will agree that wilderness rescue can be the most strenuous and demanding of all the disciplines.

WHAT WOULD YOU DO? Reflection

As a first-arriving EMS responder to a SAR call out, you will want to establish how long the subject has been missing, the subject's name, physical description, description of clothing, and any favorite places to which the subject may likely go. In addition, you will want to ascertain if the subject has any medical conditions, and what medications are prescribed for him.

Initially, EMS response personnel would want to notify resources such as a canine search team. If the subject is missing in a wilderness area, a wilderness SAR team should be contacted. Resources from the National Park Service should be utilized in location within or near national parks. In this scenario, EMS response personnel should consider utilizing a canine search, especially if the canine handler is able to find an adequate scent. If a canine search is not warranted, a hasty search of the nearby trails around the property is appropriate, with emphasis placed on those that the subject normally travels.

Review Questions

1. During a search and rescue operations, more than 75 percent of subjects are found in the first ______ hours.
2. Who is the best source of information when conducting interviews about a person possibly lost in a wilderness area?

3. What reasons contribute to the delay in alerting response personnel about a missing person?
4. What factors should be evaluated when assessing the urgency of a wilderness search and rescue operation?
5. What are the behavioral patterns that children between ages 1 and 6 years possess as related to being lost?
6. What is the advantage of initiating an accountability system during a wilderness search and rescue mission?
7. What are the typical hazards that can affect response personnel who are actively searching for a missing person in a mountainous area?
8. What type of search method involves positioning rescuers on roadway intersections, bridges, and river crossings around an outer boundary area based on the probable distance that a missing person has traveled over a certain amount of time?
9. Once a subject is found, what factors should be considered when making the decision to transport a nonambulatory subject out of the wilderness by foot or bivouac in place?
10. What rules should be adhered to when searching for a missing person with canines?

References

Federal Emergency Management Agency. (2008). "The National Response Framework." See the organization wesbite.

National Fire Protection Association. (2009). "NFPA 1670: Standard on Operations and Training for Technical Search and Rescue Incidents. Quincy, MA: National Fire Protection Association.

National Fire Protection Association. (2013). "NFPA 1006: Standard for Technical Rescuer Professional Qualifications, Confined Space Rescue." Quincy, MA: National Fire Protection Association.

National Park Service. (2011). "RM-59: Search and Rescue Reference Manual." See the organization website.

National Search and Rescue Committee. (2013). "U.S. Coast Guard Addendum to the United States National Search and Rescue Supplement (NSS) to the International Aeronautical and Maritime Search and Rescue Manual (IAMSAR)." Washington, DC: U.S. Department of Homeland Security and U.S. Coast Guard.

Pruitt, M. (2008). "Technical Rescue Awareness Level Training" [Powerpoint and Lecture Notes]. See the M.A B.A.S. 201 Tactical Rescue Team website.

U.S. Coast Guard. (2013). "SAR Manuals and Documents." See the organization website.

United States Homeland Emergency Response Organization. (2006). "Wilderness SAR Technical & Unit Leader Reference Guide." Austin, TX: United States Homeland Emergency Response Organization.

Key Terms

accountability system A system implemented within the incident command system to track the location of personnel as they arrive on the scene and continued throughout the course of an incident until it is terminated.

AMBER Alert Program AMBER is an acronym for "America's Missing: Broadcasting Emergency Response," named originally for Amber Hagerman, a 9-year-old child who was abducted and murdered in Arlington, Texas, in 1996. AMBER Alerts are broadcasted via commercial radio stations, television stations, and cable TV by the Emergency Alert System, NOAA

Weather Radio, and many Department of Transportation highway signs.

base of operation (BoO) An established location on the scene of a larger-scale incident where the most important functions of the incident command system are coordinated.

bastard search The search method in which rescuers look in obvious places while assuming that the person was not really lost. In many cases, the person being searched for either has found his own way out or has gone home without telling anyone.

choke point search The search method that uses the same principles as confinement by staging rescuers in specific locations where a subject is most likely to travel.

confinement area A bounded area set up to limit where the subject may travel undetected, or to establish that the subject has not already passed a desired boundary of the search area.

containment area A bounded area set up to confine a subject to a specific area.

despondent An individual who suffers from depression, loss of hope, confidence, or courage.

Emergency Management Agency (EMA) A U.S. government organization that provides assistance, planning, and other services on the local, state, and federal levels as related to disaster management.

grid search The process of dividing the search area into smaller grids and methodically searching each of the segments, typically using a line search.

hasty search The process of performing a quick search of an area where a subject may likely be located.

last known point (LKP) The last position a person was in determined by clues, evidence belonging to the subject, or a credible eyewitness report indicating that the missing subject was known to be at a specific location.

National Search and Rescue Committee (NSARC) A federal committee comprised of the Department of Homeland Security, Department of the Interior, Department of Commerce, Defense Department, Department of Transportation, Federal Communications Commission, and the National Aeronautics and Space Administration and designated to oversee the National Search and Rescue Plan and act as a coordinating forum for national SAR matters.

National Search and Rescue Plan (NSP) An interagency agreement providing national arrangements for coordination of search and rescue services to meet both domestic and international commitments.

point last seen (PLS) The point where the subject was last seen by an eyewitness or captured on video at a specific time and location.

public information officer (PIO) A representative for an agency or organization responsible for coordinating and providing information to the media and public.

search area The area designated to be searched.

search and rescue (SAR) incident Any situation requiring notification, alerting, and possibly activating the SAR system for an operation.

unified incident command The process of bringing together the incident commanders of all major organizations directly involved in the incident in order to coordinate an effective response, while at the same time each carries out its own jurisdictional responsibilities.

Incidents of National Consequence

14 CHAPTER

RAY BARISHANSKY

DAVID HARRINGTON

Objectives

After reading this chapter, the student should be able to:

14.1 Identify the different factors that define an incident of national consequence.

14.2 Review past incidents of national consequence that affected EMS response.

14.3 Identify the common issues faced by EMS response personnel when responding to an incident of national consequence and methods for dealing with each of them.

14.4 Explain the importance of creating an organized incident action plan when operating at an incident of national consequence.

14.5 Identify the need for and methods of establishing scene security.

14.6 Identify methods for dealing with mass casualty incidents (MCI).

14.7 Explain safety when responding to incidents of national consequence.

14.8 Explain the importance of addressing the long-term physical and mental effects that an incident of national consequence can place on an EMS responder.

Key Terms

chemical, biological, radiological, nuclear, and explosive (CBRNE)

Community Emergency Response Team (CERT) program

consequence

emergency operations plan (EOP)

incident of national consequence
local emergency planning commission (LEPC)
poisons
post-traumatic stress disorder (PTSD)
toxins
weapons of mass destruction (WMDs)

WHAT WOULD YOU DO?

It is Monday morning, just after 9:00 A.M., and you are functioning as the EMS supervisor for the shift. As you leave the ambulance operations center, you hear what sounds like a rumble of thunder. Not giving it any more thought, you crest a hill and see a large plume of heavy black smoke billowing from the skyline of the downtown area. As you pick up the radio mike to call it in, the 9-1-1 dispatcher dispatches two of the downtown units and yourself to a report of an explosion at the federal courthouse. As you approach the area, you observe multiple fire apparatus and law enforcement vehicles attempting to access the scene, which is being made difficult by civilians trying to escape the area. You are only able to get within two blocks of the federal building, which is heavily damaged and on fire. You see dozens of people with a variety of traumatic injuries emerging from the cloud of greyish dust and smoke that is coming from the building.

Questions

1. What are the indications that would define this event as a possible incident of national consequence?
2. What factors should you consider as you develop an action plan to deal with this complex event?
3. What resources would you request initially and predict that you will require if the incident continues long term?

INTRODUCTION

The emergency medical service (EMS), early in its 40-year history, typically played more of a support role to fire, rescue, and law enforcement agencies that were responsible for mitigating dynamic and challenging incidents. During this time, EMS had the primary responsibility to receive patients from the rescue team or other lead agencies and then transport them directly to the closest medical facility. Much of the decision making about the patient's future had already been made by this point. Over the past decade, through research studies and lessons learned from past incidents, EMS has recognized changes that were necessary not only to better serve communities but also to further progress the EMS industry as an equal partner to the other stakeholders in the emergency services community (police, fire, and emergency management agency (EMA)).

INCIDENTS OF NATIONAL CONSEQUENCE

An **incident of national consequence** is a situation of mass effect that has the potential to impact the entire nation either though the action itself or through the number of patients/fatalities involved. Incidents of national consequence do not respect jurisdictional boundaries, often affecting widespread areas and requiring the resources of multiple communities.

Side Bar

Factors That Define an Incident of National Consequence

- Large numbers of patients overwhelming the normal operational capability of the local emergency services
- Incidents that result in a large number of casualties and loss of life
- Incidents at public assemblies or famous landmarks
- An incident that crosses jurisdictional boundaries and requires the response of multiple agencies, up to and possibly including state and federal resources.
- Incidents of long duration, overlapping into multiple days and even weeks
- Incidents related to catastrophic weather events
- Incidents resulting from criminal or terrorist activities
- Incidents of public health that create a community health scare

The scope of an incident by itself will depend greatly on the nature of the event. Incidents can include large highway traffic accidents, air disasters, passenger train derailments, hazardous material releases, terrorist events, and breakouts of pandemic viruses and diseases. There is no community immune from any of these possible scenarios. All of these events present some common issues for the emergency services. The most common issue faced is an emergency response organization that is unprepared to adequately handle these large-scale events.

The term **consequence** is the outcome or change that results from an incident. An incident of national consequence can quickly catch the attention of the public and attain the national spotlight, especially in this age of social media. In most cases, shortly after the conclusion of a large incident, a lessons-learned phase develops. This phase of learning is taken directly from a series of after-action reports that are created from issues that surface during the incident. The lessons learned from any incident, especially in a large-scale incident, can have a long-term cause and effect that directly affect the scope of operations across the emergency services industry. This can easily create a ripple effect across the EMS, ultimately changing the way matters are mitigated during similar incidents in the future.

During the earlier history of the emergency services, most response agencies were considered stand-alone, essentially operating as independent agencies within their jurisdictions. Mutual aid was recognized and given but only under certain circumstances. Over time, several factors including budgetary constraints, limited resources, and increased demand for specific operational capabilities have required many areas to combine certain resources, especially during large-scale incidents. Since the formation of public safety 9-1-1 centers, many communities now dispatch multiple response resources simultaneously. This gives EMS units a greater opportunity to be first on scene of a wide variety of large-scale complex incidents. For this reason, EMS crews and supervisors should possess a greater knowledge and understanding of the factors that create an incident of national consequence, and the appropriate measures for dealing with these situations, some of which will have consequences that extend beyond their own limited borders.

SOME INCIDENTS OF NATIONAL CONSEQUENCE

Some events in world history are good examples of incidents of national consequence. All of these events share some similar factors, such as a large number of casualties and loss of life, and a tremendous amount of resources needed. On the other hand, these incidents differ by the way that they are managed. Some of the events were managed by the fire service or EMA, while others were managed by law enforcement. In all of these cases, though, EMS played an instrumental role that directly led to significantly reducing the potential for further loss of life.

World Trade Center Bombing, 1993

On 26 February, 1993, a terrorist truck bomb exploded on a Level B-2 parking garage that sat below the two World Trade Center towers. The explosion itself tore upward, creating a huge hole seven stories above the blast. While 1,042 persons were injured, only six persons were killed. Of the total number injured, 124 were first responders. This was one of the first recorded acts of terrorism against the U.S. mainland.

Tokyo Subway Sarin Attack, 1995

On March 20, 1995, the terrorist group Aum Shinrikyo initiated a sarin gas attack on the subway system in Tokyo, Japan, killing 12 civilians and injuring more than 5,000. Communication issues resulted in a delay in response. Only 688 patients were transported by ambulance out of the more than 5,000 victims affected by the attack. In fact, more patients were taken by taxi to the hospital than by EMS. Another major issue encountered was the lack of decontamination facilities on site. This led to contaminated patients being transported to the emergency departments and further affecting other patients and health care workers. Approximately 10 percent of the EMS providers became contaminated and suffered ill effects of the sarin (Metzger, 2004). Many of the issues encountered during this terrorist event were later looked on as learning opportunities that assisted in the development of emergency action plans for similar incidents.

Oklahoma City Bombing, 1995

On April 19, 1995, a large bomb weighing somewhere between 4,800 and 7,000 pounds made of fertilizer and ammonium nitrate placed in a rented cargo van was detonated in front of the Murrah Federal Building in Oklahoma City, Oklahoma. (See Figure 14.1.) Timothy McVeigh, seen as a right-wing extremist or in some references even as a neo-Nazi, anti-government and loss of his Christian identity, had detonated the device using a timer. The explosion directly caused a serious collapse of the upper level of the building, bringing it down onto the lower floors. Of the 361 persons in the building at the time of the collapse, 163 died. EMS and fire resources immediately responded to the scene and began search and rescue operations. Within the first hour, nearly 140 patients were transported to area hospitals. During the first 24 hours, 444 total victims were treated by on-scene responders (Metzger, 2004).

Columbine Shooting, 1999

On April 20, 1999, in Littleton, Colorado, two students, Eric Harris and Dylan Klebold, planned and carried out an attack at their high school using semiautomatic weapons and approximately a hundred improvised incendiary devices (IED). Their plans were not only to kill as many of their fellow students as they could using the weapons that they were carrying but also to inflict as many casualties among the fleeing students and first responders as possible with the IEDs. In all, 15 persons were killed, including both Harris and Klebold. On-scene EMS and fire personnel triaged an additional 160 victims. This incident became one of the

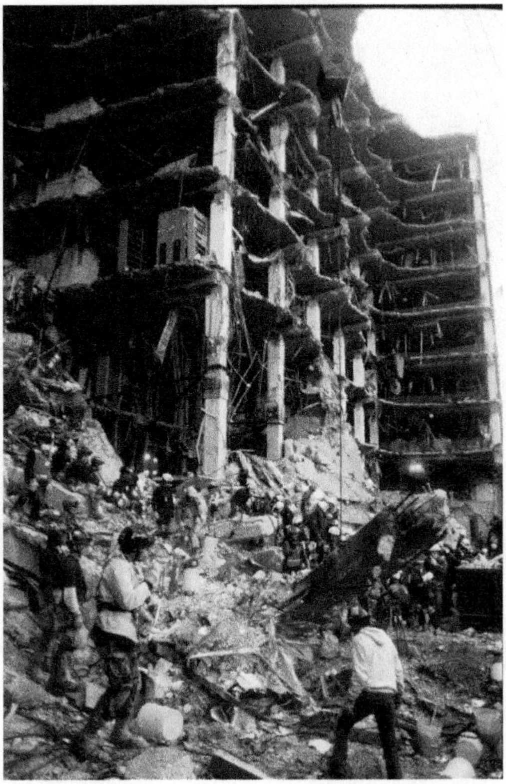

FIGURE 14.1 The Oklahoma City bombing was a domestic terrorist bomb attack on the Alfred P. Murrah Federal Building in Oklahoma City on April 19, 1995, that claimed the lives of 168 persons, including 19 children, and injured more than 680 people. *Source: FEMA News Photo.*

worse active shooter events in U.S. history and presented a number of serious issues for the EMS agencies that responded to the scene. Scene security was the greatest challenge, as responders had become direct targets of the attack. EMS operations began well before the attacks had ended, despite the significant risk to rescuers (Mell and Sztajnkrycer, 2005).

9-11 World Trade Center Attack, 2001

The attack of September 11, 2001, on the World Trade Center (WTC) towers in New York City quickly became one of the most horrific attacks on U.S. soil in history. Emergency responders from fire, law enforcement, and EMS responded immediately to find themselves becoming the victims. Over 200 EMTs and paramedics arrived on scene within 15 minutes of the event occurring. Eventually, more than 400 EMS personnel were on scene in one of the largest multiple casualty incidents in history. Many factors, such as communication breakdowns, lack of personnel accountability, and the breakdown of the command structure that occurred after the

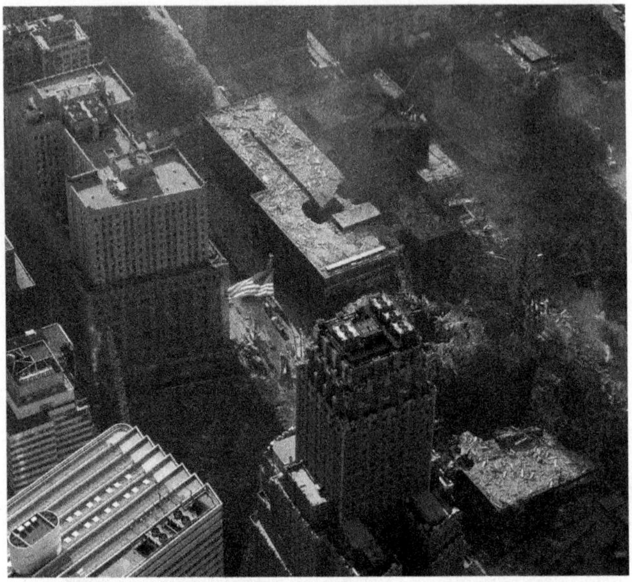

FIGURE 14.2 The attacks of 9-11 were a coordinated terrorist attack on the World Trade Center, the Pentagon, and Flight 93, which was targeted for the U.S. Capitol building. Nearly 3,000 persons lost their lives in the attack. *Source: Michael Rieger/FEMA.*

collapse of the second WTC building, led to many challenges for EMS crews. There were 2,977 fatalities; 9 of those were EMS responders. (See Figure 14.2.) More than 6,000 victims were treated in area hospitals. It is unknown how many were transported by EMS.

SARS Epidemic, 2003

In February 2003, the first cases of severe acute respiratory syndrome (SARS) were diagnosed in Toronto, Canada. By the end of March of the same year, the Ontario Ministry of Health issued a message declaring a province-wide medical state of emergency. By July 2003, more than 200 persons in Toronto had been diagnosed with SARS. Toronto's EMS resources were especially affected when it was determined that 850 of their paramedics had experienced 1,166 potential SARS exposures. This further led to a 10-day home quarantine of 436 of those paramedics, leading to a serious deficiency in the EMS system. Of the 436 potentially affected paramedics, SARS-like symptoms developed in 62 of them.

Hurricane Katrina, 2005

Hurricane Katrina quickly became one of the most deadly and destructive hurricanes in U.S. history. (See Figure 14.3.) With more than 1,800 fatalities associated with the storm, Hurricane Katrina greatly affected four states and cost $108 billion to repair the damage done. Resources responding to Katrina included federal government agencies, state and local-level agencies, National Guard troops, nongovernmental agencies, charity organizations, and private individuals.

The Federal Emergency Management Agency (FEMA) and the Department of Homeland Security (DHS) provided much of the support during this event, but response

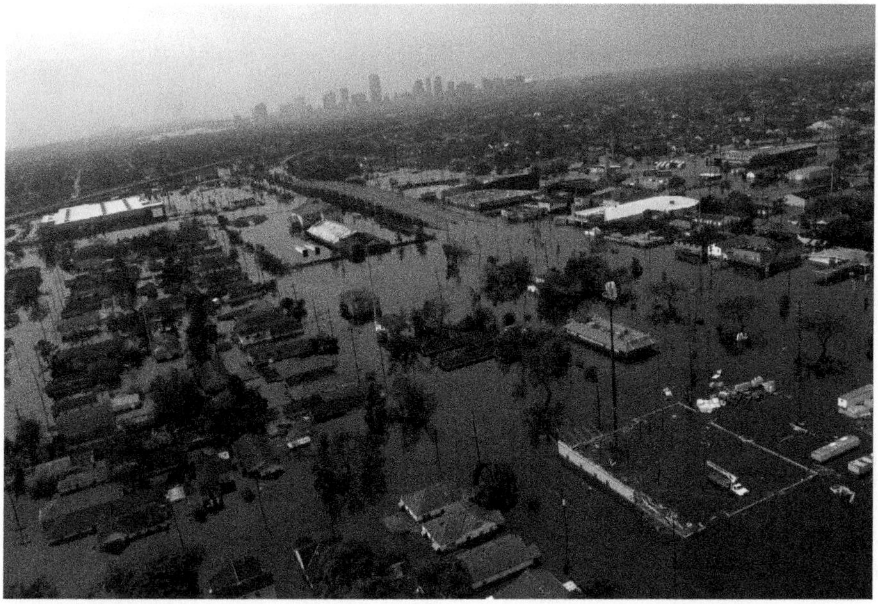

FIGURE 14.3 Hurricane Katrina was the deadliest and most destructive hurricane in U.S. history. The storm took over 1,800 lives and caused in excess of $81 billion. *Source: Jocelyn Augustino/FEMA.*

was not limited to just the federal government. In accordance with the Tenth Amendment to the U.S. Constitution, each state, during a large-scale disaster, is responsible for the health and welfare of its citizens. However, once the incident overwhelms the capabilities of a state's resources, they may call for assistance from the federal government.

In conjunction with the Emergency Management Assistance Compact (EMAC), resources from across the United States were sent to each of the affected states in the form of disaster supplies, search and rescue teams, and ambulances. Under EMAC, the state governor has the authority to request assistance in the form of resources from any of the fifty participating states to aid them during any emergency or disaster that is declared by the governor of the affected state. In addition, the U.S. Department of Defense deployed resources from the Coast Guard, Navy, and Air Force to assist in search and rescue and in aeromedical transportation. (See Figure 14.4.) The states of Florida, Louisiana, Mississippi, and Alabama activated and deployed more than 10,000 National Guard troops. Because of this disaster, many changes were made to better assist local EMS agencies with obtaining mutual aid resources more quickly and efficiently.

ISSUES IDENTIFIED DURING INCIDENTS OF NATIONAL CONSEQUENCE

With most large-scale events, response agencies collect their experiences and develop after-action reports that later become the lessons learned. This enables the emergency services community across the world to review and learn from what went well and what did not. The results from many years of research and review of case studies have identified some issues that are consistent with most incidents.

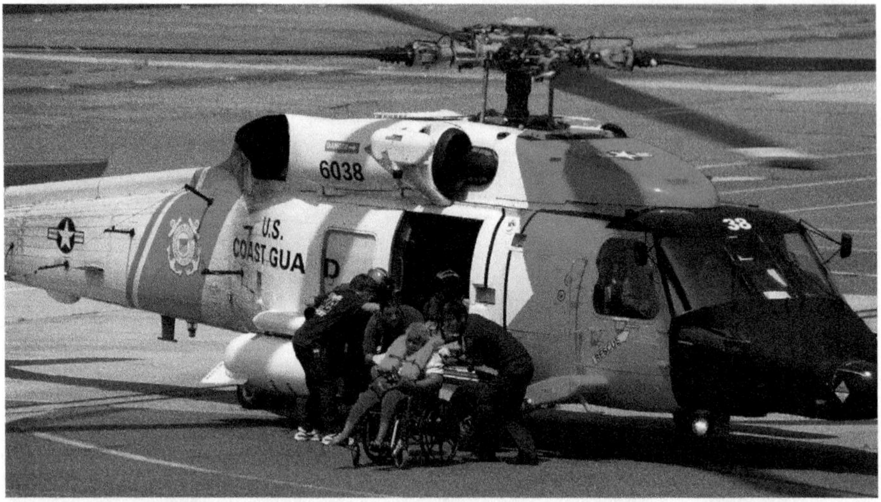

FIGURE 14.4 ■ The U.S. Coast Guard has been commended for efforts in saving and assisting in the evacuation of medical patients. *Source: Michael Rieger/FEMA.*

INADEQUATE RESOURCES AT THE LOCAL LEVEL

Many communities possess modest resources that are only capable of delivering the services required to maintain the normal demands of their community. When a large-scale incident occurs within these jurisdictions, emergency services are overwhelmed and quickly cease to effectively manage the demands of not only the incident but also the normal demands of the community. In a community of any size, this can become quite a logistical challenge. It must be understood that the normal everyday demand on a community does not cease just because a large-scale disaster strikes. To combat this imposing issue, many areas have developed a regional mutual aid agreement between all their neighboring towns as part of an **emergency operations plan (EOP)** that can be implemented and allow for resources to quickly be mobilized. This will allow for response agencies to continue meeting the demands of the community. Many states have adopted the strike team concept. The purpose of the EMS strike teams is to provide ALS or BLS transportation in areas during events where the local EMS agencies have become overwhelmed and are unable to provide services without additional resources. These teams are typically activated through a request from state or regional EMS authorities.

LACK OF KNOWLEDGE AND INFORMATION

In many larger communities, a tremendous amount of time and effort have been dedicated to creating pre-incident plans for special events and the specific locations or sites that possess the potential for a high loss of life should an event occur. These could include, but are not limited to, stadiums or arena events, amusement parks, visitor attractions, and other events that typically bring in a large number of people. Although it seems impossible to forecast every possible incident that could occur, it is feasible to plan for the most likely occurrence and develop action plans for worst-case scenarios. These plans would include evacuation procedures, communication plans, triage, treatment, and transportation plans, and, most important, security procedures that address responder safety. All of these plans should share similar strategies but also be specific for the individual venue. Not having information or knowledge of the venues can result in major problems.

TRAFFIC CONDITIONS

When creating an EOP for any incident, it must be recognized that the immediate area around an incident site will quickly shut down due to traffic congestion. This can ultimately delay and deny emergency responders' access to the incident site. The preplan must involve cooperation between the local law enforcement and other agencies to quickly gain control of the predetermined entrances and egresses from the incident location as well as the area immediately around it. Besides the issues created by the public, plans must be made to accommodate the influx of emergency vehicles. If the incident involves a fire, the fire apparatus should have clear access. The same goes for EMS. A planned route should be created where an ambulance can come into the scene, receive its patients, and then easily exit the scene toward the transport destination. (See Figure 14.5.) Apparatus staging areas can quickly resolve these issues before they begin if addressed early by incident command (IC) (U.S. Fire Administration, 2004).

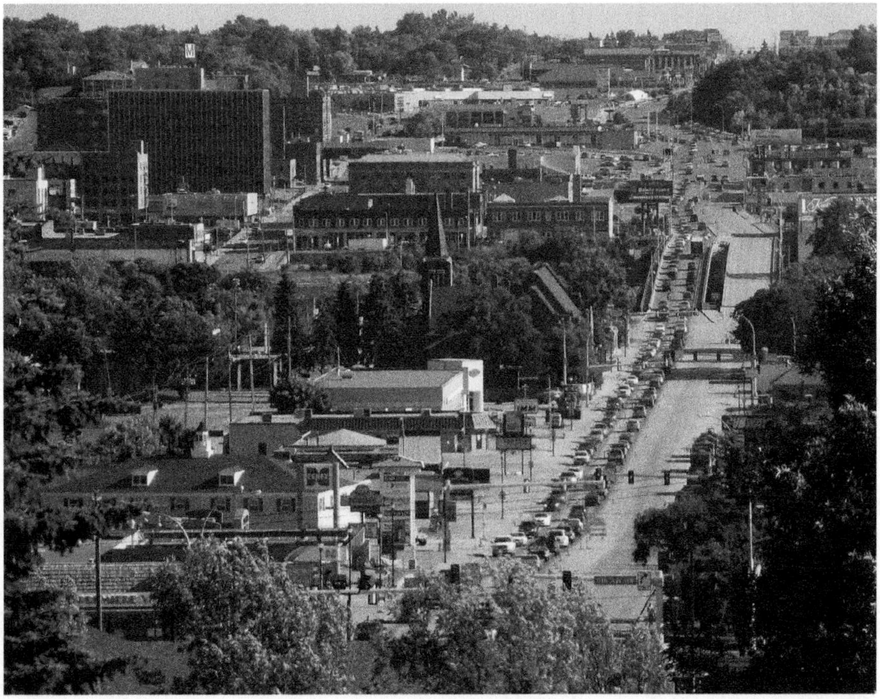

FIGURE 14.5 Proper planning must be conducted to route the evacuation traffic to where it will not interfere with inbound response resources. *Source: Brian Hvinden/FEMA.*

UNREQUESTED ASSISTANCE AND FREELANCERS

As happens during most large-scale incidents, untrained citizen responders or community groups will arrive unexpectedly and attempt to lend assistance to rescue and EMS operations. Not only does this affect an incident commander's accountability plan, but it also creates nearly unmanageable confusion leading to a higher degree of risk for the safety of the citizens, patients, and first responders. This was evident during 9-11 at the World Trade Center as well as the Pentagon. The large influx of unrequested responders and freelancers caused a slowdown of the operation due to issues related to the identity and accountability of responders. In addition, first responders not affiliated with approved or requested mutual aid resources can increase the liability for the authority having jurisdiction (AHJ) due to malpractice and insurance issues, all leading to potential lawsuits and other legal issues.

To combat this issue, securing the scene is of upmost importance and must be done early in the operation. Law enforcement should be utilized to form a security perimeter around the incident site to prevent unauthorized personnel from wandering into the scene. However, in many areas, citizen responders have played an important role in being a force multiplier when they are properly trained and utilized in an organized manner. The **Community Emergency Response Team (CERT) program** was developed by FEMA to train citizens from all walks of life to respond to large events when requested and assist in the mitigation of certain situations, and whose training is commonly at the awareness level.

Self-dispatched emergency response agencies and individuals can also bring their own source of complications to the incident scene. During any large incident, most incident commanders will agree that there cannot be enough help, but the help must be organized and brought in at the right time. Even during the most complex and widespread incidents, a specific and deliberate plan of action must be strictly implemented. Without this operational discipline, not only is safety furthered compromised, but the increased potential for redundancy of actions can lead to inefficient use of resources.

RESPONDER ACCOUNTABILITY

Accountability and responder safety are of upmost importance during any high-risk situation. It must be anticipated that emergency response resources will self-dispatch to large-scale incidents. This issue can be addressed by creating a resource staging area prior to the arrival of all response apparatus and personnel. This can be done by requesting law enforcement to establish traffic choke points to which resources can be routed. From there, all response equipment and personnel can be grouped into a single location where they can be staged until needed. It is imperative that a staging officer be assigned to this function. The use of an effective accountability system is important in keeping track of resources during any incident. Being able to track the location of on-scene response personnel will prevent freelancing and reduce the possibility of losing responders during the event itself. If a responder goes missing, every effort must be made to locate him, even if it includes stopping all operations.

COMMUNICATIONS DISRUPTIONS

During any incident, one of the most important assets is the effective communications between both local and outside emergency response agencies. Not only does this increase responder safety, but it assists with sustaining an organized effort to carry out a single coordinated action plan. Communications fail during an operation for multiple reasons, which usually fall into two general areas: technology failures and organizational failures (U.S. Fire Administration, 2004).

Technology Failures

Technology failures can involve a piece of equipment or a component failing to function properly, leaving the device inoperable. Sometimes response agencies are unable to effectively communicate with each other due to being on different frequencies and bandwidths. Many agencies do not share common frequencies due to technology incompatibilities or the lack of written agreements to utilize the frequencies of their neighboring response agencies. In the past, little thought or effort was expended to bring the different response elements together to talk to each other effectively during large-scale events by means of two-way radios. This has been evident during nearly every incident involving multiple agency responses and is still fairly common today.

Since the 9-11 terrorist attacks, FEMA and the Department of Homeland Security have made interoperable communications a national priority. The goal of this process is to enable emergency service organizations from different disciplines and jurisdictions to communicate with each other by means of common mutual aid frequencies that can be utilized during large-scale incidents. This initiative was the result of the hundreds of agencies involved in the 9-11 events being unable to effectively communicate with each other. An EMS manager should be familiar with the capability and functionality of his own radio system and those of other response agencies within his jurisdiction.

Cellular and data technologies are also vulnerable to failure. During a large-scale incident, cell phones are generally ineffective due to increased demand overloading the system. Many cell phone companies have established mechanisms for giving emergency service workers priority on the system. However, this is not entirely effective (U.S. Fire Administration, 2004).

Organizational Failures

Organizational failures are largely caused by response agencies not working together to establish response procedures for large-scale incidents. This form of communication breakdown can lead to operational disorganization due to agencies not having clear direction about how to effectively work together. To mitigate this, a coalition must be formed between these organizations that effectively establishes the roles and responsibilities of all the different players. This partnership allows for everyone involved to gain a much better understanding of what every counterpart can bring to the table and what can be expected from each in the time of need. This greatly helps to reduce the stress that is created during a response, which may lead to a further breakdown in communications. Even with these agreements and understandings in place, the best-laid plan will fail without practice. Organized drills should be conducted on a regular basis so that all participants can practice their response plans. This will ultimately lead to better communication among the major stakeholders and increase the likelihood of a much better outcome.

SCENE SECURITY

Despite the fact that emergency response personnel respond directly to dangerous situations to perform lifesaving functions, they have increasingly become targets for those who wish to inflict further harm. This was first seen during the Atlanta abortion clinic bombing committed by Eric Rudolph in 1997. In this situation, an initial explosive was detonated in order to draw responders into the scene. A second bomb was positioned in a location that was clearly designed to target first responders. The devise detonated 45 minutes later, injuring five responders and one media cameraman.

As an event occurs, it becomes important to establish clear boundaries around the inner and outer perimeters of the incident to prevent perpetrators from infiltrating the scene and inflicting further violence. It is the primary responsibility of law enforcement to secure an incident scene and deny entry to all unauthorized persons.

When responding to any event, EMS response personnel should always be observant for potential violence. If possible, crews should stage at a distance before entering the scene until law enforcement has secured and cleared the scene. Even then, security is never guaranteed (U.S. Fire Administration, 2004).

Due to the potential for violence toward first responders, FEMA has established new deployment guidelines that require urban search and rescue (USAR) teams to have an attached protection element that is deployed with each team on missions. These protective force elements are made up of law enforcement personnel from the area where the USAR team is home based. Incidents that do not have a USAR response will rely on local law enforcement for security. For this reason, law enforcement from your jurisdiction should be included in the creation of all disaster plans, which should always address scene security. If these resources are limited, other resources should be considered from neighboring jurisdictions. Obtaining resources beyond the local level, such as the National Guard, would require requests to be made to the state EMA, typically from the local EMA.

Security perimeters are based on several different factors. Are there hazardous materials or other inherent hazards that can present a danger to rescuers or the public? How large is the incident site? Does the incident site encompass only a single building or several city blocks? How many resources are available to carry out the security requirement? Is the incident site considered "sensitive" in nature (such as a government facility)? In the latter case, you should expect that state or federal security resources would eventually assume control of the site's security (U.S. Fire Administration, 2004).

Incidents that have the potential to last for multiple work periods require a base-of-operation (BoO). The BoO is the designated location where the incident command and other activities occur. (See Figure 14.6.) These

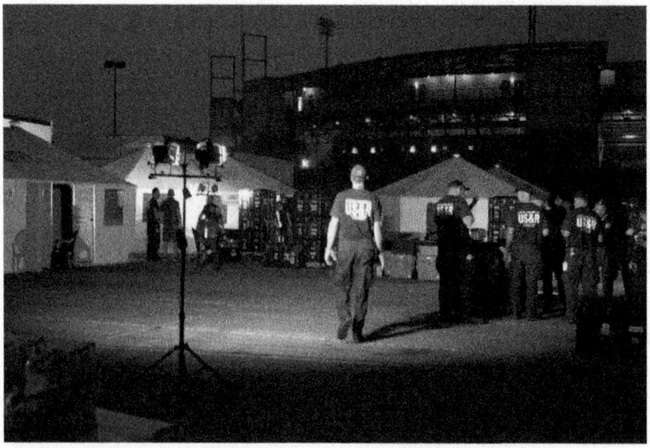

FIGURE 14.6 Bases of operation (BoO) are mobile facilities built to house the response personnel as well as the headquarters during an event. *Source: Jocelyn Augustino/FEMA.*

activities include temporary housing of response personnel, mess kitchens, staging of equipment and supplies, and medical facilities for responders. In the case of Hurricane Katrina, multiple BoO installations became targets for looters who wanted to steal the supplies. Security of the BoO and safety of the emergency responders are imperative and must be taken seriously at all times. This same security sensibility must also be in place with emergency vehicles, both in the staging areas and when in the field on a response. Emergency vehicles should never be left running with the keys inside unless special kill switch modifications have been made to them. If possible, an additional person should stay with each vehicle to deter theft. Even during normal daily operations, EMS crews have become the target of theft from armed perpetrators. If a crew is faced with this situation, resistance may lead to further violence and even death. The crew should immediately surrender the items that are being sought, even if it includes the vehicle.

Containment and security during an incident of national consequence are very fluid and challenging and should be methodically conducted under the direction of trained law enforcement officials. This type of logistics should be well thought out and planned for long before an incident occurs. Waiting until an event of a large magnitude occurs will usually create greater chances for a security breach to occur.

EXPOSURE TO HAZARDOUS CONTAMINATION

Exposure to hazardous contaminants is a risk on any incident scene. Emergency response personnel should assume that an exposure hazard exists—until proven otherwise. (See Figure 14.7.) EMS workers can be contaminated by products of weapons of mass destruction. For example, EMS workers were directly exposed to Sarin gas in the Tokyo subway when they came in close contact with patients. This type of attack would be classified as a **chemical, biological, radiological, nuclear, and explosive (CBRNE)** event. CBRNE is often related directly to **weapons of mass destruction (WMDs)** used by a terrorist with the intent of causing death and destruction. This should not be confused with a hazardous

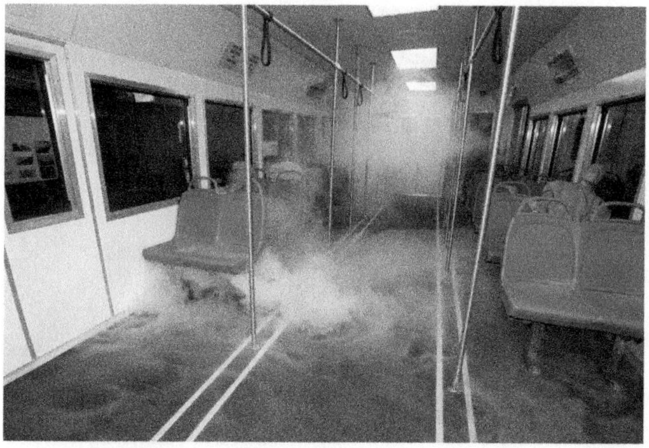

FIGURE 14.7 Response personnel should always be alert to any indication of weapons of mass destruction or hazardous materials when responding to any incident. *Source: Shannon Arledge/FEMA.*

material release, which is an event that typically results from an accidental release of a harmful substance.

Poisons or **toxins** present themselves in many different forms. Solids forms include powders and dust. Anthrax in the form of powder is an example of a solid. Liquid poisons or toxins include the by-products that are created by the production of methamphetamines. Certain chemicals by themselves may be somewhat harmless, but if mixed with other chemicals they can become dangerous. For example, when household bleach is mixed with ammonia, hydrogen sulfide gas is created. Gasses are a result of vaporization of liquids. When a solid reaches a specific temperature, it begins to off-gas vapors by the process of sublimation.

Poisons and toxins can enter the body through four routes: inhalation, absorption, ingestion, and injection. Inhalation can occur when a victim inhales a poison in the form of gas or fine powder. Absorption can occur when a victim's skin comes directly in contact with a substance, such as a liquid. The toxin can be absorbed through the skin and into the bloodstream. Ingestion of a toxin can occur when the victim touches something contaminated and then accidentally puts his hand in his mouth. Poisons can also be injected into the body by a contaminated needle or sharp object.

Performing a thorough pre-arrival size-up is necessary for response personnel to not blindly become victims. Be aware of plumes or vapor clouds that may be carried by prevailing winds. If possible, always approach a scene from upwind and uphill to allow for hazardous vapors or liquids to travel away from you. If hazardous materials are reported, do not enter. Entry should only be facilitated by response personnel trained and with equipment to mitigate these hazards.

Patients contaminated with hazardous substances should be decontaminated prior to being placed in an ambulance. If the situation involved a mass casualty incident (MCI) with multiple contaminated victims, a decontamination corridor should be created and carried out by a hazardous materials team or trained fire department. (See Figure 14.8.) Preparations must be made for emergency decontamination of emergency response personnel. After the decontamination process has been completed, the patients must be transported

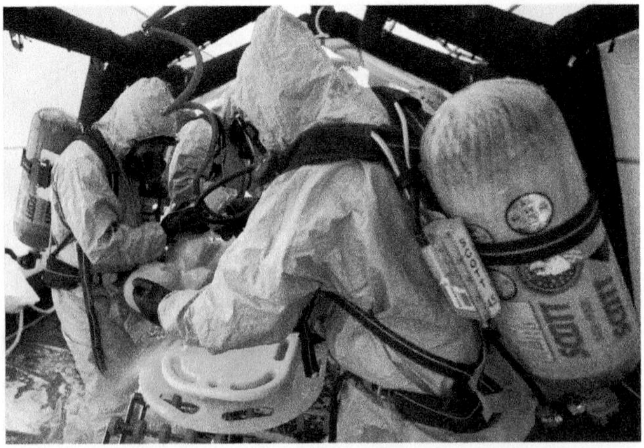

FIGURE 14.8 When mitigating an incident involving a large number of potentially contaminated victims, a decontamination corridor can be established prior to transportation. *Source: Daniells Duff/FEMA.*

to the appropriate facility. Most hospital emergency departments (EDs) now have decontamination facilities at or near the entrances to the ED. Early notification of the hospitals will allow for them to properly prepare their staff and facilities for potentially contaminated patients.

ADDITIONAL HAZARDS

During incidents of national consequence, EMS responders are just as vulnerable to being injured or killed as any other person on the scene. During the Oklahoma City bombing, 37-year-old registered nurse Rebecca Anderson, R.N., responded to the scene to assist after hearing the explosion because she wanted to do what she could to assist in the effort. Before she could help anyone, she was struck in the back of the head by a heavy piece of falling debris, and she later died in the hospital from her injuries. Would-be rescuers make up the large percentage of casualties during large-scale incidents. Much of this is due to the lack of knowledge on the rescuers' part of the existing and potential hazards that are associated with the incident.

Lack of discipline is another contributing factor to the high number of associated rescuer casualties. Response personnel should possess a high level of self-discipline when functioning at these types of event. This is accomplished by rescuers understanding and accepting their training and capability limitations. Without personal discipline, rescuers are likely to take greater risks than is proportional to the benefit.

In addition, compassion should be considered the number-one potential killer of emergency service providers. Compassion for patients is something everybody in EMS is taught from the very first day in training. Although this is a very admirable value to possess, it also is something that is not regularly recommended in the rescue field. The place and time for compassion to lead a rescuer's thought process come after the patient has been freed from the rubble and safely delivered to the care of the EMS providers in the back of the ambulance. Compassion should not drive a decision to take a tremendous risk that has little or no benefit.

Safety during an incident of national consequence should begin from the time a request for response is received. This starts with the 9-1-1 call takers asking specific and thorough questions about the incident and relaying this information to the responders. Responders should always be cautious about total reliance on the accuracy of this information. During a large event, emotions are running high and exaggeration is common. By expecting the worse-case scenario, response personnel can better prepare themselves against a false sense of security.

Response personnel should always conduct a windshield survey before exiting their vehicles. On approach to the scene, they should observe for smoke or cloudy plumes that might indicate a fire or hazardous material release. If the incident is a result of an earthquake, EMS must watch for disrupted utilities such as downed electrical lines, undermined roadways due to water main breaks, and scattered debris. No one should attempt to drive through high water. Even rushing water at 1 foot in depth has enough force to wash away a car. In addition, unstable structures or other objects could collapse. (See Figure 14.9.) In the event of a partial building collapse or a fire, emergency vehicles should not be parked any closer than 1.5 times the height of the involved structure. In situations involving the release of hazardous materials, parking uphill and upwind of the release is best. Upon exiting the vehicle, the process of sizing up a scene should be a continual process and not end until the operation has been terminated. Emergency scenes, especially those of a larger magnitude, are very fluid in nature and can dramatically change without much warning.

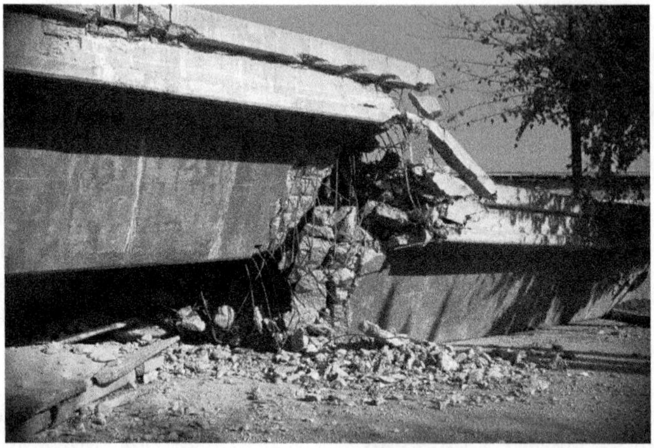

FIGURE 14.9 ■ Responders to earthquakes should be observant of unstable structures, disrupted above- and below-ground utilities, undermined roadways due to water main breaks, and scattered debris. *Source: FEMA News Photo.*

MASS CASUALTY INCIDENTS

The most challenging issue with any large-scale incident is the logistics of caring for a large number of patients. If an emergency response provider arrived first on the scene of an MCI event, it is the responsibility of that EMS provider to activate the established MCI protocol or procedures. Additional help must be summoned immediately. Although that provider may not

Best Practice

An Action Plan and Mutual Aid Resources Save Lives

On July 19, 1989, United Flight 232, a DC-10 with a complement of 300 passengers and crew, took off from Stapleton Airport in Denver, Colorado, bound for Chicago. A catastrophic failure and disintegration of the fan rotor in the rear tail engine resulted in severance of the three hydraulic lines that controlled the aircraft's avionics. The aircraft was diverted to Sioux City airport some 70 miles from its position. During this time, resources in Sioux City, including fire, police, and EMS—immediately implemented a well-designed and practiced disaster plan. At 4:01 P.M., during landing, the left wing of the aircraft struck the ground, causing the aircraft to break into two pieces and erupt into a huge fireball. Resources, already in place, immediately began fire suppression and rescue operations. EMS units quickly converged on the scene and began triaging, treating, and transporting victims. Within 16 minutes of the crash, the first patient arrived at the hospital, where doctors and nurses had already activated their MCI plan. Even more amazing, by 4:40 P.M., just 39 minutes into the incident, the last injured patient arrived at the hospital.

Prior to this event, the local EMS agency had worked diligently with local hospitals, fire departments, and ambulance services from around the region to prepare for a large MCI event. Because of the great amount of effort that was put into their emergency action plan and the utilization of area mutual aid resources, 186 lives were spared.

have the ability to establish incident command, he will need to have the ability to communicate the specific situation and needs to other responding units. Incident command should be transferred to the first-arriving fire official.

In the event that the number of potential victims overwhelms the abilities for the local hospitals, plans should be in place to affectively deal with the patient overload. Many jurisdictions rely on predetermined alternate care sites for this purpose. (See Figure 14.10.) Alternate care sites have been used in many communities. These facilities can be used as makeshift hospitals or temporary care sites for overflow patients. Schools, climate-controlled warehouses, community centers, and other such buildings are excellent facilities to accommodate this need. The success of this lies with trained medical personnel, such as doctors and nurses, to staff these facilities. Many hospitals have in-house field teams that can deploy with the equipment needed to treat patients during these events. These types of arrangements are logistically challenging and must be included within the disaster planning for the local jurisdiction.

Another vital part of mitigating a large-scale MCI is to have an efficient system for bringing in arriving ambulances to a staging area without creating congestion. The units must be able to easily access the transport area where the patients are brought to them from the treatment areas. From there, the crews are given a patient and immediately directed to the appropriate medical facility by the transport officer, who is similar to an air traffic controller in organizing the chaos of multiple arriving and departing resources.

In situations where the incident has a large number of ambulatory stable patients, school or transit busses have been successful for transporting these patients to a medical facility. Prior arrangements can be made through the **local emergency planning commission (LEPC)** or EMA to be utilized during a disaster. Once requested, these services, whether private or government, will send their vehicles along with a driver to the location requested. A trained responder should be assigned to the bus to provide care for these patients until they are safely delivered to a medical facility.

The dissemination of patients is typically conducted by a local or regional medical control center that has the ability to access databases

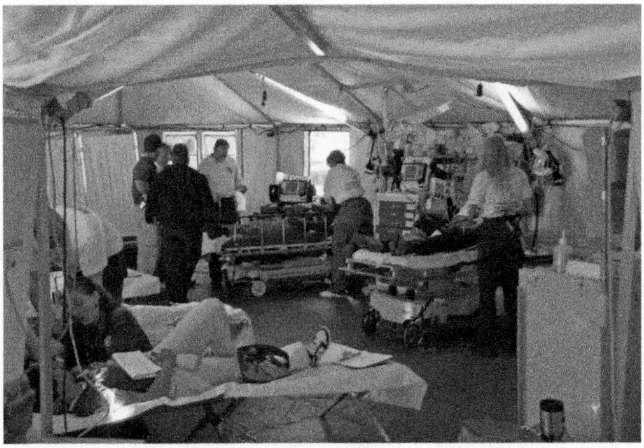

FIGURE 14.10 Disaster medical teams may use predetermined alternate care sites to treat mass numbers of victims. *Source: Marvin Nauman/FEMA.*

which establish the number of empty beds at specific area hospitals based on the patient demand. This information is sent to the transport officer, who then directs the ambulance crew on their transport destination.

Preplanning for these types of events can greatly add to the successful mitigation of an MCI event. Along with preplanning, regularly scheduled MCI drills should be conducted on both the local and regional levels. This type of cooperation among different agencies ensures that everyone is working together more effectively when a real incident occurs.

LONG-TERM EFFECTS ON RESPONSE PERSONNEL

As an event occurs and response personnel arrive to perform their duties, the main focus is the rescue operation. Once the hazards have been mitigated and the last patient has been transported to the hospital, little thought is given to the emergency workers responsible for providing the rescue and patient care. Many studies have been conducted to identify the medical and mental effects caused by the stress of working a large-scale incident. Medical conditions, such as lung and heart diseases, have been directly attributed to exposure to certain contaminants on the scene.

The 9-11 attack on the World Trade Center is an example of response personnel being affected both physically and mentally. The total number of response workers who were affected by the "WTC cough" is still unknown. This condition has been blamed for an unknown number of deaths of WTC 9-11 workers, as well as tens of thousands of other workers who have claimed chronic respiratory problems due to breathing in the contaminated dust from the debris pile of the World Trade Center buildings. Within a year of the disaster, mental health studies started to identify that response workers to the WTC disaster were experiencing the same **post-traumatic stress disorder (PTSD)** as soldiers returning from Afghanistan. This mental health condition can contribute to depression, panic disorders, and a greater likelihood of substance abuse. It can also create a greater chance for disruption of a person's family, work, and social life. It cannot be overlooked that incidents of this magnitude can create additional victims far beyond the conclusion of the event itself. Fire, rescue, and EMS response workers are just as likely to be affected by an incident of national consequence; however, symptoms of this victimization may not be obvious until long after the event. It has been recommended by many mental health professionals that response personnel be given long-term mental health screenings and associated treatment to address these effects (Babbel, 2011).

Forgotten victims of these large-scale incidents are the family members of the response personnel who are suffering from PTSD. When a traumatic event affects one member of the family, other family members can also be affected. In response to their family member suffering from the stress of an event, family members may feel many different emotions, including sympathy for their loved one. Although this is a normal reaction, it can also have negative emotional effects, including the loved one feeling that they are not strong enough to overcome the event. Over time and given the lack of understanding about PTSD, family members can begin suffering from depression, fear and worrying, guilt and shame, anger, and other negative feelings. All of these strong emotions can lead to drug and alcohol abuse, sleep issues, and other health problems. It is important for family members to learn about PTSD and its effects. Most communities have resources through which families can obtain treatment for this disorder.

Many communities train and utilize personnel in critical incident stress debriefings.

These unique teams travel from outside areas to give rescuers the opportunity to talk about their experiences and vent their stress. Although this alone may not prevent PTSD, it does serve to identify those individuals who may need additional assistance. If the rescue and recovery event spans several hours or days, these teams may be brought to the scene.

CHAPTER REVIEW

Summary

An incident of national consequence can strike any community at any time. Such events can vary in scale and present multiple challenges for EMS responders, including lack of response resources, communication breakdowns, exposure to contaminants, and long-term health effects.

There is no realistic way to predict when and where a disaster will strike. For this reason, EMS organizations, along with other emergency response agencies, should be as prepared as possible for mitigating these types of events. This is accomplished by consistent training in and practicing of incident management in both the classroom and in live training exercises involving all of the response agencies within the local and regional jurisdictions. EMS agencies should also review the local and regional response and evacuation procedures for large-scale disasters, including MCI events.

The dynamics of emergency management have changed significantly over the past several decades due to the complexities of large-scale incidents. No one response organization has the ability or resources to effectively manage an incident of national consequence. It requires the cooperation of all of these resources and their unique talents in these times of need to bring a disaster to the best possible conclusion.

WHAT WOULD YOU DO? Review

The event described is an explosion in a federal building that is occupied by a large number of people. The fact that this is a high-profile facility, along with the potential for a high loss of life and large numbers of injured, attracts greater attention from the national media. As you develop an action plan to deal with this event, responder safety should be a top priority. This would include consideration of scene security, existing and potential hazards to responders from debris, contaminants, and secondary devices. In addition, the availability of EMS resources from local and regional agencies, along with the available beds in the area hospitals, should be considered. Adequate communications and an incident command structure should be considered a necessity to successfully mitigate this event.

Initially additional transport units should be requested. A staging area, along with a staging officer should be requested, to organize the incoming units. If the community possesses a regional medical control center, this resource should immediately be activated to initiate the community's MCI plan. Busses may be requested to transport large numbers of ambulatory stable patients. If the event spans over several hours, efforts should be made to recall off-duty personnel to relieve exhausted response personnel. Personnel qualified to deal with critical incident stress should be notified and possibly utilized to begin the initial mitigation for PTSD.

Review Questions

1. What factors define a potential incident of national consequence?
2. What are the issues that may be faced by EMS response personnel when operating at an incident of national consequence?
3. What can be done to reduce the traffic problems that can plague the incident site?
4. What procedures should be employed to create more scene security for response personnel?
5. Why should the first-arriving EMS response unit not immediately begin patient care?
6. Why should response personnel only approach a scene with potential hazardous material from the upwind/uphill direction?
7. What are the advantages of using an established responder accountability system?
8. As an EMS response unit approaches the scene of a large-scale incident, what should the crew be observant for prior to exiting the vehicle?
9. If faced with multiple patients contaminated with a hazardous material, what methods could be employed to conduct decontamination?
10. What is the best approach to reducing the likelihood of organizational failures on the scenes of incidents of national consequence?

References

Babbel, S. (2011, September 12). "Post Traumatic Stress Disorder After 9/11 and Katrina." *Psychology Today.* See the organization website.

Mell, H. K., and M. D. Sztajnkrycer. (2005). "EMS Response to Columbine: Lessons Learned." *The Internet Journal of Rescue and Disaster Medicine*, 5(1). See the organization website.

Metzger, L. R. (2004, September 30). *Emergency Response for Homeland Security: Lessons Learned and the Need for Analysis* (Center for Risk and Economic Analysis of Terrorist Events). Los Angeles, California: University of Southern California.

U.S. Fire Administration, Federal Emergency Management Agency. (2004, May). *Responding to Incidents of National Consequence: Recommendations for America's Fire and Emergency Services Based on the Events of September 11, 2001.* Washington, DC: Federal Emergency Management Agency.

Key Terms

chemical, biological, radiological, nuclear, and explosives (CBRNE) The four hazards terrorists may use to inflict mass destruction.

community emergency response team (CERT) A federal government program that educates people about disaster preparedness for hazards that may impact their community and trains them in basic disaster response skills, such as fire safety, light search and rescue, team organization, and disaster medical operations.

consequence The result that follows an action or event.

emergency operations plan (EOP) The plan maintained by various jurisdictional levels for responding to a wide variety of potential hazards.

incident of national consequence An incident of mass affect that has the potential to impact the entire nation either through the action itself or through the number of patients/fatalities involved.

local emergency planning commission (LEPC) A body made up of officials from law enforcement, fire service, EMS, hospitals, public health, private industry, Red Cross, Salvation Army, military, emergency management agency, and members of the public who are responsible for identifying and cataloging potential hazards, identifying available resources, and creating emergency plans.

poisons Substances that when introduced into the body by inhalation, ingestion, absorption, or injection can cause harm or death.

post-traumatic stress disorder (PTSD) A mental health condition described as a severe anxiety disorder that can be the result of exposure to an event that results in psychological trauma.

toxins Poisonous substances produced by living cells or organisms capable of causing diseases when introduced to the body.

weapons of mass destruction (WMDs) Weapons designed to kill and bring substantial harm to large numbers of people or cause massive destruction.

CHAPTER 15

Developing an EMS-Related Special Operations Team

Eric Powell

Objectives

After reading this chapter, the student should be able to:

15.1 Consider the variables involved in developing an EMS-related special operations team.

15.2 Discuss the different types of EMS-related special operations teams and their primary missions.

15.3 Search and find resources to assist in creating a needs assessment for an EMS-related special operations team.

15.4 Foster advocacy and develop support for the creation of an EMS-related special operations team.

15.5 Explain the variables involved in selecting personnel for an EMS-related special operations team.

15.6 Assess and evaluate training standards and execute initial and annual compulsory training for an EMS-related special operations team.

15.7 Find funding streams to assist in implementing an EMS-related special operations team.

15.8 Discuss the aspects of human resources-related practice with respect to an EMS-related special operations team.

Key Terms

Equal Employment Opportunity Commission (EEOC)
funding streams
mixed methods
needs assessment
Statistical Package for the Social Sciences (SPSS)

WHAT WOULD YOU DO?

You are the operations chief for an EMS department that serves a municipality of approximately 65,000 people. For years, the volunteer rescue squad has performed the vehicle extrication and technical rescue role for your jurisdiction. With the recent downturn in the economy, the local rescue squad has lost a substantial amount of funding and has had to cut back much of their technical capability. Political pressure has motivated the municipal council to contact your EMS chief and have selected technical rescue duties to be transferred to your EMS department. The chief has tasked you to select personnel for the new rescue service provision and to create a budget and standard operating guidelines specific to the rescue role.

Questions

1. With respect to guidance and resources, where would you begin?
2. What considerations should you address in the selection process for the personnel?
3. How would you go about selecting equipment and training?

INTRODUCTION

Developing an EMS special operations team requires the EMS manager to do a great deal of research and develop a solid planning method. (See Figure 15.1.) The ability to be meticulous and think strategically about program and team goals and objectives will position the project manager for success. Team leaders should consider contingencies that might be needed to meet challenges while allowing for compromise when necessary and holding to critical standards when required. The planning process for any emergent service provision is dynamic and fluid; a manager should be ready for changes throughout the endeavor. Economic conditions in the United States may be slow to improve, and the EMS manager involved in this process must be knowledgeable about funding mechanisms as well as imaginative to overcome budgetary challenges.

This chapter will examine the types of EMS-related special operations teams as well as a project manager's major considerations for the development of an EMS-related special operations team. The following are the six major considerations:

1. Needs assessment methodology
2. Advocacy and support development
3. Team selection methods
4. Training
5. Financing
6. Human resources standards

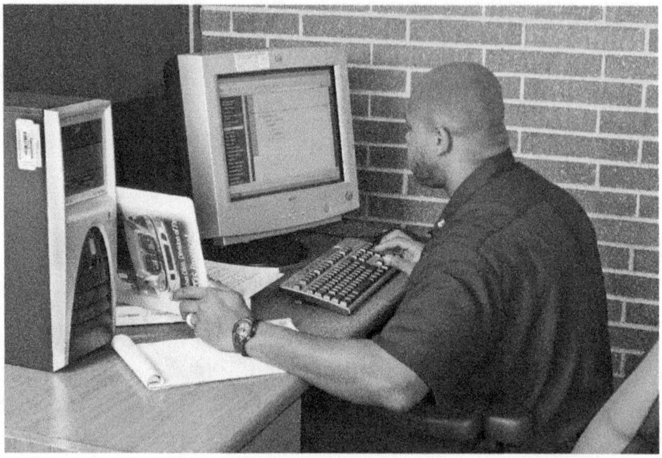

FIGURE 15.1 ■ As the EMS manager you will be responsible for many decisions.

EXAMPLES OF EMS-RELATED SPECIAL OPERATIONS TEAMS

The EMS special operations mission offers opportunities for different types of people to practice within environments/venues that match their personal interests. (See Figure 15.2.) Differences within the special operations teams exist with respect to levels of physicality, proficiency, and work environments. The common component for working within EMS special operations is the commitment to the mission. The missions will vary among EMS departments as needs and resources allow. (See the "Skill Sets for Special Operations" sidebar for prerequisites for most EMS-related special operations teams.)

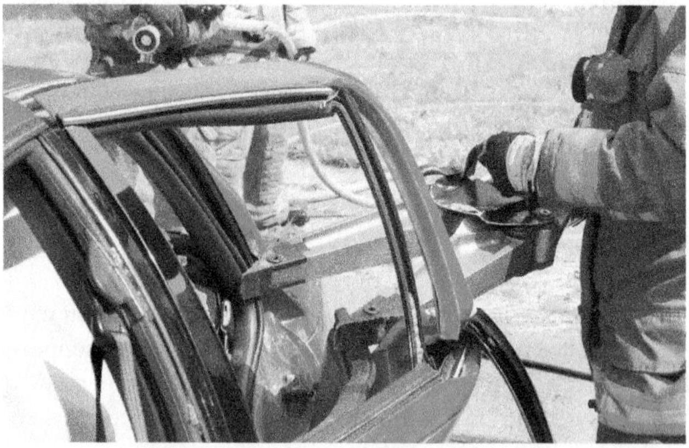

FIGURE 15.2 ■ EMS personnel can take on many roles providing special operations at incident scenes.

Side Bar

Skill Sets for Special Operations

Most EMS-related special operations teams seek the following skill sets:

- Task-specific physical fitness (physical strength, flexibility, and cardiovascular endurance)
- Ability to work in high-stress, high-acuity environments
- Ability to practice with limited/depleted resources to accomplish the mission
- Emotional and psychological stability

VEHICULAR AND MACHINERY RESCUE

Vehicular and machinery rescue involves motor vehicle collisions, industrial machinery entrapment, and farm rescue situations. Members of this type of team will utilize extrication equipment and hand tools. Physical fitness, physical strength (especially the upper body), endurance, and the ability to work in austere, extreme noise and weather environments are considerations for any applicants to position themselves for success. This type of EMS-related special operations team is one of the more common examples.

TACTICAL EMERGENCY MEDICAL SERVICES

Tactical EMTs and paramedics provide a unique and valuable service to law enforcement across the United States by their ability to treat injured and ill tactical team members, civilian victims, and perpetrators. (See Figure 15.3.) This service provision is commonly referred to as tactical emergency medical services (TEMS). TEMS assists in decreasing the liability of law enforcement agencies in specialized and high-risk tactical operations by providing emergent care to those requiring it. In many such operations, a typical EMS response is not feasible due to lack of scene security and external threats.

TEMS personnel should be screened psychologically for fitness of duty. EMS agencies may choose to allow personnel to cross-train as sworn law enforcement officers of various degrees. Capabilities, rules, and regulations vary among agencies. Currently, issues of liability, use of force, and funding are providing challenges for TEMS across the United States.

SWIFTWATER RESCUE OPERATIONS

Swiftwater rescues are specialized operations in river, creek, canal, and dam-release situations. Most of these operations involve flash flooding and severe weather. Candidates for this job go through stringent industry-accepted training and certification. Proficiency with rope rescue skills is of particular value for the EMS swiftwater specialist. Some agencies utilize motorized boat operations as part of their swiftwater rescue service. (See Figure 15.4.) National Fire Protection Association (NFPA) 1006: Standard for Technical Rescuer Professional Qualifications (NFPA, 2013) is a good resource for an interested candidate to review. In addition, personnel selection criteria should include swimming and water endurance examinations.

LIFEGUARD OPERATIONS

Lifeguard operations are prevalent in coastal areas, but there are opportunities for this type of service throughout the United States. This position is different from the swiftwater component as day-to-day lifeguard operations typically utilize less equipment and focus on preventive water safety. The EMS lifeguard may also have responsibilities for rule enforcement (e.g., littering, surfing zone infractions, alcohol, etc.). Prevention is another important

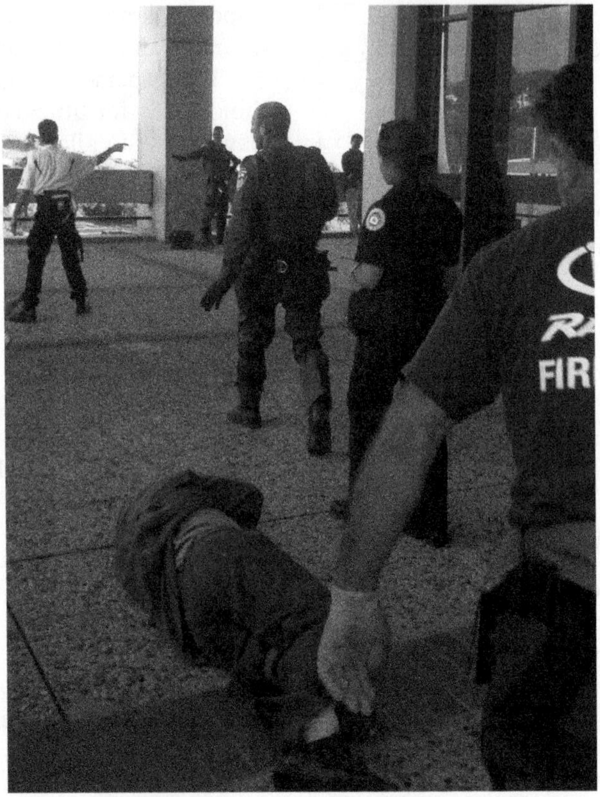

FIGURE 15.3 ■ Some agencies have EMS personnel participating in SWAT incidents providing tactical medicine. *Source: Sam Bradley, Urban Shield, 2011.*

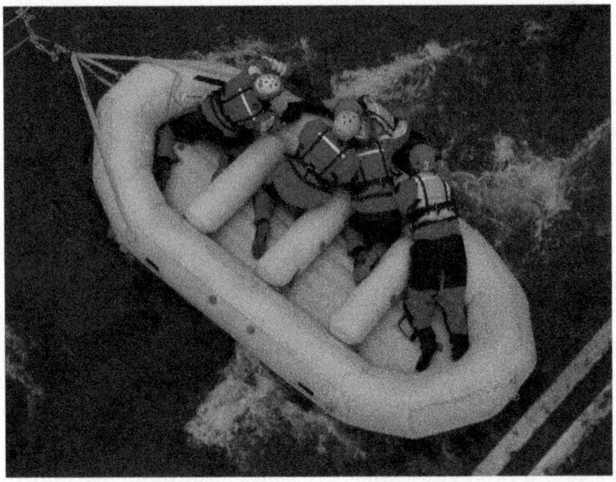

FIGURE 15.4 ■ Water rescue can occur in virtually any location. Personnel need to be trained to effect a rescue in such conditions. *Source: Specialized Figure and Rescue.*

role for the EMS lifeguard. Educating the public on water hazards prior to entering the water or answering questions on rules, swimming areas, and such can minimize problems before they develop. Observation of crowds in and out of the water is a critical task. In addition, personnel selection criteria should include swimming and water endurance examinations that differ from the swiftwater examinations by the use of different equipment and rescue techniques.

HAZARDOUS MATERIALS AND TECHNICAL RESCUE

Common examples of technical rescue include hazardous materials teams, trench rescue, confined-space rescue, and high-angle rescue. Hazardous materials and technical rescue teams are two of the most common teams of EMS special operations examples and offer EMS agencies many daily incidents across the United States. (See Figure 15.5.) Certification

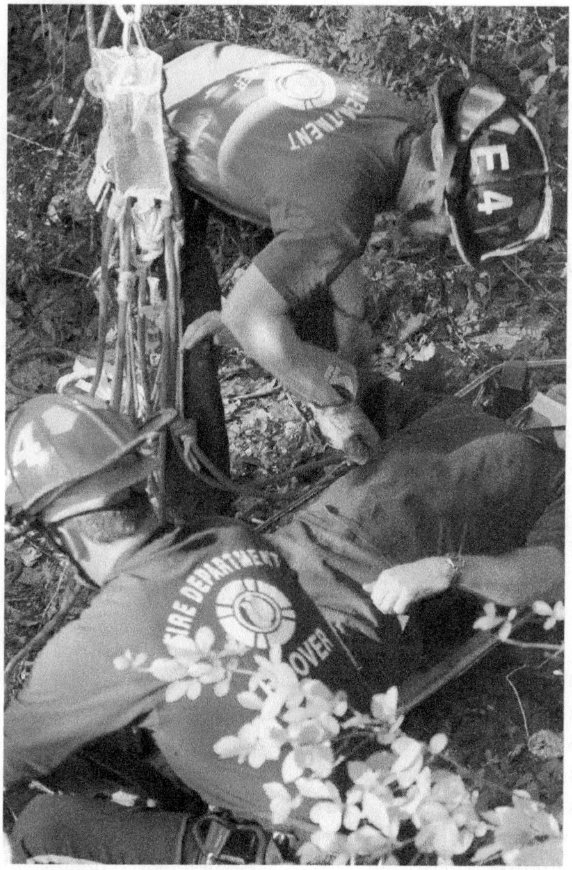

FIGURE 15.5 ■ EMS may perform or assist with various specialized teams.

courses for these types of operations can be measured in weeks in some situations. With respect to hazardous materials, National Fire Protection Association (NFPA) 473: Standard for Competencies for EMS Personnel Responding to Hazardous Materials/Weapons of Mass Destruction Incidents (NFPA, 2013) is a good resource for an interested candidate to review. Continuing education with these specialties is mandatory and must be adhered to strictly. In addition, personnel selection criteria should include specific screening for phobias associated with use of self-contained breathing apparatus, confined spaces, and heights.

AEROMEDICAL OPERATIONS

Of all the specialized teams listed in this section, this particular endeavor will be cost-prohibitive for almost all EMS agencies when considering capital outlays for aircraft, maintenance, parts, insurance, ancillary equipment, and more. (See Figure 15.6.) Selection criteria should include medical screening as appropriate and mandated by the Federal Aviation Administration.

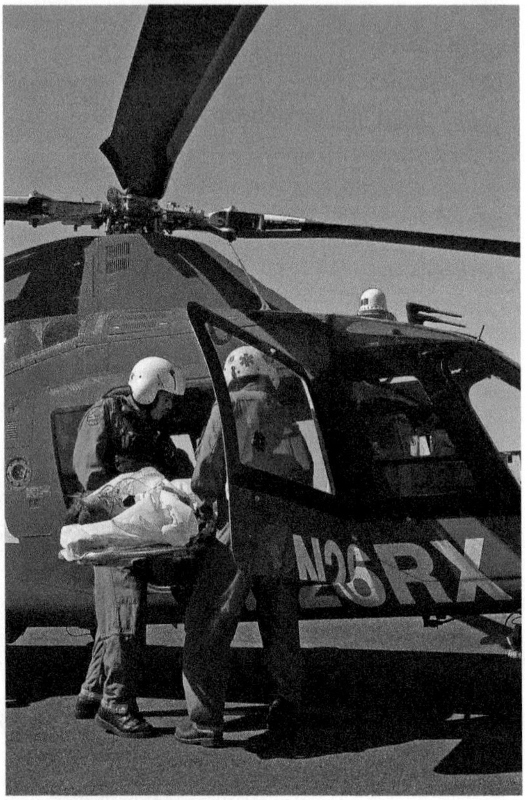

FIGURE 15.6 ■ Flight medicine is considered special operations in EMS.

SPECIAL EVENTS TEAMS

Special events teams cover situations such as sporting events, concerts, fairs, political protests, and attractions. This work environment does not typically have as high a level of physical and/or mental stressors as the other special operations teams listed in this section. However, this team can be a valuable asset as the general public will be interacting with them in nonexigent environments. Team selection criteria should include clinical proficiency testing and an assessment center utilizing instrumentation to measure interpersonal interactions. Special events response can involve major stressors and challenges as experienced in 2013 at the Boston Marathon IED bombing.

COMMUNITY-BASED PARAMEDIC

Community-based paramedics typically possess an exceptional clinical proficiency. This work environment typically does not have any additional physical requirements beyond what is typical in the EMS profession. Community-based paramedics deal more with the chronically ill and/or minor/routine provision of medical care such as caring for influenza/colds, wound care, and providing immunizations.

Community-based paramedics may be considered to be advanced-practice paramedics.

CRITICAL CARE PARAMEDIC

Critical care paramedics have additional skill sets for working with ventilator patients, balloon pumps, and expanded pharmacological formularies. These team members may work on ground-based advanced life support units or aeromedical services. Team selection should focus on clinical proficiency and quality assurance and improvement histories. Critical care paramedics also may be considered advanced-practice paramedics.

Critical care paramedics are not needed for every service, as that level of patient care has to be established. Reimbursement streams for critical care can be complex or nonexistent. The resources required for critical care service provision include a strong medical direction component, a committed health care system, and a stringent quality improvement process. Critical care paramedics also carry a higher degree of liability due to their increased skill set. Maintenance of skills proficiency is

Best Practice

Guilford County Bicycle Emergency Response Team

The Guilford County (North Carolina) EMS (GCEMS) Bicycle Emergency Response Team (BERT) began in the 1993–1994 timeframe with the demands of the Greater Greensboro Open PGA Golf Tournament (now known as the Wyndham Championship). At the time, EMS coverage was necessary, but there were significant restrictions on motorized vehicles. The bicycle EMS team was born, offering the agency many more applications as time passed.

GCEMS Captain/Paramedic Mike Hudspeth, the current BERT team leader, has been in charge of the team since 2000. His leadership has been exemplary as the team follows the most stringent public-safety bike standards in the United States through the International Police Mountain Bike Association (IPMBA). The standard IPMBA course for the EMS providers is 32 hours in length and focuses on bicycle safety, defensive cycling, slow-speed skills, and balance technique; all are critical skills when working among highly populated public venues. In addition, qualified applicants are indoctrinated in public relations skills as the paramedics assigned to the team are very approachable to the general public when on duty. The prerequisites for candidates for the BERT team are 1 year of service, a stringent review of employment and clinical proficiency history, a strong recommendation from the candidate's supervisor, and a successful attempt during the tryout phase, which is typically held in October of each year.

During the tryout phase, candidates must complete a 6-mile ride with equipment within 30 minutes. Afterward, they must perform 5 minutes of CPR while answering scenario questions to elicit correct responses under stress. The preceptors are graded under a standard to assess clinical proficiency, efficacy, and the ability to communicate with family members and the public during exigent patient care. In addition, the candidates must successfully navigate three significant obstacle courses that evaluate balance, coordination, and time restrictions.

The team members offer Guilford County EMS the ability to reach areas that are not conducive to ambulance or all-terrain vehicle use. In crowded urbanized areas, the team members can quickly navigate and traverse areas that would take additional EMS units much longer. Bridging the gap between traveling by ambulance and by foot is a value-added component to traditional EMS service provision.

an added component for this role. In addition, there is no national standard and very few state standards for critical care paramedic certification/licensure.

DEVELOPMENT OF AN EMS-RELATED SPECIAL OPERATIONS TEAM

The EMS manager tasked with developing an EMS special operations team has a substantial number of variables to consider. This development process cannot be completed alone. The successful EMS manager will seek out counsel and feedback from stakeholders inside and outside of the organization. The six major considerations that an EMS project manager should consider during the development process are as follows:

- Needs assessment
- Advocacy and support development
- Team selection
- Training
- Financing
- Human resources considerations

THE NEEDS ASSESSMENT

An EMS-related special operations team must be proven necessary for a specific municipality or county in order for it to be implemented and appreciated. Local government leadership may view an EMS-related special operations team with some disdain, especially if there is not an articulated need for it. As the United States experiences a continued downturn in the economy, **funding streams** for new projects and programs will be highly competitive. The idea for a special operations team will be competing with other human services, transportation, law enforcement and fire service, and public works projects. Provision of a **needs assessment**, with statistically accurate data sets and projected outcomes, will be critical to the success. By proving that an EMS-related special operations team will improve public safety, public health, and morbidity and/or mortality-related outcomes will aid in the success and implementation of this team.

Fortunately, for the project manager who is creating an EMS-related special operations team, there are many textbook and Internet resources to assist them in performing a statistically valid and factually accurate needs assessment. The needs assessment will establish the facts needed to bring forward the idea for the project. Some needs assessments will be short, with limited groups, and others will be comprehensive and include the provision of a community/advanced practice paramedic who may have a broad spread of stakeholders.

The University of Kansas website has a program entitled *The Community Toolbox*, which provides guidance on how to carry out a comprehensive needs assessment via the following seventeen specific steps (University of Kansas, 2013):

1. *What are our reasons for choosing to do this survey?* As the EMS project manager with responsibilities for developing a special operations team, the manager will either recognize a situation that requires an intervention, such as adding another operational mission task such as vehicular and machinery rescue, or a task will be appointed to the manager from the command staff, administration, or municipal/county government.
2. *What are our goals in doing this survey?* The main goal of the survey is to find out if a specialized team is needed and/or feasible. Remember, it is just as valuable to find out that creation of an EMS-related special operations team is not needed or is not feasible as it is otherwise. No matter what, if the needs assessment is carried out correctly and is valid, the data will be of use to the EMS manager.
3. *Are we ready to conduct this survey?* Make sure there are resources to conduct the survey.

The project manager should be ready for a lot of work and motivation to see the project completed in a comprehensive manner. The public demands the best effort for EMS provision.

4. *Decide how much time you have to do the survey, from start to finish.* Establish timeframes and deadlines during the needs assessment process and try to meet benchmarks. As the EMS manager, being a good time manager will increase your chances of success.
5. *Decide how many people are going to be asked.* How many people will it take to provide the leadership and constituency with valid, reliable data? Establishing relationships with people who are experts in research or data collection methods is an ideal undertaking in this situation. The manager's first attempts at establishing these relationships might be at the local college, university, or public health department.
6. *Decide what kinds of people are going to be asked.* This is marginally easier than deciding how many people are going to be asked. In the beginning, the EMS manager may include command staff and the medical director in order to keep everyone informed about the project. Other examples include the general public, public health officials, transportation officials, primary care providers, law enforcement officials, elected local/state leadership, and so on. A particular agency's situation will dictate who is included in the needs assessment data collection.
7. *Decide what questions will be asked.* One of the best ways to approach this situation is to brainstorm or perform a free-writing exercise to get thoughts on paper. Allow those initial questions to be reviewed by knowledgeable colleagues who are exposed to the actual or perceived need. The EMS project manager should not be afraid to receive constructive criticism or revision; it will make for a stronger assessment.
8. *Decide who will ask the questions (or write the questions).* The EMS manager needs to select the right person or author who understands that different people have different perceptions, understanding, intellectual acuity, cultural norms, language, and so on.
9. *Create a draft of the full survey.* Remember, the first draft is the first draft. Almost 100 percent of the time, the manager will be making changes to the needs assessment instrumentation in the beginning.
10. *Try out the survey on a test group.* Always perform a pilot test or two. All needs assessments will benefit from having the bugs worked out a time or two. Not doing a pilot test almost guarantees some untoward event happening in the assessment process.
11. *Revise the survey on the basis of your test group feedback.* As noted in this list, the EMS manager wants to get things right in the real-time distribution. Do not be afraid of changing things.
12. *When you are satisfied that all necessary revisions have been made, administer the survey to the people you have chosen.* At this point, go ahead and take a short amount of time to review the selected persons or groups to receive the survey. The EMS project manager may want to revise the distribution slightly to provide accurate data.
13. *Tabulate your results.* There are many different ways to tabulate data. The EMS manager can search out means of central tendency by hand and calculator, utilize computer programs such as the **Statistical Package for the Social Sciences (SPSS)**, or perform content or narrative analysis on focus group comments.
14. *Interpret your results.* The EMS project manager should not be afraid to get expert help with interpreting results. Invariably, a good statistician may find relevant data that might otherwise be overlooked. Ask several colleagues, a supervisor, and the medical director to take a look at the data and identify trends. Be mindful if the needs assessment project is sensitive in nature. In that case, make it a need-to-know distribution.

15. *Plan future actions.* The EMS manager begins problem solving to meet the challenge of what is needed. Throughout this process, objectivity needs to be maintained, and the EMS manager can compromise and negotiate with stakeholders, decision makers, and any opposition.
16. *Implement your actions.* The level of detail in this phase needs to be just as good as it was in the development process. Remember, every good plan for implementation is perfect, until it is implemented. Expect that there will be revisions along the way.
17. *Repeat your assessment at regular intervals.* The EMS manager must investigate the data to look for positive outcomes. For example, if a community-based paramedic team is created, the manager might investigate data on targeted morbidity statistics, patient satisfaction, reduction of emergency department overcrowding situations, impacts on medical accessibility for underserved populations, and so on. The most important outcome EMS practitioners want to impact is the decrease of morbidity and mortality.

A needs assessment does not have to be a numerical data set by itself. In fact, a qualitative method, such as personal interviews or focus groups can be of considerable value as well as valid in their application. Another type is a **mixed methods** survey, using both quantitative and qualitative data. This method is gaining popularity as well as scientific acceptance.

ADVOCACY AND SUPPORT DEVELOPMENT

Good EMS administrators know that any substantive operational implementation idea needs support on many different levels. Those EMS administrators who recognize political opportunities and know how to collaborate can pull off projects that otherwise would have been short lived. The EMS manager must be detail oriented and have some level of political prowess. Four traits that will be beneficial to the EMS manager when seeking advocacy and support will be the ability to communicate, collaborate, negotiate/compromise wisely, and lead.

Communication

When an EMS project manager develops a special operations team, it helps to recognize that a good communication skill set will be a critical component to the success of the endeavor. Therefore, thoughtful and clear interactions will be to their advantage.

Communication, whether written or oral, reaches all of the constituents of the special operations team. The EMS project manager must provide cogent information to a varied number of people in many forms of clarity and complexity. For example, speaking to a community group will be much different than writing a briefing to your county's administrative and financial team.

Listening to all of your constituents will be just as important, if not more so, than your oral and written directives. If the EMS project manager is perceived as not listening to suggestions or counsel, then he should expect more challenges and push-back to his efforts.

EMS practitioners communicate on many different levels. With such a diverse array of stakeholders and with proper planning, they can position themselves for success. Subsequently, during the selection process for special operations team members, communications skills should be assessed as work responsibilities will differ from field practitioners in traditional roles. Consider the importance of an EMS special operations team member working at a special event with the opportunity to interact with the general public on a continuous basis for an 8-hour shift.

Collaboration

As EMS personnel work together daily to maintain operational rhythm and provide a standard of care to their patients, one can reason that the EMS project manager with the task of developing a special operations team may possess this skill set to some degree. However, bringing in diverse groups, political affiliations, and interests into the mix of team development can be a considerable challenge. Diverse special interests in a project demand a creative and effective collaborative facilitator.

In their research, Snead and Wycoff (1997) indicated the presence of collaboration barriers among team members. A partial list of their findings is directly applicable to EMS project management and what the EMS manager may face as the team is developed. This list includes:

- Need to know policies
- Rigid hierarchical structure
- Chain of command communication restrictions
- Separation of functional areas
- Shiftwork (*Source: Excerpt from To Do Doing Done: A Creative Approach to Managing Projects & Effectively Finishing What Matters Most by G. L. Snead and J. Wycoff. Published by Simon & Schuster, © 1997, p. 213.*)

Other collaboration barriers that are well known to EMS and public safety are turf guarding, political sensitivities, apathy, antagonism, and fatigue or burnout. The EMS project manager must create enthusiasm for the special operation team's development.

Negotiation and Compromise

When creating an EMS Special Operations team, negotiation and compromise go hand in hand. The EMS project manager and his staff may have a vision for development of a special operations team, but it could end up looking nothing like what was envisioned if negotiation skills are not properly used.

Common strategies used in negotiation of projects are readily available to the EMS project manager. These strategies may include:

- Constantly seek opportunities for collaboration, even issues that seem contentious may be worked through
- Find shared opportunities for accomplishments between groups
- Clearly express your group or organizational goals
- Actively listen to different viewpoints
- Never intentionally misinform or hide information; integrity issues will end the process
- Seek out information if an issue or question is incomplete

The ability to thoughtfully and effectively compromise when needed is another positive trait of a negotiator. Knowing what battles are winnable, when to acquiesce, and when to compromise and still effectively get the job done will position the special operations team development project for success.

Leadership

Within a given textbook, a section on leadership could be well over 150 to 200 pages in length. We will focus here on what leadership traits might be helpful in the project manager aspect of EMS special operations team creation. (Refer to the "Traits of a Leader" sidebar for some universally accepted traits of a leader.)

Side Bar

Traits of a Leader

Active listener	Honest	Even tempered
Objective	Rational	Self-motivated
Compassionate	Serves others	Emotionally mature
Energetic	Team player	Competent
Communicates well	Fair minded	Moral
Proficient	Empathetic	Ethical
Consistent in actions		

TEAM SELECTION

An EMS special operations team must have the proper human resources capital to staff the team. The team members, their proficiencies, and their commitment to the team mission are just as important as planning, implementation, and policy development. In addition, during team selection, standardized human resources principles should be followed at all times. The considerations for EMS special operations team selection are physical fitness/physical fitness assessments, psychological fitness/psychological fitness assessments, assessment center utilization with standardized criteria, clinical skills assessment, and criminal background/workplace disciplinary record check. Some team selection activities may have significant costs associated with them (e.g., physical fitness equipment, time scheduled for fitness assignments, etc.).

Physical Fitness Assessments

The agency may already have a physical fitness assessment instrument/evaluation program. If so, this is a great starting point for a particular special operations team. The physical fitness assessment must be functional in order to be valid. Having candidates complete a timed long-distance run for a TEMS position without assessing their upper body strength would not meet the criteria for a functional assessment. The physical fitness assessment must assess the functional work responsibilities of the team member's roles and responsibilities. In addition, command staff/administration must review the prospective physical fitness assessment with the human resources department before administering it to candidates. Consistency in application of the assessment to the candidates is also important. The EMS manager may be asked to develop or distribute a liability waiver to each candidate prior to the assessment. Prospective EMS managers should also follow the agency's policies and operational guidelines.

Psychological Fitness Assessments

Some EMS-related special operations teams will require a psychological examination by a psychologist (i.e., TEMS). This could include both a written examination and an interview. These assessments can be expensive and be mandated yearly by some agencies. Counsel with the human resources department and/or legal counsel should be sought for any questions about this type of evaluation and the agency's involvement.

Assessment Center Utilization

A standardized assessment center may be a good idea when evaluating candidates for a special operations role. Typically, training bureaus of the agency involved run these centers. Standardized instrumentation, scenarios, time frames, and interrater reliability are fostered in these types of environment. These centers project a fair and equal opportunity to the candidates, and they decrease liability and otherwise untoward events for the agency involved.

Clinical Skills Assessment

A clinical skills assessment may be warranted for any of the special operation team candidates. After all, the main role, no matter what team a candidate is selected for, is patient care. The major consideration for a clinical skills assessment is the alignment of the assessment to the functional work responsibility of the particular team member and his role. Two evaluators per station are recommended to enhance interrater reliability.

Criminal Background/Workplace Disciplinary Record Check

The criminal background investigation criterion is most likely used by the agency for new hires. Having the ability to review disciplinary records will vary from agency to agency, so relevant operational guidelines and policies should be followed. The ability to review a candidate's record for untoward or repetitive disciplinary infractions will be of value in the overall assessment of the candidate. In the case of a TEMS candidate, this may be of significant importance to the agency and the law enforcement agency with which the department is partnering.

TRAINING

When planning for the training aspect of an EMS special operations team, there are many elements to consider. The following are some of the most important elements:

1. Cost/capital equipment
2. Reputation/proficiency of the training cadre and the curriculum
3. Ability of personnel to successfully complete training
4. Mandatory/compulsory continuing education to maintain specialty training certifications

Training costs can be substantial, and when the increased costs associated with an EMS special operations team are added in, the financial consideration alone can stop the EMS manager from developing a special operations team.

FINANCING

Financing an EMS special operations team may be one variable that provides a barrier that cannot be overcome easily. The EMS manager must have a considerable number of tasks completed and/or considered before seeking funding. In addition, the EMS manager must avail himself to difficult and exacting questions and fact finding to bring the project forward to implementation. The start-up costs will be one of the aspects to consider when bringing forward the project proposal to decision makers who can make the project happen. Accuracy with start-up cost projections will be critical to the success of the project. A small measure of overestimation of funding is better than having cost overruns. The consequences of a significant cost overrun could cause the EMS special operations team to be cancelled.

Public Sector Grants and Foundations

Public sector grants comprise a type of funding stream that is typically sought after by public safety agencies when they have a substantial capital need and a municipal budget that does not meet the need. Many types of grants are available. Although there may not be an existing public sector grant guide specific for EMS, other resources may be helpful in grant writing and submission. Here are several examples:

1. The Federal Emergency Management Agency (2012) has a "Grants & Assistance Program for Emergency Personnel" section on its website that provides a good starting point for the EMS project manager seeking funding for their special operations team.
2. The International Chiefs of Police (IACP) has a "Best Practice Guide: Grant Writing" (Bridget Newell, n.d.). Even though the publication was written for the law enforcement profession, the guide still provides valuable information for the EMS manager.
3. The Department of Homeland Security (n.d.) grant funding information is comprehensive in its scope and is another worthwhile starting point for the EMS manager.
4. Third-party grant assistance also may be obtained, as there are many different private companies that assist in the grant process. Some assist with grant writing; others assist in the application process. Please note that these companies are for-profit and can incur a cost to your agency. Be thorough and ask as many

questions as you can of the company regarding costs, requirements, and contractual issues. Key terms to use during an Internet search are *grant writing, grant writing assistance,* and the like.

Municipal/County Budgeting

An EMS manager will generally have an above-average working knowledge of the budget in its entirety, but do not hesitate to find a mentor to use as a guide through this process. The current and past budgets can be used to establish the baseline for the financial requirements. An EMS-related special operations team's impact on the agency budget will be one of the first questions asked by decision-making leadership. Be ready to address their questions and anticipate what questions may be asked. This is a good strategic-thinking tactic that can be used with staff or interested parties with whom you may be working.

Special Taxation

In some situations, a special tax may be established to assist or fully fund a public safety endeavor. An example of this type of legislation is California Proposition 30, which guarantees funding for public safety services that have been aligned from state to local status. Although this example does not specifically address EMS-related special operations team, it does impact the continued service of existing teams within that framework.

Donations

Donations are effectively utilized by volunteer organizations and should not be dismissed as an option if it is legal for the EMS agency to accept them. Being able to articulate a need for a special operations team to stakeholders in the volunteer or combination delivery model is just as important as the paid career model.

Legal Considerations

When considering pursuit of a funding stream(s), the project manager must be cognizant that some legal restrictions exist that may prevent access or be illegal. Situations exist that prohibit municipal/county agencies from accessing certain types of funds. A legal representative/liaison can assist in this situation.

HUMAN RESOURCES CONSIDERATIONS

The EMS manager will want to work very closely with the human resources department and command staff with respect to any condition related to personnel working within the EMS special operations context. Being familiar with **Equal Employment Opportunity Commission (EEOC)** guidelines and practices must be one of the first things to consider, and those guidelines and standards must be adhered to throughout the entire process, even into operations. Specialized medical screening and physical examinations may be warranted for special operations personnel; these screenings may be over and above what is typically done for other EMS personnel and be recurrent in their application. Be receptive to real or perceived human resources issues as you plan for and solicit feedback from stakeholders.

CHAPTER REVIEW

Summary

The EMS manager responsible for the development of an EMS special operations team will have substantial tasks and will need to create positive working relationships with many different types of stakeholders, both internal and external to their agency. Understanding the needs assessment process is a critical trait for the EMS manager as it allows for a structured process to prove or disprove the project. Learning about team selection and sustainability factors from EMS agencies with similar and successful teams will help the EMS manager a great deal during team implementation. In addition, a working knowledge of human resources policies and procedures as well as a prudent and accurate approach to budgeting will round out the basic foundation that will position the EMS manager and the special operations team for success.

WHAT WOULD YOU DO? Reflection

In your role of operations chief for an EMS department, you have been tasked to create a technical rescue extrication team for your agency. There are several places to begin in order for you to meet this task from your municipal leadership and citizens. The following is a preliminary listing of places and resources you could consider:

- Data from your dispatch center as to the number of rescue squad responses that list types of response and locations of response. These data should be correlated with response reports generated from the rescue squad. Look specifically for technical rescue situations.
- Inventory of types of rescue squad equipment (i.e., apparatus, specialized equipment, and supplies) as well as their utilization history. You may or may not be able to acquire any existing rescue squad equipment for use, so be ready to purchase needed equipment and justify why you need it.
- Assess your personnel as to their ability to perform the new mission tasking as well as the cost for training to update skill sets to perform the new mission. Make sure that any training is taught by those with the appropriate expertise, certification/licensure, and regulatory compliance.
- Identify funding streams to assist in cost-deflection of the new team.

The candidates for the new team should have the following mandates/traits: be physically fit in order to perform the new task, be willing to attend and successfully complete training, be willing to maintain proficiency in this new role via recurrent training if needed, and be willing to work in the austere/diverse environments of EMS special operations. The agency must follow accepted Equal Employment Opportunity Commission (EEOC) and human resource standards at all times during the selection process and implementation. The appropriate life safety equipment should be provided to all team members, and specialized medical and psychological screening should be conducted if warranted for any EMS special operations team member.

There are many agencies and expertise in public safety from which to seek counsel. Begin with your state's EMS or public safety commission/division. Identify agencies and departments that have performed the type of specialized operation with success and gather information about their standard operating guidelines, human resources procedures, and apparatus/equipment lists. If there is an existing regulatory agency that has jurisdiction over your new mission, make contact with that agency, find out how your agency can be compliant, and ask about training standards and delivery. You may want to have an experienced agency and personnel provide training to your department.

Review Questions

1. What aspects of your EMS agency or outside variables would you consider in the early stages of developing an EMS-related special operations team?
2. As you consider your stakeholders in the development of EMS-related special operations team, list those people/entities from whom you would seek advocacy. Provide reasons why you selected those people/entities.
3. Go back to question 1 and select an EMS-related special operations teams, or two teams, that would provide benefit to the people of your community. From that, what considerations would you make with selection of team members?
4. What equipment and support materials will you require for your team?
5. What do you as the project manager envision with respect to training needs for the personnel selected for your team? Will there be a need for any recurrent and/or mandatory/regulated training? What cost is associated with these variables?
6. If possible, obtain a copy of the current and past year's operational budget for your EMS agency. What are some line items and trends that would be barriers to developing your team as well as line items and trends that may assist you in developing your team?
7. From the previous question, what funding streams would you seek and why? If you were the project manager for a volunteer EMS agency, how would you market a fund-raising strategy to implement an EMS special operations team?
8. For the selection of your EMS-related special operations team members, what characteristics of the selection process will provide a fair, accurate, and effective process?
9. Ultimately, what should be the end goal for the creation of your EMS-related special operations team?
10. What barriers to communication and collaboration in your agency need to be changed in order for you to successfully develop a special operations team?

References

Berkowitz, W. R. (1982). *Community Impact: Creating Grassroots Change in Hard Times.* Cambridge, MA: Schenkman Publishing.

Cox, F. M., J. L. Erlich, J. Rothman, and J.E. Tropman (eds). (1987). *Strategies of Community Organization: Macro Practice,* 4th ed. Itasca, IL: F. E. Peacock Publishers.

Fawcett, S. B., A. Paine-Andrews, V. T. Francisco, K. P. Richter, R. K. Lewis, et al. (1994). "Preventing Adolescent Pregnancy: An Action Planning Guide for Community Based Initiatives." Lawrence, KS: University of Kansas.

Federal Emergency Management Agency. (2012). "Grants & Assistance Program for Emergency Personnel." See the organization website.

National Fire Protection Association. (2013). "Standard for Technical Rescuer Professional." See the organization website.

Neuber, K. A. (1980). *Needs Assessment: A Model for Community Planning.* Beverly Hills, CA: Sage Publications.

Newell, B. (n.d.). "Best Practice Guide: Grant Writing." Alexandria, VA: International Association of Chiefs of Police.

Snead, G. L., and J. Wycoff. (1997). *To Do, Doing, Done.* New York: Fireside/Simon & Schuster.

Taylor, J. (2006). *A Survival Guide for Project Managers,* 2nd ed. New York: American Management Association.

University of Kansas. (2013). "Conducting Needs Assessment Surveys." *The Community Tool Box.* See the Community Tool Box website.

U.S. Department of Homeland Security. (n.d.). "DHS Financial Assistance." See the organization website.

Key Terms

Equal Employment Opportunity Commission (EEOC) An agency responsible for enforcing federal laws that make it illegal to discriminate against a job applicant or employee due to the person's race, color, religion, sex, national origin, age, disability, or genetic information.

funding streams The identified and available funding prospects for a project or cause.

mixed methods A data collection/research strategy that uses both quantitative (numbers) and qualitative (narrative) methods.

needs assessment A methodical process of focusing on needs.

Statistical Package for the Social Sciences (SPSS) Computer program for tabulating data.

Glossary

accountability system A system implemented within the incident command system to track the location of personnel as they arrive on the scene and continued throughout the course of an incident until it is terminated.

access and egress equipment The equipment utilized by confined-space rescue teams to enter into and exit from a confined space.

air management officer An attendant who is assigned to oversee and track the time in and air usage by entry personnel while operating within a confined space.

AMBER Alert Program AMBER is an acronym for "America's Missing: Broadcasting Emergency Response," named originally for Amber Hagerman, a 9-year-old child who was abducted and murdered in Arlington, Texas, in 1996. AMBER Alerts are broadcasted via commercial radio stations, television stations, and cable TV by the Emergency Alert System, NOAA Weather Radio, and many Department of Transportation highway signs.

anchors A natural or manmade object that is used as part of a system to anchor the ropes and rigging devices used in a rope rescue system.

anthrax An infectious disease due to a bacterium called *Bacillus anthracis*. Infection in humans most often involves the skin, gastrointestinal tract, or lungs.

antibiotics Types of medication used to damage or destroy bacteria, thus allowing the body to ward off an infection.

antivirals A broad application that is developed to target either a specific virus or in certain instances.

approach hazard A hazard that may be encountered EMS personnel while responding to the scene of an incident.

attendant Someone trained in permit-required confined-space entry and surface rescue who remains outside of the confined space and monitors the safety of the authorized entrant or entry team.

Authority Having Jurisdiction (AHJ) The organization, office, or individual—such as a fire chief; fire marshal, chief of a fire prevention bureau, labor department, or health department; building official; or electrical inspector—who is responsible for approving equipment, an installation, or a procedure.

awareness level The minimum capability of a responder who could be called upon to respond to, or could be the first on the scene of, a technical rescue incident. This level can involve search, rescue, and recovery operations.

bacterium One-celled, living things. When seen under a microscope they look like balls, rods, or spirals.

barricaded subjects Criminal suspects who are holding ground in a physical location, are refusing to submit to police requests to surrender, and are in possession of, or have access to, weapons.

base of operation (BoO) An established location on the scene of a larger-scale incident where the most important functions of the incident command system are coordinated.

basic rescue teams A group of individuals who provide rescue at incidents and who have a minimal level of education and training to perform said services.

bastard search The search method in which rescuers look in obvious places while assuming that the person was not really lost. In many cases, the person being searched for either has found his own way out or has gone home without telling anyone.

Black Death/Plague One of the oldest identifiable diseases known to man; a disease of wild rodents spread from one rodent to another by flea ectoparasites and to humans either by the bite of infected fleas or when handling infected hosts.

blackwater diving The act of diving in low visibility conditions.

bulk A type of packaging that may hold a liquid capacity greater than 119 gallons (450 liters), a solid net mass greater than 882 pounds (400 kg), or a gas capacity greater than 1,001 pounds (454 kg).

canine search teams Search dog teams trained for search and rescue operations for living and deceased victims in a variety of environments and conditions.

carabiners An oval or D-shaped metal, load-bearing connector with a self-closing gate, used to join components of a rope system.

caves A natural, underground space that is large enough for humans to enter.

chemical, biological, radiological, nuclear, and explosives (CBRNE) The four hazards terrorists may use to inflict mass destruction.

choke point search The search method that uses the same principles as confinement by staging rescuers in specific locations where a subject is most likely to travel.

cholera An infection of the small intestine that causes a large amount of watery diarrhea, caused by the bacterium *Vibrio cholerae.*

collapse patterns The expected characteristics that are demonstrated by a structure during a specific type of collapse.

command staff The personnel who are in charge of an incident and report directly to the incident commander.

communicable disease An infectious disease that can be passed from one person to another person.

community emergency response team (CERT) A community-level program administered by the Federal Emergency Management Agency that educates people about disaster preparedness for hazards that may impact their community and trains them in basic disaster response skills, such as fire safety, light search and rescue, team organization, and disaster medical operations.

complexity analysis A combination of involved factors that affect the probability of control of an incident.

concentrated load A load that is applied to a structural component at one single point rather than being distributed uniformly across a span.

concentration Quantity of a substance dissolved in, or mixed with, a specific quantity of another substance.

confinement area A bounded area set up to limit where the subject may travel undetected, or to establish that the subject has not already passed a desired boundary of the search area.

consequence The result that follows an action or event.

containment area A bounded area set up to confine a subject to a specific area.

control zones An area created on an incident scene outside of an established perimeter that surrounds an area determined to be extremely hazardous.

counter-sniper operations Tactics used by a sniper to mitigate damage or disable another sniper.

cribbing The filling of void spaces to prevent the movement a vehicle.

cultures of unnecessary risk An environment that encourages participants to take on risk that is not necessary and can or does harm or kill them.

cutting tools A type of tool used to cut through the different types of materials found at an extrication scene.

dead load The total weight of the building materials, equipment, and fixtures that are permanently attached to the building itself.

decontamination The physical and/or chemical process of reducing and preventing the spread of contamination from people, animals, the environment, or equipment.

design load The maximum load that a structure and its components are designed to handle.

despondent An individual who suffers from depression, loss of hope, confidence, or courage.

dignity protection Tactical assignment to mitigate the threat of violence against an important person.

disaster medical assistance teams (DMAT) Voluntary medical personnel units organized and equipped to provide austere medical care in a disaster area or medical services at transfer points or reception sites associated with patient evacuation.

disentanglement The removal of debris and vehicle parts that trap a person in a vehicle.

distributed load An external force or load that is spread over a region of length, surface, or area as opposed to a single point.

diving or marine operations SWAT teams that specialize in marine or maritime operations.

emergency incident rehabilitation The process of providing rest, rehydration, nourishment, and medical evaluation to responders who are involved in extended and/or extreme incident scene operations.

Emergency Management Agency (EMA) A U.S. government organization that provides assistance, planning, and other services on the local, state, and federal levels as related to disaster management.

emergency operations plan (EOP) The plan maintained by various jurisdictional levels for responding to a wide variety of potential hazards.

engulfment An event during which a liquid or fine granular solid substance converges in surrounding and/or burying the victim.

entrant An employee or rescuer who is trained to enter a permit-required confined space.

entrapment A condition in which a victim cannot self-rescue due to being trapped by debris, soil, or other product.

epidemic Outbreaks of a disease in a community or region that is more than usual.

Equal Employment Opportunity Commission (EEOC) An agency responsible for enforcing federal laws that make it illegal to discriminate against a job applicant or employee due to the person's race, color, religion, sex, national origin, age, disability, or genetic information.

event A planned activity.

excavation Any manmade cut, cavity, trench, or depression in an earth surface that is formed by earth removal.

extrication The process of removing or disentangling a victim from an entrapment.

extrication teams A group of individuals who are trained and equipped to remove and disentangle patients from a vehicle.

extrication tools A type of equipment used to remove and disentangle a patient from a vehicle.

facility containment systems The packaging, containers, and containment systems that are part of a fixed facility's operation.

facility paperwork Plans that document facility layouts, emergency contact information, chemical data, and any planning necessary for handling facility emergencies.

fall factor A ratio used to describe the force exerted on a rope when it stops a falling person. The ratio of the total length of rope compared to the distance of the fall.

Federal Emergency Management Agency (FEMA) An independent agency of the United States government that is responsible for federal emergency preparedness and mitigation and response activities.

FEMA Resource Typing System The categorization and description of resources commonly utilized in large incidents to assist emergency management personnel to identify, locate, request, order, and track outside resources to the jurisdiction that needs them.

FinForm boards A heavy-duty plywood that is generally 4 feet × 8 feet × 1 foot in dimension.

flash fire A sudden, intense, but very short in duration fire caused by the ignition of a mixture of a flammable substance such as dust, a flammable or combustible vapor, or a flammable gas dispersed in air.

force The strength or energy of the different types of loads that bear upon the components of a structure.

funding streams The identified and available funding prospects for a project or cause.

fungi An organism that can be found throughout nature in plants, soils, trees, vegetation, and in and on animals, including humans; can be beneficial or deadly to humans.

fusion center(s) A set point for the receipt, analysis, gathering, and sharing of threat-related information between the federal, state, and local governments and private sector partners.

gate-valve lockouts Devices used to cover a control valve that denies access to unauthorized personnel preventing them from opening the valve.

grid search The process of dividing the search area into smaller grids and methodically searching each of the segments, typically using a line search.

ground pads Pads that are generally made of plywood, but can be made of any material, and are used to distribute the weight of workers and equipment in the area of a trench to prevent a possible collapse.

hand tools A type of tool used during extrication; these tools are the same as those used in structural firefighting and other emergency or rescue work.

harness A system of material that creates a belt, seat, and sometimes chest strap to be used as a tool to connect a person (rescuer or victim) into a rope system.

hasty search The process of performing a quick search of an area where a subject may likely be located.

hazardous materials A dangerous product in the form of a solid, liquid, or gas that can harm people, other living organisms, property, or the environment.

Hazardous Materials Information System (HMIS) A methodology designed to place a simple label on individual containers.

hemostatic agents Material that assists in stopping bleeding and promoting clotting; applied to or mixed into a trauma dressing.

hepatitis An inflammation of the liver, most commonly caused by a viral infection. There are five main types: hepatitis A, B, C, D, and E. (*Source: Definition on Hepatitis from http://www.who.int/csr/disease/hepatitis/en/index.html, accessed September 20, 2013. Used by permission of the World Health Organization.*)

Human Immunodeficiency Virus (HIV) A virus that damages a person's body by destroying specific blood cells: CD4+ T cells. It can lead to acquired immune deficiency syndrome (AIDS).

hydraulic tools A type of tool in which force is exerted by a high-pressure liquid.

ice rescue The rescue of victims having fallen through or stranded on ice.

immediately dangerous to life and health (IDLH) A condition that poses an immediate or delayed threat to life or that would cause irreversible adverse health effects.

impact load A dynamic load that results from the forces created by the movement of operating machinery, elevators, cranes, vehicles, heavy winds, seismic activity, and similar moving forces.

incident An unexpected occurrence that happens in connection with something else.

incident action plan (IAP) A formalized document that includes the incident goals, operational period objectives, and response strategy defined by incident command during the response planning phase.

incident commander The person responsible for overseeing every aspect of an emergency response, including development of incident objectives, managing all incident operations, and management of resources.

incident command post (ICP) The field location at which the primary tactical level, on scene incident command functions are performed.

incident command system (ICS) Allows for organizations to work together effectively by establishing common terminology and advocates a management-by-objectives philosophy.

incident of national consequence An incident of mass affect that has the potential to impact the entire nation either through the action itself or through the number of patients/fatalities involved.

influenza A contagious respiratory illness caused by viruses. It can cause mild to severe illness, and at times can lead to death.

influenza-like illness (ILI) The flu until proven otherwise.

interoperability The ability of different organizations to work together to promote efficiency, effectiveness and safety in an operation.

last known point (LKP) The last position a person was in determined by clues, evidence belonging to the subject, or a credible eyewitness report indicating that the missing subject was known to be at a specific location.

light and medium tactical rescue task forces Teams of trained first responders that can be placed into action after a natural disaster and, if warning allows, should be predeployed.

live load The forces created by the weight from the items that furnish a structure.

loads A weight or a mass that is supported.

local emergency planning commission (LEPC) A body made up of officials from law enforcement, fire service, EMS, hospitals, public health, private industry, Red Cross, Salvation Army, military, emergency management agency, and members of the public who are responsible for identifying and cataloging potential hazards, identifying available resources, and creating emergency plans.

lockout hasps Scissor-like lockout devices with multiple slots for padlocks; attached to a switch, panel, or other loop to prevent access by unauthorized personnel.

lower explosive limit (LEL) The minimal concentration of a gas or vapor in air capable of producing an explosion in the presence of an ignition source.

manual hydraulic tools A type of tool powered by someone operating a pump lever to activate the tool.

mass casualty incident (MCI) An event in which there are more patients than resources immediately available. This can vary be geographic regions depending on the availability local resources.

material safety data sheets (MSDSs) The document that includes the name, address, and phone number of the manufacturer, the chemical name of the substance and any synonyms, the chemical and physical properties of the substance, personal protective equipment necessary for contact with the substance, any potential health effects if an exposure occurs, and any handling, disposal, and storing procedures.

medical ambulance bus A specially designed medical bus to accommodate a large amount of patients for transport. These vehicles are designed to hold litters and administer oxygen with medically trained providers on board.

medical intelligence Gathering of medical information about conditions, suspects, and other data that may have an impact on a tactical operation.

Medical Reserve Corps (MRC) A federally established, community-based, organized group of volunteers (medical and non-medical) intended to supplement existing community medical and emergency response systems.

medical team officer A role performed by a tactical provider that would include gathering and monitoring information to ensure the health of tactical team members.

medical threat assessments Identification of threats that can have negative consequences to the physiologic and psychological health of a tactical team.

mixed methods A data collection/research strategy that uses both quantitative (numbers) and qualitative (narrative) methods.

National Fire Protection Administration (NFPA) An international nonprofit organization whose mission is to reduce fire and other hazards by providing and advocating codes and standards, research, training, and education.

National Incident Management System (NIMS) A comprehensive, national approach to incident management that includes the incident command system, multi-agency coordination systems, and public information systems.

National Response Framework A national guide or framework for an all-hazards approach to mitigating crisis situations.

National Search and Rescue Committee (NSARC) A federal committee comprised of the Department of Homeland Security, Department of the Interior, Department of Commerce, Defense Department, Department of Transportation, Federal Communications Commission, and the National Aeronautics and Space Administration and designated to oversee the National Search and Rescue Plan and act as a coordinating forum for national SAR matters.

National Search and Rescue Plan (NSP) An interagency agreement providing national arrangements for coordination of search and rescue services to meet both domestic and international commitments.

needs assessment A methodical process of focusing on needs.

nonbulk A type of packaging that may hold a liquid capacity of 119 gallons (450 liters) or less, a solid net mass of 882 pounds (400 kg) or less, or a gas capacity of 1,001 pounds (454 kg) or less.

novel virus A virus that has never previously infected humans, or has not infected humans for a long time.

Occupational Safety and Health Administration (OSHA) A part of the U.S. Department of Labor that works to ensure safe and healthy working conditions for men and women by setting and enforcing standards and by providing training, outreach, education, and assistance.

operational capacity An agency's ability to perform at a specific operational level based upon its ability to meet specific requirements and standards.

operational period A set period of time specified for an incident (e.g., 6 hours, 8 hours, 12 hours, etc.).

operations level The capability of hazard recognition, equipment use, and techniques necessary to safely and effectively support and participate in a technical rescue incident. This level can involve search, rescue, and recovery operations, but usually operations are carried out under the supervision of technician-level personnel.

outbreak When a communicable disease is recognized to be spreading at rates that are unusually high or is atypical in nature in a given location.

packaging The process of preparing a patient for removal from a confined space with the use of specially designed equipment to protects a patient's cervical spine, torso, and extremities.

pandemic An outbreak of a disease in a community or region that is more than usual.

parasite An organism that lives in or on and off of a host.

parts per million (ppm) The concentration by volume of one part of a gas or vapor, or by weight of a liquid or solid, per million parts of air or liquid.

personnel accountability report (PAR) A systematic process conducted by incident command and used to account for all response personnel on the scene of an operation.

persons with special needs Patients or victims who require additional services in order to maintain their quality of life.

physical search team A team that specializes in conducting a physical search for victims in a collapse environment without the use of specialized search equipment.

pipe blanks Disks or flanges placed on the end of or within a pipe connection that prevents liquid product from flowing through the pipe.

planning meeting A meeting held as needed throughout the duration of an incident, to select specific strategies and tactics for incident control operations, and for service and support planning.

pneumatic lifting tools A type of tool used to lift or displace objects that cannot be lifted by conventional means.

point last seen (PLS) The point where the subject was last seen by an eyewitness or captured on video at a specific time and location.

poisons Substances that when introduced into the body by inhalation, ingestion, absorption, or injection can cause harm or death.

polio A crippling and potentially fatal infectious disease with no cure, but there are safe and effective vaccines.

post-incident review (PIR) An important process for looking at the MCI from a retrospective view. This is utilized to identify the strengths and weaknesses of the operations of any incident.

post-traumatic stress disorder (PTSD) A mental health condition described as a severe anxiety disorder that can be the result of exposure to an event that results in psychological trauma.

power-driven hydraulic tools A type of tool that has a wide range of uses and power and speed superior to manual hydraulic tools.

primary triage The first phase of immediately identifying those critically injured patients so that you formulate your action plan to treat and transport patients from the scene of the incident.

prying tools A type of tool used to provide leverage and mechanical advantages by multiplying the force applied; used to open hoods, trunks, and doors.

public information officer (PIO) A representative for an agency or organization responsible for coordinating and providing information to the media and public.

pulley A tool used either to increase mechanical advantage in a rope system or to decrease friction when ropes change direction in a rope system.

quarantine The act of isolating a person from the public to stop or limit the spread of disease.

resources A variety of assets, such as personnel equipment, teams, and supplies, utilized to meet the needs of an incident.

rigging A technique used to further stabilize the vehicle.

rinsate A type of water, containing low concentrations of contaminants, that results from the cleaning of containers.

risk avoidance Not performing or doing in order to prevent an incident from occurring.

risk control A concept that is divided into risk avoidance, risk reduction, and risk transfer.

risk evaluation The act of determining the potential of the severity of loss and the probability of occurrence.

risk identification The process through which safety officers attempt to recognize and assess potential problems.

risk management A coordinated set of activities and methods that is used to direct an organization and to control the many risks that can affect its ability to achieve objectives.

risk reduction A situation in which risk is minimized because of actions taken.

risk transfer The transfer of risk to another person or agency or the purchase of insurance to reduce the cost of the risk.

search and rescue (SAR) incident Any situation requiring notification, alerting, and possibly activating the SAR system for an operation.

search area The area designated to be searched.

secondary collapse An additional partial or complete collapse initiated from the damage inflicted by a primary event.

secondary triage The process in which patients receive another assessment to identify if their condition has changed. It is done when the patient is moved from one location to another.

Severe Acute Respiratory Syndrome (SARS) A syndrome that appeared in 2003 with symptoms including fever, malaise, chills, headache, myalgia, dizziness, rigors, cough, sore throat, and runny nose.

shims Thinner cribbing pieces used to fill the gaps between the bigger pieces.

shipping papers The proper documentation that must accompany the shipment when chemicals are transported.

shoring A technique often utilized when cribbing cannot be accomplished in a practical way due to the opening or span being too large.

situational awareness The process through which rescuers grasp what is going on around them on the emergency scene, convert that information into a format that is useful for making decisions, logically think through the consequences of the decisions that they make, and determine the measures that are needed to mitigate the incident.

size-up The steps taken when first arriving on scene to help set up the immediate incident objectives.

SLUDGEM A mnemonic for the signs of organophosphate poisoning: *s*alivation, *l*acrimation, *u*rination, *d*efecation, *g*astrointestinal problems, *e*mesis, and *m*iosis (contracted pupils).

smallpox An acute contagious disease caused by variola virus. It was one of the world's most feared diseases until it was eradicated by a collaborative global vaccination program led by the World Health Organization. The last known natural case was in Somalia in 1977. (*Source: Definition of Smallpox from http://www.who.int/csr/disease/smallpox/en/index.html, accessed September 20, 2013. Used by permission of the World Health Organization.*)

SMART objectives An acronym used in incident planning to describe five characteristics to create an effective plan. These are *smart*, *measurable*, *action oriented*, *realistic*, and *time sensitive*.

special operations Teams that provide patient care, technical rescue, and specialized services at major events, specialized incidents, and mass casualty incidents.

special weapons and tactical (SWAT) teams Specialized units of law enforcement that focus on mitigating high-risk incidents such as barricaded suspect, hostage rescue, incidents with high-powered firearms, drug enforcement, high-risk warrants, and dignitary protection.

standard operating procedure (SOP) An established departmental procedure or process that should be carried out in response to a specific operation or in a given situation.

Statistical Package for the Social Sciences (SPSS) Computer program for tabulating data.

Stokes basket A device used as a part of a rope system to secure sick or injured victims as they are moved through the system.

strike team A specified combination of the same type and kind of resources (generally three to five similar units), with common communications and a leader.

striking tools A type of tool that includes axes, hammers, mallets, battering rams, punches, and picks.

structural collapse The loss of the load-carrying capacity of a component or member within a structure due to the material being stressed beyond its strength limit, resulting in a fracture or excessive deformations and subsequent structural failure.

surge capacity The ability to manage a large volume of patients unexpectedly at any given time.

surveillance The collection and analysis of health-related data to assist in preventing a serious adverse clinical event.

swiftwater rescue A type of rescue in environments with fast currents, such as rivers or floods.

tactical emergency medical support A group of people providing medical support in a tactical law enforcement environment.

tactical medicine Emergency medical services support to the SWAT team provided by specially trained medical providers.

tactical tourniquets A device used in a tactical setting to control hemorrhage from bleeding.

tactics meeting The time set to review the tactics developed by the operations section chief.

task force A group of resources (generally mixed in type) with common communications and a leader that may be preestablished and sent to an incident or formed at an incident.

technician level The capability of hazard recognition, equipment use, and techniques necessary to safely and effectively coordinate, perform, and supervise a technical rescue incident. This level can involve search, rescue, and recovery operations.

toxins Poisonous substances produced by living cells or organisms capable of causing diseases when introduced to the body.

trench A narrow excavation made below the ground surface. In general, the depth is greater than its width, and the width is not greater than 15 feet.

trench box A prefabricated shoring/shielding device that is placed into a trench to protect workers from a collapse.

triage A concept based upon the French word meaning "to sort out" and is the process of identifying the status of a patient during an MCI.

tularemia An infection common in wild rodents that is passed to humans through contact with infected animal tissues or by ticks, biting flies, and mosquitoes.

typing of incidents A way of defining a major incident.

unified incident command The process of bringing together the incident commanders of all major organizations directly involved in the incident in order to coordinate an effective response, while at the same time each carries out its own jurisdictional responsibilities.

Universal Precautions OSHA's required method of control to protect employees from exposure to all human blood and other potentially infectious material (OPIM).

unsafe practices Those actions, whether intentional or not, that pose either a direct or indirect threat the physical well-being of a provider.

upper explosive limit (UEL) Highest concentration of a gas or vapor in air capable of producing an explosion in the presence of an ignition source.

urban search and rescue (USAR) The location, rescue (extrication), and initial medical stabilization of victims trapped in confined spaces.

U.S. National Grid (USNG) A ground-based gridded coordinate system designed and implemented to provide a seamless, standardized system of reference for nationwide use during times of crisis.

ventilation The process of purging a contaminated atmosphere within a confined space with fresh air by the use of specially designed fans or blowers.

viral hemorrhagic fever A group of illnesses caused by several distinct families of viruses. The term is used to describe a severe multisystem syndrome in which, characteristically, the vascular system is damaged, the body's ability to regulate itself is impaired, and hemorrhage is present.

water rescue A type of rescue of victims in a water-related situation.

weapons of mass destruction (WMDs) Weapons designed to kill and bring substantial harm to large numbers of people or cause massive destruction.

webbing A type of soft, flat woven material used in rope systems to secure loads.

windshield survey The assessment of the scene that personnel do as they arrive on the scene of an incident.

World Health Organization (WHO) A United Nations agency established to coordinate international health activities and to help governments improve health services.

Index

I

J

K

L